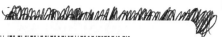

MW01065027

Intensive Care

a
practical
manual

Obstetric Intensive Care

a practical manual

EDITOR

MICHAEL R. FOLEY, MD

Director, Obstetric Intensive Care
Associate Director, Maternal Fetal Medicine
Good Samaritan Regional Medical Center and
Phoenix Perinatal Associates
Phoenix, Arizona
Clinical Associate Professor
Department of OB/GYN
University of Arizona
Tucson, Arizona

ASSISTANT EDITOR

THOMAS H. STRONG, JR., MD

Associate Director
Maternal-Fetal Medicine
Good Samaritan Regional Medical Center
Phoenix Perinatal Associates
Phoenix, Arizona

W.B. SAUNDERS COMPANY

A Division of Harcourt Brace & Company
Philadelphia   London   Toronto   Montreal   Sydney   Tokyo

W.B. SAUNDERS COMPANY

A Division of Harcourt Brace & Company

The Curtis Center
Independence Square West
Philadelphia, Pennsylvania 19106

Library of Congress Cataloging-in-Publication Data

Obstetric intensive care: a practical manual / editor, Michael R. Foley; assistant editor, Thomas H. Strong, Jr.

p.   cm.

ISBN 0–7216–1317–9

1. Obstetrical emergencies.   I. Foley, Michael R.   II. Strong, Thomas H., Jr.   [DNLM: 1. Pregnancy Complications.   2. Intensive Care—in pregnancy.   WQ 240 0134 1997]

RG571.0266   1997   618.2′025—dc20

DNLM/DLC   96–41406

OBSTETRIC INTENSIVE CARE: A PRACTICAL MANUAL   ISBN 0–7216–1317–9

Printed in the United States of America.

Last digit is the print number: 9   8   7   6   5   4   3   2   1

each other, so the mean pressure is taken. The normal resting mean right atrial pressure is 2 to 6 mm Hg. Elevated right atrial pressures may occur in the following conditions: right ventricular failure, tricuspid stenosis and regurgitation, cardiac tamponade, constrictive pericarditis, pulmonary hypertension, chronic left ventricular failure, and volume overload.

The phases of systole and diastole in the right ventricular pressure tracing can be divided into seven events (Fig. 1–2B). Systolic events include (1) isovolumetric contraction, (2) rapid ejection, and (3) reduced ejection. Diastolic events include (4) isovolumetric relaxation, (5) early diastole, (6) atrial systole, and (7) end diastole.

The pulmonary artery pressure tracing is illustrated in Figure 1–2C. A sharp rise in pressure is followed by a decline as the volume decreases. When the right ventricular pressure falls below the level of the pulmonary artery pressure, the pulmonary valve snaps shut. This sudden closure of the valve leaflets causes the dicrotic notch in the pulmonary artery pressure tracing.

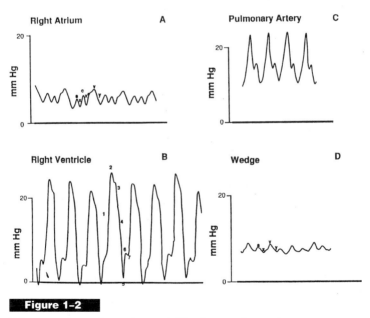

Figure 1–2

Pulmonary artery catheter placement. Waveforms and normal pressures. (Adapted from Daily EK, Schroeder JP: Hemodynamic Waveforms: Exercises in Identification and Analysis. St. Louis, C.V. Mosby, 1983.)

Normal pulmonary artery systolic pressure is 20 to 30 mm Hg. Normal end-diastolic pressure is 8 to 12 mm Hg.

The following box helps to illustrate cardiac chamber pressures:

5 mm Hg Right atrium	10 mm Hg Left atrium
25 mm Hg Right ventricle	100 mm Hg Left ventricle

$$\text{Pulmonary artery pressure} = \frac{\text{right ventricle}}{\text{left atrium}} = \frac{(25)}{(10)}$$

Elevated pulmonary artery pressures are seen in pulmonary disease, primary pulmonary hypertension, mitral stenosis or regurgitation, left ventricular failure, and intracardiac left-to-right shunts. Hypoxia increases pulmonary vascular resistance and pulmonary artery pressure.

When a small branch of the pulmonary artery is occluded by inflation of the balloon on the Swan-Ganz catheter, the pressure tracing reflects left atrial pressure. The waveform looks similar to the right atrial pressure tracing described above (see Fig. 1–2A). The a wave of the wedge pressure is produced by left atrial contraction followed by the x descent (see Fig. 1–2D). The c wave is produced by closure of the mitral valve but usually is not seen. The v wave is produced by filling of the left atrium and bulging back of the mitral valve during ventricular systole. The decline following the v wave is called the "y descent." The normal resting mean wedge pressure is 6 to 12 mm Hg. Elevated wedge pressure is seen with left ventricular failure, mitral stenosis or regurgitation, cardiac tamponade, constrictive pericarditis, and volume overload.

■
Determining the Hemodynamic Profile

Cardiac output is measured by the thermodilution cardiac output computer using five (10-mL) injections of iced saline. Highest and lowest values are discarded, and the mean of the three remaining values is recorded. The value for the first injection is usually high because of heat gained by the injectate in cooling the catheter. The following measured hemodynamic variables are then used to calculate the rest of the hemodynamic profile: heart rate, blood pressure, pulmonary artery pressure, pulmonary capillary wedge pressure, central venous pressure, cardiac output, and height and weight. The derived variables include cardiac index, stroke volume and index, systemic vascular resistance and index, pulmonary vascular resistance and index, and left and right ventricular stroke work and indices (Table 1–4 provides formulas).

■
Oxygen Transport

Arterial oxygen content (CaO_2) is the sum of the oxygen bound to hemoglobin and that dissolved in plasma as described by the equation:

$$CaO_2 = (Hgb \times 1.36 \times SaO_2) + (PaO_2 \times 0.003)$$

where 1.36 is the amount (in milliliters) of oxygen bound to 1 gm of hemoglobin (Hgb); SaO_2 is the arterial oxygen saturation; and 0.003 is the solubility coefficient of oxygen in human plasma. If SaO_2 is 1.0, or 100% saturated, Hgb is 15 g/dL, and PaO_2 is 100 mm Hg, then:

$$
\begin{aligned}
CaO_2 &= (15 \times 1.36 \times 1.0) + (100 \times 0.003) \\
&= 20 + 0.3 \\
&= 20 \text{ mL/dL}
\end{aligned}
$$

The amount of oxygen dissolved in the plasma usually does not make a significant contribution to CaO_2.

Mixed venous blood gives an estimate of the balance between oxygen supply and demand. For example, in low cardiac output states with a high rate of peripheral oxygen extraction, mixed venous oxygen tension ($P\bar{v}O_2$) is low. Normal $P\bar{v}O_2$ ranges from 35 to 45 mm Hg, and mixed venous oxygen saturation ($S\bar{v}O_2$) ranges from 0.68 to 0.76. Clinical concern for tissue hypoxia arises when the $P\bar{v}O_2$ falls below 30 mm Hg and/or the $S\bar{v}O_2$ falls by 5 to 10% over 3 to 5 minutes or to a value below 0.60. Mixed venous oxygen content is measured on blood drawn from the pulmonary artery rather than from the superior vena cava or the right atrium. This is necessary because oxygen saturation in the inferior vena cava is higher than in the superior vena cava because drainage of coronary sinus blood into the right atrium contaminates the chamber with markedly desaturated blood, owing to the high myocardial oxygen extraction

Table 1–4
Derived Hemodynamic Parameters

Parameter	Abbreviation	Formula	Units
Pulse pressure	PP	$BP_{syst} - BP_{diast}$	mm Hg
Mean arterial pressure	MAP	$BP_{diast} + 1/3\ PP$	mm Hg
Cardiac index	CI	$\dfrac{CO}{BSA}$	$L/min/m^2$
Stroke volume	SV	$\dfrac{CO \times 1000}{HR}$	mL
Stroke index	SI	$\dfrac{SV}{BSA}$	$mL/beat/m^2$
Systemic vascular resistance	SVR	$\dfrac{MAP - CVP}{CO} \times 80$	$dyne/sec/cm^{-5}$
Systemic vascular resistance index	SVRI	$SVR \times BSA$	$dyne/sec/cm^{-5}/m^2$
Pulmonary vascular resistance	PVR	$\dfrac{\overline{PAP} - PCWP}{CO} \times 80$	$dyne/sec/cm^{-5}$
Pulmonary vascular resistance index	PVRI	$PVR \times BSA$	$dyne/sec/cm^{-5}/m^2$
Left ventricular stroke work	LVSW	$SV \times MAP \times 0.136$	gm/m
Left ventricular stroke work index	LVSWI	$\dfrac{LVSW}{BSA}$	$gm/m/m^2$
Right ventricular stroke work	RVSW	$SV \times \overline{PAP} \times 0.136$	gm/m
Right ventricular stroke work index	RVSWI	$\dfrac{RVSW}{BSA}$	$gm/m/m^2$

Key: BP_{syst}, systolic blood pressure; BP_{diast}, diastolic blood pressure; CO, cardiac output; HR, heart rate; BSA, body surface area; $\overline{PAP}$, mean pulmonary artery pressure; PCWP, pulmonary capillary wedge pressure.

rate. After blood from the three sources passes through the right ventricle into the pulmonary artery it is thoroughly mixed, resulting in a true "mixed venous" sample.

Mixed venous oxygen content is calculated as follows:

$$C\bar{v}_{O_2} = (Hgb \times 1.36 \times S\bar{v}_{O_2}) + (P\bar{v}_{O_2} \times 0.003)$$

If Hgb = 15 gm, $S\bar{v}_{O_2}$ = 0.75, and $P\bar{v}_{O_2}$ = 40 mm Hg, then:

$$C\bar{v}_{O_2} = (15 \times 1.36 \times 0.75) + (40 \times 0.003)$$
$$= 15 + 0.12$$
$$= 15 \text{ mL/dL}$$

The arterial-venous oxygen content difference is described by the equation:

$$A - \bar{V}_{O_2} = Ca_{O_2} - C\bar{v}_{O_2}$$

Substituting the above calculations:

$$A - \bar{V}_{O_2} = 20 - 15 = 5 \text{ mL } O_2/dL$$

The normal range of the arterial-venous oxygen content difference is 3.5 to 5.0 mL/dL.

Oxygen delivery ($\dot{D}_{O_2}$) is the product of arterial oxygen content (Ca_{O_2}) and cardiac output (CO) as expressed by the equation:

$$\dot{D}_{O_2} = CO \times Ca_{O_2} \times 10$$

If cardiac output equals 5 L/min, then:

$$\dot{D}_{O_2} = 5 \times 20 \times 10 = 1000 \text{ mL/min.}$$

Oxygen delivery is normally about 1000 mL/min. Oxygen consumption ($\dot{V}_{O_2}$) is the amount of oxygen that diffuses into the tissues and is expressed by the equation:

$$V_{O_2} = CO \times (Ca_{O_2} - C\bar{v}_{O_2}) \times 10$$
$$= 5 \times 5 \times 10 = 250 \text{ mL/min.}$$

Oxygen consumption is normally about 250 mL/min.

■
Oxyhemoglobin Dissociation Curve

Basic familiarity with the oxyhemoglobin dissociation curve is necessary to understand oxygen transport and the influence of shifts in the curve. Acidosis, increased red cell 2,3-diphosphoglycerate (DPG), and fever shift the curve to the right, thus

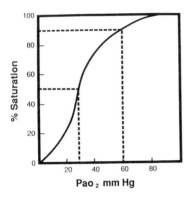

Figure 1–3

The oxyhemoglobin dissociation curve of normal blood. Hemoglobin is 50% saturated at a Pa_{O_2} of 27 mm Hg. Pa_{O_2} of 60 mm Hg correlates with oxygen saturation of about 90%. (From Gabbe SG, Niebyl JR, Simpson JL (eds): Obstetrics: Normal and Problem Pregnancies, 2nd ed. New York, Churchill Livingstone, 1991.)

reducing the hemoglobin's affinity for oxygen and increasing oxygen unloading in the tissues. Alkalosis, reduced red cell 2,3-DPG, and hypothermia cause the curve to shift to the left with the opposite effects on tissue oxygenation. As seen in Figure 1–3, hemoglobin is 50% saturated (P_{50}) at a Pa_{O_2} of 27 mm Hg. Pa_{O_2} of 60 mm Hg correlates with oxygen saturation of about 90%. Thus, little is gained in oxygen saturation by increasing Pa_{O_2} much higher than 60 mm Hg. On the other hand, below Pa_{O_2} of 60 mm Hg, small changes in Pa_{O_2} result in large changes in oxygen saturation. A Pa_{O_2} less than 20 mm Hg is incompatible with life.

■ Hemodynamic Support

Cardiac output is determined by four factors: preload, afterload, rate, and contractility. According to the Frank-Starling principle, the force of striated muscle contraction varies directly with the muscle's initial length. The relationship between myocardial fiber length and fiber shortening can be graphically described by the curve in Figure 1–4. Fiber length can best be equated with preload or filling volume of the ventricle. To allow clinical estimation of preload, the pressure correlate of the filling volume is used (i.e., right or left ventricular end-diastolic pressure). Varying compliance alters the pressure-volume relationship. For example, a poorly compliant left ventricle resulting from myocardial hypertrophy or ischemia requires higher intracavitary pressure to achieve a specific end-diastolic volume or fiber stretch.

Afterload is defined both as the wall tension of the ventricle during ejection and the resistance to forward flow in the form of vascular resistance (vasoconstriction). In the absence of aortic or pulmonary stenosis, vascular resistance in the appropriate bed—systemic or pulmonary—determines the afterload for that side of the heart. The effect of afterload on ventricular output is shown in Figure 1–5.

Heart rate has a marked effect on cardiac output (i.e., cardiac output is the product of heart rate and stroke volume). Increases in heart rate are achieved at the expense of diastolic filling time, systolic emptying time being rate independent. Marked increases in heart rate may lead to circulatory depression when they cause myocardial ischemia or when reduced diastolic filling or loss of atrial "kick" prevents adequate ventricular preload. As a general rule, a heart rate that exceeds the difference of 220 and the patient's age in years reduces cardiac output and myocardial perfusion.

Contractility is defined as the inherent force and velocity of ventricular contraction when preload and afterload are constant. An increase in contractility is associated with an increase in stroke volume despite "fixed" preload. Factors that affect contractility include sympathetic impulses, catecholamines, acid-base and electrolyte disturbances, ischemia, loss of myocardium,

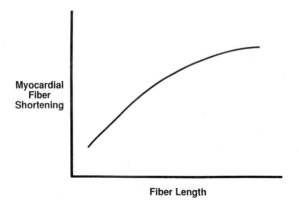

Figure 1–4

Starling curve relates myocardial fiber length to fiber shortening. (From Rosenthal MH: Intrapartum intensive care management of the cardiac patient. Clin Obstet Gynecol 24:789, 1981.)

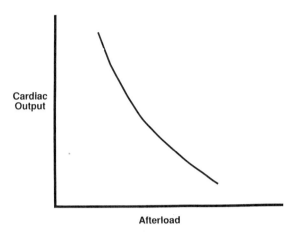

Cardiac
Output

Afterload

Figure 1–5

Relationship of afterload to cardiac output at a constant preload. (From Rosenthal MH: Intrapartum intensive care management of the cardiac patient. Clin Obstet Gynecol 24:789, 1981.)

hypoxia, and drugs or toxins. A third heart sound, distant heart sounds, and a narrow pulse pressure suggest impaired contractility. Radionuclide ventriculograms and two-dimensional (2D) echocardiography allow determination of ventricular size and contractile state. Effects of altered myocardial contractility on cardiac output at a given preload are shown in Figure 1–6.

Figure 1–7 uses the Starling curves to summarize the effects on ventricular function of increases and decreases in preload, afterload, and contractility. The agents used to treat hemodynamic instability are grouped in Table 1–4. The therapeutic rationale for supporting the cardiovascular system based on the Frank-Starling relationship is illustrated in Figure 1–8.

The primary adjustment to improve low cardiac output is to optimize preload using volume expansion. Because of the lack of correlation between measurements on the right and left sides of the heart in patients with significant cardiopulmonary disease, pulmonary capillary wedge pressure (PCWP) is monitored to optimize left ventricular preload and to avoid pulmonary edema. If blood pressure and cardiac output do not respond to fluids (i.e., a PCWP of approximately 15 mm Hg), then a positive inotropic agent may be needed to increase myocardial contractility. Usually, dopamine is the drug of choice. It is utilized because its activity is modified at different doses. At a dose of 2 to 3 μg/

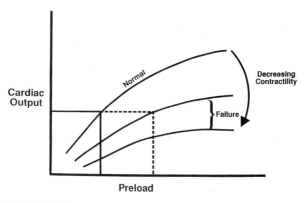

Figure 1–6

Cardiac function curves demonstrate downward displacement secondary to decreased contractility and failure. Dotted line represents increased preload demands in failure. (From Rosenthal MH: Intrapartum intensive care management of the cardiac patient. Clin Obstet Gynecol 24:789, 1981.)

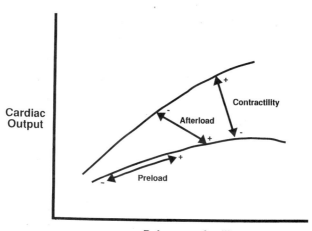

Figure 1–7

Alteration in Starling curve of ventricular function caused by increases and decreases in preload, afterload, and contractility. (From Rosenthal MH: Intrapartum intensive care management of the cardiac patient. Clin Obstet Gynecol 24:789, 1981.)

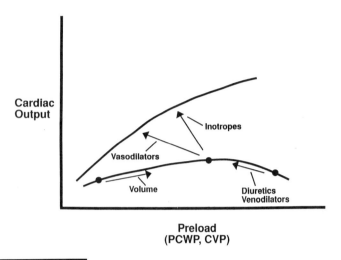

Figure 1-8

Treatment approaches for altered hemodynamic states based on Starling's law of the heart. Key: PCWP, pulmonary capillary wedge pressure; CVP, central venous pressure. (From Rosenthal MH: Intrapartum intensive care management of the cardiac patient. Clin Obstet Gynecol 24:789, 1981.)

kg/min, renal and splanchnic vasodilatation occur; up to 10 µg/kg/min, positive inotropy occurs; and over 10 µg/kg/min, vasoconstriction predominates. These dose ranges reflect predominance of action only. There is a great deal of overlap and individuality of response. The usual therapeutic range for dopamine in clinical practice is 1 to 10 µg/kg/min. When the requirement exceeds this, a more potent vasopressor such as norepinephrine is added and the dopamine is decreased to renotonic doses in the hope that renal blood flow will be preserved.

Afterload may be manipulated with vasodilators in cardiac failure or in low cardiac output states secondary to severe hypertension. Vasodilators have varying effects on arterial and venous resistance. Nitroglycerin, which is predominantly a venodilator, may cause a greater reduction in preload than in afterload. Nitroprusside, which equally dilates arteries and veins, may be preferred; however, marked decreases in systemic vascular resistance result in hypotension, poor perfusion, and myocardial ischemia. The use of a vasodilator requires careful observation of the adequacy of intravascular volume and the net effect on cardiac output.

Table 1-5

Invasive Hemodynamic Findings During the Third Trimester of Normal Pregnancy

Author (yr)	Method of Determination	Number of Patients	MAP (mm Hg)	HR (bpm)	SV (mL)	CO (L/min)	SVR (dyne/sec/cm^{-5})	CI (L/min/m²)	SVRI (dyne/sec/cm^{-5}/m²)	PCWP (mm Hg)	CVP (mm Hg)
Hamilton (1948)	Fick		99	83	71	4.6					
Werko (1954)	Fick	11	90	96	58	6.5				5	
Bader et al. (1955)	Fick	11		78	79	5.5	1244	3.4			
Walters et al. (1966)	Dye dilution	15	86	84	76	6.2					
Kerr (1968)	Fick	5	79			6.3	1119				
Smith (1970)	RIHSA	10				4.5					
Ueland et al. (1972)	Dye dilution	13	86	86	79	6.7	1056				
Lim & Walters (1979)	Dye dilution	23	85	80	93	7.8	1540				
Lees (1979)	Thermodilution	14	95	84		5.9	1145				
Groenendijk et al. (1984)	Thermodilution	4		84			886	4.5		9	
Walenburg (1988)	Thermodilution	7	83	80				4.0	1629	6	4
Clark et al. (1989)	Thermodilution	10	90	83		6.2	1210			8	4

Key: MAP, mean arterial pressure; HR, heart rate; SV, stroke volume; CO, cardiac output; SVR, systemic vascular resistance; CI, cardiac index; SVRI, systemic vascular resistance index; PCWP, pulmonary capillary wedge pressure; CVP, central venous pressure.

17

Table 1–6

Normal Hemodynamic Parameters for the Third Trimester of Pregnancy

Parameter	Normal Range
Heart rate	60–100 bpm
Mean arterial pressure	70–100 mm Hg
Pulmonary capillary wedge pressure	6–12 mm Hg
Central venous pressure	1–7 mm Hg
Cardiac output	5.0–7.5 L/min
Cardiac index	3.0–4.6 L/min/m^2
Stroke volume	60–90 mL
Systemic vascular resistance	800–1500 dyne/sec/cm^{-5}
Systemic vascular resistance index	1360–2550 dyne/sec/cm^{-5}/m^2
Pulmonary vascular resistance	50–150 dyne/sec/cm^{-5}
Pulmonary vascular resistance index	85–255 dyne/sec/cm^{-5}/m^2

Hemodynamics of Normal Pregnancy

Table 1–5 summarizes several invasive hemodynamic studies in normal pregnancy. These data are representative of patients in the third trimester lying in the lateral recumbent position. As previously noted, the mean values for each parameter are quite variable and there is a broad range; for example, Ueland and coworkers found a mean cardiac output of 6.7 L/min (range, 3.7 to 8.4 L/min). Three of the more important recent studies done with the Swan-Ganz catheter are those by Groenendijk and colleagues, Wallenburg, and Clark and associates. Groenendijk's group and Wallenburg reported cardiac index; Clark's group, reported cardiac output. Using 1.7 m^2 as the mean body surface area to convert cardiac index to cardiac output results in mean outputs of 7.6 L/min and 6.8 L/min, respectively, for the two Dutch studies, as compared with 6.2 ± 1.0 L/min in Clark's study. Corresponding systemic vascular resistances are slightly lower in the Dutch studies, although among the three investigations wedge pressures and central venous pressures "agree." After synthesizing the hemodynamic data reported in Table 1–5, I proposed a normal range for hemodynamic parameters in the third trimester of pregnancy (Table 1–6).

■ Bibliography

Benedetti TJ, Cotton DB, Read JC, et al.: Hemodynamic observations in severe preeclampsia with a flow-directed pulmonary artery catheter. Am J Obstet Gynecol 1980;136:467.

Clark SL, Cotton DB, Lee W, et al.: Central hemodynamic assessment of normal term pregnancy. Am J Obstet Gynecol 1989;161:1439.

Daily EK, Schroeder JP: Hemodynamic Waveforms: Exercises in Identification and Analysis. St. Louis, C.V. Mosby, 1983.

Invasive Hemodynamic Monitoring in Obstetrics and Gynecology. ACOG Technical Bulletin No. 175. Washington, DC, American College of Obstetricians and Gynecologists, 1992.

Mabie WC: Critical care obstetrics. *In* Gabbe SG, Niebyl JR, Simpson JL (eds): Obstetrics: Normal and Problem Pregnancies, Ed 2. New York, Churchill Livingstone, 1991.

Mabie WC, Sibai BM: Treatment in an obstetric intensive care unit. Am J Obstet Gynecol 1990;162:1.

Matthay MA, Chatterjee K: Bedside catheterization of the pulmonary artery: Risks compared with benefits. Ann Intern Med 1988;109:826.

Rosenthal MH: Intrapartum intensive care management of the cardiac patient. Clin Obstet Gynecol 1981;24:789.

Snyder JV: Oxygen transport: The model and reality. *In* Snyder JV, Pinsky MR (eds): Oxygen Transport in the Critically Ill. Chicago, Year Book, 1987.

Swan HJ, Ganz W, Forrester J, et al.: Catheterization of the heart in man with the use of a flow-directed balloon-tipped catheter. N Engl J Med 1970;283:447.

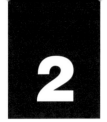

THOMAS H. STRONG, JR.

Transfusion of Blood Components and Derivatives in the Obstetric Intensive Care Patient

Although historically whole blood has been the mainstay of blood transfusion therapy, the past two decades have seen increasing use of and preference for blood components. As a result, transfusion of whole blood is now an uncommon practice, usually indicated only for rapid, simultaneous replacement of blood volume and oxygen-carrying capacity. Since 1 U of whole blood consists of roughly 500 mL of fluid, there is a significant risk of circulatory overload when many units are used. After 24 hours of extravascular storage, platelets and granulocytes are completely lost from whole blood and 2,3-diphosphoglycerate is depleted. Without this important compound, the oxygen-carrying capacity of red blood cells is significantly compromised. After one week's storage, the labile clotting factors (factors V and VIII) are also lost. The changes that occur in whole blood during storage outside the body are known as "storage lesion." Other changes include increases in the plasma levels of potassium and ammonia. In contemporary medical practice, blood component therapy is recommended in almost all clinical situations. Blood component therapy allows the physician to treat the specific derangement in the patient's blood. There are many blood components and derivatives that may be transfused during pregnancy; however, many are so infrequently indicated that they fall outside the scope of this book. The blood products that are more commonly used in pregnancy are generally subdivided into cellular and plasma components.

■ Cellular Components (Table 2–1)

Red Blood Cells

- Most patients who require replacement of red blood cells (RBCs) should receive packed RBCs.

Table 2-1

Blood Components

Component	Contents	Indications	Approximate Volume (mL)	Risk of Hepatitis	Approximate Shelf Life	Expected Effect
Packed RBCs	Red cells, some plasma, few WBCs	Increase red cell mass	300	Same as whole blood	21 d	Increase Hct 3%/U, Hgb 1 gm/U
Leukocyte-poor blood	RBCs, some plasma, few WBCs	Prevent febrile reactions, increase red cell mass	250	Same as whole blood	21–24 d	Increase Hct 3%/U, Hgb 1 gm/U Reduce febrile reactions
Platelets	Platelets, some plasma, RBCs, few WBCs	Bleeding due to thrombocytopenia	50	Same as whole blood	Up to 5 d	Increase total platelet count 7500/mm^3 per unit
Fresh-frozen plasma	Plasma, clotting factors	Treatment of coagulation disorders (only source of factors V, XI, XII)	250	Same as whole blood	2 hr thawed, 12 m frozen	Increase total fibrinogen 10–15 mg/dL per unit
Cryoprecipitate	Fibrinogen, factors V, VIII, XIII, von Willebrand's factor, fibronectin	Hemophilia A, von Willebrand's disease, fibrinogen deficiency	40	Same as whole blood	4–6 hr thawed, 12 m frozen	Increase total fibrinogen 10–15 mg/dL per unit

- One unit of packed RBCs contains roughly 250 mL of RBCs and 50 mL of plasma and has a hematocrit of approximately 80%. The decreased plasma volume of packed cells minimizes the risk of fluid overload.
- Transfusion of 1 U of packed RBCs into a 70-kg person usually increases the hemoglobin level by 1 gm/dL.
- Like whole blood, packed RBCs have a shelf life of approximately 6 weeks when stored at 1° to 6°C.
- Frozen RBCs can be stored at −70°C for years; however, the freezing process destroys white blood cells (WBCs), which may be present in the unit of blood.
- When WBCs have been removed from a unit of blood, the blood is considered "leukocyte poor" and carries less risk of febrile transfusion reactions.
- Gravidas who exhibit cardiovascular instability, a hemoglobin value below 8 to 9 gm/dL, or evidence of fetal compromise should be considered as candidates for RBC transfusion.

Autologous Blood

Autologous transfusion is the collection and reinfusion of the patient's own blood; therefore, the donor and recipient are one. Exclusive or supplemental use of autologous blood can reduce or eliminate many transfusion reactions and/or exposure to transfusion-associated infections. Until recently, pregnant women were not allowed to donate blood because the effects on the fetus of intravascular volume changes were unknown. A growing data base now suggests that it is safe for a pregnant woman to donate blood in the third trimester.

It is not unreasonable to encourage pregnant patients at increased risk for blood transfusion (i.e., with placenta previa) to consider autologous blood donation; however, the obstetric care provider should not deny the option of autologous donation to low-risk patients. The recommended guidelines for autologous blood donation during pregnancy are as follows:

- A minimum predonation hemoglobin value of 11 gm/dL.
- Because RBCs may be refrigerated in liquid form for only 6 weeks, initiation of autologous blood donation generally occurs approximately 6 weeks before their anticipated use. The last donation should be given at least 2 weeks before the estimated date of confinement.
- One week should elapse between donations.

- Autologous blood donation should be used selectively. Autologous transfusions should not be used indiscriminately in asymptomatic patients. Unnecessary transfusion of autologous blood increases the risk of circulatory overload.
- Owing to the special logistics of autologous blood, the potential autologous donor should be aware that this technique is more costly than homologous transfusions.
- The patient should be aware that autologous blood donation does not completely eliminate the possibility of homologous transfusion.

Platelet Concentrates

Platelets are separated from whole blood and suspended in small amounts of plasma. They can be collected from a single donor or from multiple ones. Platelet concentrates are indicated for the treatment of hemorrhage due to thrombocytopenia or platelet dysfunction (thrombocytopathia). Thrombocytopenia and thrombocytopathia must be defined. For example, in the presence of immune thrombocytopenic purpura (ITP) when platelets are destroyed via an antibody-mediated process, corticosteroids rather than platelets probably represent the best therapy. Additionally, patients taking aspirin preparations can experience potentially serious bleeding despite absolutely normal platelet counts.

- In pregnant patients thrombocytopenia is considered to be present when the platelet count falls below $100,000/mm^3$. Bleeding following major surgery or trauma rarely occurs when the platelet count is $50,000/mm^3$ or greater, assuming normal platelet function. When the platelet count ranges from 20,000 to $50,000/mm^3$, bleeding with major surgery or trauma occasionally occurs. Platelet transfusion may be performed prophylactically in nonbleeding patients whose platelet count is $20,000/mm^3$ or less. When the platelet count falls to $10,000/mm^3$, bleeding with trauma or surgery is likely. Spontaneous bleeding can occur once the platelet count drops below $10,000/mm^3$.
- Patients who receive massive transfusions within a short period of time can develop dilutional thrombocytopenia. Following replacement of one blood volume, 35 to 40% of a patient's platelets usually remain. Most patients who receive rapid replacement of one to two blood volumes do

not develop hemorrhage problems, however. Platelets should not be given in the setting of massive transfusion unless significant thrombocytopenia or clinically abnormal bleeding occurs.

- One unit of platelets is equivalent to the number of platelets typically found in 1 U of whole blood and in a 70-kg patient typically increases the platelet count by approximately 7500 platelets/mm^3. Typically, the platelet count equilibrates within 10 minutes of transfusion. Owing to this rapid equilibration the platelet count can be assessed immediately following completion of the transfusion.

- Platelet concentrates contain sufficient numbers of serum-bound RBCs to cause alloimmunization to red cell antigens. Therefore, the possibility of Rh immunization by red cells in female recipients should be considered.

■
Plasma Components (see Table 2–1)

Fresh-Frozen Plasma

Fresh-frozen plasma (FFP) is plasma extracted from whole blood within 6 hours of collection and then frozen. The typical volume of a unit of FFP is 250 mL and contains 700 mg of fibrinogen. FFP is indicated to correct deficiencies of multiple clotting factors in bleeding patients. The clotting factor deficiencies can be secondary to liver disease, vitamin K deficiency, or disseminated intravascular coagulation (DIC). FFP may also be used for specific factor deficiencies (factors II, V, VII, IX, X, and XI) when specific component therapy is not available. FFP is also indicated when rapid reversal of warfarin's effects is indicated. Warfarin causes a deficiency of the vitamin K–dependent factors (II, VII, IX, and X). The administration of vitamin K eventually reverses this deficiency, but FFP effects more rapid recovery, when needed.

- One unit of FFP typically increases the fibrinogen level by approximately 10 to 15 mg/dL. When FFP is indicated, 15 mL/kg is a reasonable guideline for the initiation of FFP therapy (target posttransfusion serum fibrinogen value is ~100 mg/dL).
- When use of FFP is anticipated, it should be kept in mind that 30 minutes is required to thaw FFP in the blood bank.
- When only factor VIII, von Willebrand's factor, or

fibrinogen is needed, cryoprecipitate is a more appropriate therapeutic choice. Inappropriate uses of FFP include volume expansion and nutritional supplementation.

Cryoprecipitate

Cryoprecipitate is extracted from whole blood that has been frozen and then allowed to thaw at "refrigerator temperatures." The product is a cold-insoluble fraction of FFP that precipitates under these conditions. Cryoprecipitate is rich in factor VIII (80 to 120 U) and fibrinogen (200 mg) and contains von Willebrand's factor and factor XIII. As 1 unit of cryoprecipitate consists of only 40 mL of fluid, it more efficiently raises the fibrinogen level than FFP does (250 mg/U). The indications for the use of cryoprecipitate include treatment of von Willebrand's disease, factor VIII deficiency, and fibrinogen deficiency. Since cryoprecipitate is a single-donor product, it carries less risk than "pooled" clotting factor concentrates for hepatitis and human immunodeficiency virus (HIV) transmission.

■
Risks of Transfusion

Infection

The risk of disease transmission increases with the number of donor exposures. The most common causes of transfusion-associated infections are the human hepatitis viruses. Among these viruses, the hepatitis C virus had been diagnosed most often.: it was present approximately once in every 100 U of blood transfused. Until recently, no screening test was available to identify this virus in donated blood. On the other hand, a screening test has long existed for the hepatitis B virus. Therefore, the incidence of this infection has been lower, historically, (1 per 300 U transfused) than that for the C variety. With the development of hepatitis C screening, it is anticipated that the incidence of hepatitis C among transfusion recipients will decline.

As is widely known, the HIV virus is uniformly fatal. The risk of acquiring this virus ranges from 1 in 40,000 to 1 in 1 million units of transfused blood products, depending on which part of the United States one is in. While a screening test is available for HIV infection, the HIV antibody screen can take 6 months or more to convert following infection. Blood donated by an HIV-infected person during this "window" would give a false-negative antibody screen result.

Clinically significant cytomegalovirus (CMV) infections usually occur in immunocompromised patients; however, a small but significant portion of "healthy" persons in the population have never been exposed to CMV and thus have no natural immunity to it. While CMV infection in the adult is usually a benign, subclinical process, primary infection in a fetus can have devastating effects. Therefore, only seronegative blood products should be administered to seronegative patients.

On rare occasions, bacterial and endotoxic contamination can occur in donated blood products. Bacterially infected blood could potentially lead to septicemia in the patient who receives it. Other organisms that are less frequently transmitted through transfusion include the agents of malaria, parvovirus, Epstein-Barr virus, *Babesia* organism, and T-cell viruses.

Immune-Mediated Reactions

Transfusion reactions typically are triggered by antigens on RBCs and WBCs. There are two types of transfusion reactions: hemolytic and nonhemolytic. The hemolytic variety occurs in 1 of every 6000 transfusions and is fatal in 1 of every 100,000 units of blood transfused. The ABO-system antigens are usually responsible for hemolytic reactions. Nonhemolytic transfusion reactions are much more common (1 per 100). Usually characterized by febrile or urticarial reactions, the incidence of nonhemolytic reactions can be reduced by using leukocyte-poor products. Alloimmunization can result in platelet antibodies that may prevent therapeutic response in the thrombocytopenic patient who receives platelet transfusion. Rarely graft-versus-host disease can occur following transfusion of some blood components (e.g., platelets, white blood cells) into an immunocompromised person.

■ Colloid Solutions

Intravenous fluids containing particles that will not pass through a semipermeable membrane and are larger than 10 kd are known as colloids (Table 2–2). Compared to crystalloid solutions, colloids are more expensive, less readily available, and may be associated with anaphylactoid reactions; however, they

Table 2-2			
Colloid Infusions			
Colloid	Dose (mL)	Crystalloid Volume Expansion Equivalent	Estimated Duration of Effect (hr)
Albumin			
5%	500–750	Similar	Half-life 12–16
25%	100–200	450 mL over 1 hr (100 mL dose)	Half-life 12–16
Hetastarch	500–1000	Similar	24–36
Dextran 40	500	750 mL over 1 hr 1050 mL over 2 hr	24

tend to produce greater elevations in colloid oncotic pressure than crystalloids. Colloids also tend to produce greater increases in plasma volume.

Effective management of hypovolemic shock depends more on successful fluid resuscitation than on what fluid actually is used. Which solution is used is a function of medical philosophy and risk-benefit analysis.

Albumin

Albumin solutions may rapidly restore intravascular volume, especially if serum albumin levels are less than 2 gm/dL. Albumin is available in concentrations of 5% and 25%. When 25 gm of albumin is infused, intravascular volume increases by roughly 450 mL over 60 minutes, as a result of albumin's considerable oncotic activity. However, the benefits are transient and may result in complications, such as pulmonary edema, if excessively administered. Supplemental albumin is rapidly redistributed throughout the extracellular space, disappearing from the circulation at a rate of up to 8% per hour. In the setting of shock or sepsis, the rate can approach 30% per hour. Other potential benefits of supplemental albumin include (1) limitation of lipid peroxidation by scavenging free radicals, (2) binding free fatty acids and lysozymes, (3) inhibition of pathologic platelet activation, and (4) inhibition of factor Xa by antithrombin III.

Dextran

Dextran is a large, glucose polymer solution available with polymers having mean molecular weights of 40,000 (dextran 40) or 70,000 (dextran 70). A 500-mL infusion of dextran 40 produces intravascular volume expansion of 1050 mL over 2 hours and improves capillary blood flow by reducing viscosity and red cell aggregation. As with albumin, dextran's effects are temporary and may be associated with pulmonary edema if used too aggressively. Dextran may also foster hemorrhage by reducing platelet and clotting factor activation and by binding with fibrin to produce less stable clots. Additionally, dextran can induce renal failure and anaphylactoid reactions. Dextran may also interfere with laboratory cross-matching of blood by reducing RBC aggregation. Therefore, blood typing and cross-matching should be performed before administering dextran.

Hetastarch

Hydroxymethyl starch is a synthetic molecule available in a 6% solution in normal saline. Like albumin and dextran, it possesses considerable oncotic activity and can induce intravascular fluid expansion; however, hetastarch increases colloid oncotic pressure even more effectively than albumin. The volume-expanding effect of hetastarch may last 24 to 36 hours. Hetastarch may also prolong prothrombin and partial thromboplastin times, decrease platelet counts, and reduce clot tensile strength; moreover, hetastarch may artifactually increase serum amylase levels.

Red Blood Cell–Saving Devices

The salvage of shed blood has been a topic of research since early in the nineteenth century. The first reported case of autologous transfusion occurred more than 100 years ago. Since that time, transfusion of blood shed during surgery or following trauma has become an accepted practice. Autologous blood, collected preoperatively or intraoperatively, offers a variety of advantages over homologous blood. As a perfectly compatible source, autologous blood eliminates the risk of infectious disease transmission and isoimmunization. The appropriateness of this modality during cesarean delivery is less clear, owing to the potential risk of infusing amniotic fluid or debris. Moreover, intraoperative autotransfusion is contraindicated when the patient's shed blood has been exposed to bacteria or malignant cells. As cesarean deliveries are frequently clean-contaminated or frankly contaminated procedures, intraoperative autotransfusion of shed blood may not be prudent. Nevertheless, anecdotal reports have suggested the potential utility of this technique in selected cases when cesarean delivery is complicated by hemorrhage.

■
Bibliography

Consensus Conference: Fresh-frozen plasma: Indications and risks. JAMA 1985;253(4):551.

Consensus Conference: Perioperative red blood cell transfusion. JAMA 1988;260(18):2700.

Consensus Conference: Platelet transfusion therapy. JAMA 1987;257(13):1777.

Kruskall MS, Leonard S, Klapholz H: Autologous blood donation during pregnancy: analysis of safety and blood use. Obstet Gynecol 1987;70:938.

McVay PA, Hoag RW, Hoag SM, et al.: Safety and use of autologous blood donation during the third trimester of pregnancy. Am J Obstet Gynecol 1989;169:1479.

Oberman HA: Transfusion therapy. *In* Laros RK (ed): Blood Disorders in Pregnancy. Philadelphia, Lea & Febiger, 1986; 195.

Transfusion alert: Indications for the Use of Red Blood Cells, Platelets and Fresh-Frozen Plasma. NIH Publication No. 89-2974a, May 1989.

THOMAS H. STRONG, JR.

Obstetric Hemorrhage

Occurring in approximately 5% of all pregnancies, obstetric hemorrhage is a major cause of maternal morbidity and mortality. Hemorrhage most commonly occurs in the third trimester or immediately post partum. During the third trimester, the placenta is involved in most of the bleeding that is life-threatening to mother or fetus. In the postpartum period, the uterus itself accounts for the majority of ominous bleeding events. Table 3–1 summarizes the most common causes of third trimester bleeding.

Third Trimester Bleeding

- Until the proper diagnosis is determined, it is prudent to assume that any vaginal bleeding during pregnancy is potentially life threatening.
- Digital examination of the cervix is absolutely contraindicated until placenta previa has been ruled out.
- Owing to the physiologic adaptations of pregnancy, the mother may not show significant changes in her vital signs until 25 to 30% of her intravascular volume has been lost. Often the fetus demonstrates fetal heart rate changes before the gravida shows clinical signs of significant intravascular depletion.
- Left lateral displacement of the uterus can increase maternal cardiac output and improve uteroplacental perfusion. This maneuver is always warranted when third trimester bleeding occurs.
- In the Rh-negative woman with third trimester bleeding who undergoes expectant management, administration of Rh immune globulin should not be deferred until delivery.
- Women with placenta previa or abruptio placentae are at increased risk for postpartum hemorrhage.

Table 3–1	
Causes of Third Trimester Bleeding	
Bloody show	Placenta previa
Cervical neoplasm	Placental abruption
Cervicitis	Vaginal neoplasm
Circumvallate placenta	Vasa previa
Genital tract trauma	

Placenta Previa

When placentation occurs in the lower uterine segment so that the placenta extends below the presenting part of the fetus and impinges on or completely covers the internal cervical os, placenta previa is present. Among all episodes of third trimester hemorrhage, approximately 20% are due to placenta previa. There are three types of placenta previa: (1) complete, in which the internal os is completely covered by the placenta; (2) partial, in which the internal os is partially obstructed by the overlying placenta; and (3) marginal, in which the placental edge comes up to, but does not encroach upon, the internal os. The vast majority of placentas (90%) that implant in the lower uterine segment are located in the upper half of the uterus by term. "Placental migration" relates to the progressive lengthening ("development") of the lower uterine segment that occurs late in pregnancy.

Risk Factors

Any process that prevents placental migration increases the risk for placenta previa. As the multiparous uterus undergoes less development of its lower segment than a nulliparous one, it is not surprising that increasing parity is a risk factor for placenta previa. Increasing maternal age is another risk factor but likely is a reflection of increased parity. Prior cesarean delivery is also a risk for placenta previa. The uterine scar left by cesarean delivery has been hypothesized to impede development of the lower uterine segment.

Diagnosis

The diagnosis is suggested by painless vaginal bleeding that is bright red, with or without clots. Typically, onset is sudden and without apparent provocation; however, in approximately 25% of cases uterine contractions are present. The initial episode of blood loss usually occurs in the late second or early third trimester of gestation, and incidence peaks at the 30th to 34th weeks. The first bleeding event is infrequently life threatening unless provoked by digital examination. Often the patient experiences multiple, small bleeding episodes before a major, life-threatening event occurs. A pelvic examination, douching, or intercourse can sometimes induce bleeding of a previously undiagnosed placenta previa. Ultrasonography is a highly accurate method for diagnosing placenta previa. At present, it is the diagnostic tool of choice for this problem. In experienced hands, the accuracy of abdominal sonography exceeds 90%. Since placenta previa occupies the lower uterine segment, fetal malpresentation is often present. Therefore, the obstetrician should be suspicious of placenta previa whenever a transverse lie or breech presentation occurs late in the third trimester.

Management

Uterine contractions and cervical dilatation predispose the parturient with placenta previa to significant blood loss. Cesarean

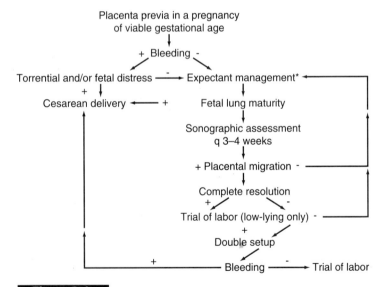

Figure 3-1

Management of placenta previa. *Hospitalize, type and cross-match blood, large-bore IVs, bed rest, tocolysis as needed, fetal lung maturity studies q 1–2 wk at 36 ± 1 wk gestation.

delivery is the standard approach for this complication of pregnancy. In the presence of a low-lying placenta or marginal placenta previa, a "double set-up" can be tried. A double set-up examination is simply a digital examination of the cervix performed in the delivery room with full preparation for cesarean delivery. In the event that significant vaginal bleeding is provoked, rapid delivery can be accomplished. If the placenta is determined to be clear of the cervical os, a trial of labor may be attempted.

Within the context that the abdomen will be the route of delivery, the key to successfully managing a gravida with placenta previa rests in the timing of delivery (Fig. 3–1). Expectant management of placenta previa typically improves the outcomes for both mother and fetus. The mother benefits from cesarean delivery of a fetus that cannot safely be delivered vaginally, and the fetus benefits from the delay in delivery until its lungs are functionally mature. Furthermore, expectant management may allow placental migration, thus affording some patients a trial of labor. Conservative management of placenta previa is a reasonable option based on the notions that (1) mothers rarely die from unprovoked vaginal bleeding and (2) prematurity is the major cause of perinatal death.

When choosing expectant management, four assumptions are made:

- The mother is stable.
- Vaginal bleeding has stopped.
- The fetus has a reassuring fetal heart rate tracing.
- Cesarean delivery can be performed immediately at any time, should emergent delivery be warranted.

Once the diagnosis of placenta previa has been confirmed, strict bed rest is the mainstay of management. Bed rest is recommended because of the traditional but unproven perception that it reduces preterm uterine contractions. Bed rest may be associated with greater fetal growth, something that may benefit the fetus should preterm delivery be necessary.

It is a matter of course that bleeding will recur. With enough blood loss, the gravida will eventually become anemic and her condition unstable. Keeping in mind the infectious potential of blood products, it is reasonable to use a maternal hemoglobin value of approximately 8 to 9 gm/dL as the limit below which transfusions should be considered in the antepartum period. Maintenance of hemoglobin in this range should provide maternal cardiovascular stability and allow adequate fetal oxygenation for a patient at bed rest. Throughout the antepartum period, appropriately typed and screened (or cross-matched) blood should be readily available. In the gravida who requires repeated transfusions, the obstetric care provider must determine if continued expectant management is prudent. Table 3–2 summarizes the maternal and fetal indications for discontinuing expectant management of placenta previa.

As gestation advances, placental migration may occur. Therefore, sonographic reassessment of the placenta is recommended every 2 to 3 weeks. It is also advisable to assess fetal growth at 2- to 3-week intervals, since intrauterine growth retardation occurs more frequently with placenta previa. When indicated, nonstress testing and fetal biophysical assessment are the preferred methods for evaluating fetal well-being. Contraction stress testing is contraindicated in the setting of placenta previa.

In the presence of uterine contractions without severe hemorrhage, tocolytic therapy is reasonable; however, the use of beta-sympathomimetics in this setting is relatively contraindicated. In hypovolemic patients sympathomimetics may worsen cardiovascular instability by producing unwanted vasodilatation. A safer tocolytic agent in the presence of uterine contractions and placenta previa is magnesium sulfate. The use of betamethasone is advocated between 24 and 34 weeks to accelerate fetal lung maturation. In a stable patient, delivery should be effected when fetal lung maturity is documented. Therefore, amniocentesis no later than 36 weeks is advocated. In the event that the fetal lungs are not mature, amniocentesis should be repeated in 7 to 14 days or at an appropriate interval to identify fetal lung maturity at its earliest appearance.

Table 3–2

Indications for Discontinuing Expectant Management of Placenta Previa

Fetal indications
    Anomalies incompatible with life
    Distress
    Death
    Pulmonary maturity
Maternal indications
    Labor that fails tocolysis
    Excessive bleeding
    Other obstetric indications (e.g., preeclampsia)

Complications

The lower uterine segment is less muscular than the fundus and therefore is less contractile. Since tonic myometrial contraction is the primary hemostatic mechanism in the postpartum period, placental implantation sites in the lower uterine segment are at increased risk for postpartum hemorrhage. Placenta accreta, the abnormal adherence of placenta to the underlying uterine wall, is associated with placenta previa (see Chapter 23). Placenta accreta is due to the absence of decidua basalis and Nitabuch's layer at the implantation site. As a result, the anchoring villi of the placenta attach directly—and irreversibly—to the myometrium. Placenta accreta is like placenta previa in that it also tends to occur at the site of old uterine incisions such as those caused by cesarean delivery. It can be quite difficult to remove adherent placental segments, and significant blood loss can result. Thus, the tendency of placenta previa to separate from the uterus can be paradoxically accompanied by areas of the placenta that are morbidly adherent to the myometrium. The standard treatment for placenta accreta with intractable hemorrhage is hysterectomy.

Placental Abruption

The placenta does not usually separate from its implantation site until after delivery of the fetus. Earlier separation of the placenta produces a potentially life-threatening situation for both mother and fetus. "Abruptio placentae" occurs in 0.5 to 2.5% of pregnancies and accounts for 30% of all third trimester hemorrhage. Its rate of recurrence in subsequent pregnancies is approximately 10%.

Because the placenta provides fetal nutrition and gas exchange, it occupies a central role in the well-being of the fetus. Disruption of placental implantation risks fetal compromise by disrupting fetal metabolic and intravascular homeostasis. As the placental implantation site is disrupted, blood can rapidly and forcefully escape. Maternal blood from these vessels can separate the layers of myometrium, dissect into the amniotic fluid, or collect as a hematoma behind the placenta or in the broad ligament. In these instances, little or no vaginal bleeding is noted. A "concealed-occult abruption," which occurs in as many as 20% of all abruptions, can produce maternal cardiovascular instability that is out of proportion to the observed amount of vaginal bleeding. Often, retroplacental bleeding dissects a path to the edge of the placenta, allowing some blood to reach the cervix and pass out of the vagina. In contrast to the bright red clotting blood associated with placenta previa, the blood passed vaginally during abruption typically is dark and nonclotting, suggesting that it is old, sequestered blood.

Risk Factors
Maternal hypertension is a significant risk factor for abruption. Occurring in almost 50% of women who eventually abrupt, hypertension may be chronic or acutely induced through the use of illicit drugs, especially cocaine. Women who have experienced abruptio placentae in previous pregnancies are at increased risk. Trauma to the maternal abdomen is also commonly associated with abruption.

Diagnosis
Since ultrasound is much less accurate at detecting abruption than placenta previa, the diagnosis of placental abruption is based largely on the patient's history and physical examination. Table 3–3 summarizes the differentiation of abruption from placenta previa. Patients with placental abruption will frequently present with a history of trauma or hypertension. Typically, the gravida complains of vaginal bleeding in concert with very strong, painful uterine contractions. A rapid increase in the height of the uterine fundus may suggest an expanding hematoma. Port wine–colored amniotic fluid may be noted at the time of membrane rupture, suggesting dissection of a hematoma into the amniotic cavity. The uterus can be hyperactive or even

Table 3–3
Differentiating Placental Abruption from Placenta Previa

	Abruption	Previa
Risks	Hypertension, trauma, prior abruption, smoking, advanced maternal age, fibroids	High parity, prior cesarean delivery
Diagnosis	Clinical	Sonographic
Pain	Yes	No
Bleeding	Dark, nonclotting (may be occult)	Bright red, clotting
Sequelae	Disseminated intravascular coagulation, postpartum hemorrhage	Placenta accreta, postpartum hemorrhage

tetanically contracted; uterine rupture is occasionally a consequence. Excessive uterine activity may precede the actual abruption and, in many instances, may contribute to the initiation of placental separation. Separation of the placenta from its implantation reduces its usefulness as an organ of gas exchange. Typically, a 30% abruption of the placenta results in significant fetal heart rate changes. The intense, "rapid-fire" contraction pattern of an ongoing abruption can contribute to fetal compromise by reducing uterine blood flow. Fetal demise results when approximately 50% of the placental surface has "abrupted." *An abruption that results in fetal demise near term is usually associated with maternal blood loss that can approach 2000 mL.* Therefore, in the presence of abruptio placentae with fetal demise, the mother should be monitored closely for evidence of hypovolemic shock. Inspection of the placenta that has undergone some degree of abruption reveals clot adherent to the site of placental disruption. Owing to the vigor of uterine contractions, fragments of placental tissue can enter the maternal circulation during abruption. On entering the maternal system, placental thromboplastin can trigger the coagulation cascade, with disseminated intravascular coagulation (DIC) a potential result. Some degree of coagulopathy occurs in approximately 20% of all severe abruptions. The uterine serosa often demonstrates a petechial, marbled pattern known as "Couvelaire uterus." This striking finding represents the hemorrhagic dissection of myometrial tissue planes mentioned earlier. Uterine atony with secondary hemorrhage is not uncommon following a significant placental abruption.

Management

In the setting of fetal distress or any contraindication to ongoing labor, cesarean delivery is recommended. The advantages of abdominal delivery include (1) rapid delivery and (2) direct access to the uterus and its vascular supply in the event that postpartum hemorrhage occurs. The disadvantages of cesarean delivery in the setting of abruption include (1) the increased risk of a major surgical procedure in a patient whose cardiovascular status may not be stable and (2) the increased hemorrhagic potential of abdominal surgery in a woman at increased risk for coagulopathy. Assuming stable maternal cardiovascular status, vaginal delivery is the preferred route for the patient with a dead fetus secondary to abruption. Fortunately, labor proceeds relatively rapidly in most active abruptions, as a result of uterine hyperactivity.

Management of women with placental abruption includes frequent monitoring of hemoglobin and hematocrit, clotting studies (prothrombin and partial thromboplastin times [PT/PTT], platelets, fibrinogen and fibrin split products), vital signs, and hourly urine output. For an unstable or oliguric patient, Swan-Ganz monitoring may be indicated. In the acute setting, continuous electronic fetal heart rate monitoring is necessary to assess fetal well-being.

Two units of packed red blood cells (PRBCs) should be cross-matched if the fetus is alive. At least 4 units should be readied if the fetus is dead. Clinical evidence of severe DIC includes persistent bleeding from sites of minor trauma (intravenous sites, minor cuts). Blood collected in a nonheparinized tube that does not clot within 6 to 8 minutes suggests clinically significant coagulopathy and typically is associated with fibrinogen levels below 100 mg/dL. Transfusion of fresh-frozen plasma (FFP) or cryoprecipitate replaces the clotting factors destroyed by consumptive coagulopathy. The goal is to achieve a fibrinogen level above 100 mg/dL. Figure 3–2 summarizes the management of placental abruption.

Chronic Abruption

At least as frequently as severe abruption, "marginal sinus separation" or "partial/chronic abruption" may initially present with signs and symptoms as acute as those of its catastrophic counterpart; however, the clinical picture stabilizes and the abruption process fails to progress, thus allowing a more conser-

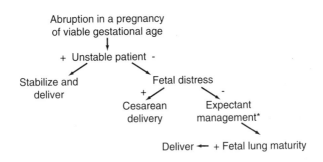

Figure 3–2

Management of placental abruption. *Hospitalize, type and cross-match blood, large-bore IVs, bed rest, tocolysis as needed, monitor for evidence of coagulopathy, twice weekly fetal assessment of well-being and fetal lung maturity studies q 1–2 wks at 36 ± 1 wk gestation.

vative approach to management. While the issue of tocolysis is controversial with any type of abruption, some advocate tocolytic therapy for women with stable, nonacute abruption, to prolong gestation until fetal lung maturity can be ensured. Interestingly, placental abruption is occasionally an undiagnosed cause of preterm labor. In these instances, tocolysis appears to do no harm. The obstetrician who expectantly manages the patient with a nonacute abruption should be aware that even the "stable" abruption is at risk for further placental detachment at any time.

Periodic assessment of hematologic status should be performed in the patient with a chronic abruption. Additionally, twice weekly nonstress testing or fetal biophysical assessment is appropriate for the gravida in this situation. Sonographic monitoring of fetal growth should be done at intervals of 2 to 4 weeks until delivery. Indications for delivery are the same as for placenta previa.

Vasa Previa

The vessels in the umbilical cord typically attach to the central portion of the placenta, arborize across its surface, and then plunge deeply to supply the placental cotyledons. The vessels do not normally extend into the amnion or chorion. With vasa previa, however, the umbilical vessels are widely dispersed across the fetal membranes at the level of the internal cervical os. In the event of membrane rupture, the vessels may be lacerated. The vaginal bleeding encountered is exclusively fetal; identification of nucleated red blood cells on microscopy strongly suggests the diagnosis. Unfortunately, there is rarely time for such diagnostic procedures before fetal exsanguination occurs. Palpation of blood vessels in the bulging fetal membranes during a cervical examination mandates cesarean delivery if the fetus is of viable gestational age and immediate vaginal delivery is not possible. Although vasa previa occurs in fewer than 1% of all deliveries, the associated fetal mortality rate approaches 90%.

■ Postpartum Hemorrhage

Postpartum hemorrhage is present when more than 500 mL of blood is lost following a vaginal birth or when bleeding at

---

Table 3–4

Origins of Postpartum Hemorrhage

Contractile tissue
    Upper uterine segment placental implantation site
Noncontractile or poorly contractile tissue
    Broad ligament
    Lower uterine segment placental implantation site
    Cervix
    Vagina (fornices, hymen, septa [anomalous], side walls)
    Perineum (periclitoral, perineal body, periurethral, rectum)
    Lower urinary tract (bladder, ureter, urethra)

---

cesarean delivery exceeds 1000 mL. Approximately 4% of all deliveries are complicated by excessive postpartum blood loss, but severe hemorrhage occurs in fewer than 1%. Not all postpartum hemorrhages are torrential. Steady flow, if neglected, is also dangerous. Table 3–4 summarizes the most common anatomic origins of postpartum hemorrhage.

Causes

Upon delivery of the placenta, bleeding is controlled by a "tourniquet effect" through tonic uterine contraction. Any process that alters the normal anatomy or physiology of the uterus interferes with efficient myometrial contractions, thus predisposing to hemorrhage. Inability of the uterus to contract ("uterine atony") is responsible for 80% of severe postpartum hemorrhages. A number of factors predispose the woman to postpartum hemorrhage secondary to atony. Table 3–5 summarizes common risk factors for postpartum hemorrhage.

Genital tract trauma is the second most common cause of excessive postpartum blood loss. Lacerations of the lower uterine segment, cervix, or vagina can be caused by a variety of obstetric procedures, including forceps or vacuum delivery, improper fetal scalp electrode or intrauterine pressure catheter placement, and manipulations for the reduction of fetal shoulder dystocia.

Management

Figure 3–3 summarizes the management of postpartum hemorrhage. Women with risk factors for postpartum hemorrhage

---

Table 3–5

Risk Factors for Postpartum Hemorrhage

Altered maternal anatomy
    Cesarean or myomectomy scar (dehiscence, rupture)
    Myomas
    Retained placental fragments
    Trauma (Duhrssen's incisions, intrauterine pressure catheter/fetal scalp
      electrode injury, occiput posterior or compound delivery, operative
      delivery, precipitous delivery—abruptio, shoulder dystocia)
    Uterine anomalies
    Uterine inversion
Altered uterine contractility
    Chorioamnionitis/endometritis
    Grand multiparity
    Magnesium sulfate administration
    Myasthenia gravis
    Placenta previa
    Prolonged or tumultuous labor
Other
    Coagulopathy
    History of postpartum hemorrhage

---

should have blood typed and held at the outset. Recognition of an active postpartum hemorrhage must prompt an immediate, systematic search for the bleeding site. Additional vascular access with a large-bore intravenous (IV) catheter should be secured. Oxytocin concentrations above 30 to 40 U per liter of IV fluid do not promote more effective uterine contractions and increase the risk of fluid overload secondary to the antidiuretic effects of this hormone.

In the absence of severe coagulopathy, a well-contracted uterus does not bleed significantly. Persistent, heavy vaginal bleeding in the face of a firm, globular uterus suggests ongoing hemorrhage from noncontractile tissue, namely, the lower uterine segment, cervix, or vagina. Identification of bleeding at one site does not obviate the search for bleeding at other sites, especially in the setting of maternal birth trauma. The search for bleeding sites is best started in the more superior aspects of the genital tract, since heavy downward flow of blood makes visualization of the more inferior landmarks difficult. As actual visualization of the upper uterus is not possible, palpation of the myometrium and manual exploration of the uterine cavity must suffice in most cases. Ultrasound may be useful in de-

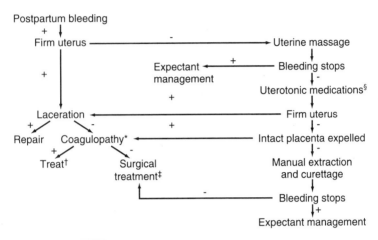

Postpartum bleeding

Figure 3–3

*Laboratory: hemoglobin/hematocrit, fibrinogen, bleeding time (optional: fibrin split products, D-dimer, PT, PTT).

†Thresholds for treatment   Treatment (see Chapter 2)
 Hemoglobin/hematocrit < 7.0 gm/21%   Packed RBCs
 Fibrinogen < 100 mg/dL   Fresh-frozen plasma or
                     cryoprecipitate
 Platelets <50,000/mm³   Platelet concentrates
 Bleeding time >8 min   Platelet concentrates
 Optional: Maternal venous blood may be collected in an unheparinized tube
      (whole blood clotting time). Failure of gross clotting within 6–8
      minutes suggests high likelihood of disseminated intravascular
      coagulation.

‡Uterine artery ligation, utero-ovarian arterial anastomosis ligation, oversew of
 placental implantation site, bilateral hypogastric artery ligation,
 fluoroscopically directed embolization and/or hysterectomy.

§Uterotonic meds (in temporal sequence)

 A. Oxytocin (Do not give as a direct IV bolus.)
    i. 10–30 units/L IV. May infuse up to 500 mL in 10 min.
    ii. 10 units via transabdominal intramyometrial injection.
 B. Methergine, 0.2 mg IM. May repeat in 5–10 min. (Do not give as a direct
    IV bolus.)
 C. Prostaglandin $F_{2\alpha}$ (Do not give as a direct IV bolus.)
    i. 0.25 mg IM then q1–2° as needed.
    ii. 0.25 mg via transabdominal intramyometrial injection.
 OR
 C. Prostaglandin E_2, 20-mg suppository per vagina or rectum.

termining the presence or absence in the uterine cavity of large placental fragments. Identification of retained placental tissue warrants manual extraction and/or curettage.

A worrisome situation is hemorrhage from the lower uterine segment, which is less responsive to uterotonic medications and difficult to suture from the vagina. Management of excessive bleeding from this area can require laparotomy. Likewise, repair of cervical or upper vaginal lacerations can be vexing. Several points must be remembered:

- Adequate exposure and visualization of the laceration are paramount.
- Avoid perforation of the bowel or bladder during suture placement.
- When suturing near the urethra, insert a catheter to prevent inadvertent ligation of this structure.
- Always use absorbable suture in the cervical, vaginal, and perineal areas.
- Avoid prolonged or excessive packing of the vaginal canal. Packing may prevent egress of ongoing blood loss and provide a false sense of security. When packs are used, always leave a "tail" protruding from the vagina.

Firm but gentle massage often reverses uterine atony. Care must be taken to avoid massage so vigorous that it injures the large vessels in the broad ligament. Uterine exploration, placental extraction, and curettage may be necessary. Should fundal massage and intravenous oxytocin fail to reverse uterine atony, ergot drugs (ergonovine, methylergonovine), 0.2 mg intramuscularly, are indicated. As ergots are potent vasoconstrictors, they are contraindicated in the presence of hypertensive disorders. Prostaglandin $F_{2\alpha}$ is a potent stimulator of uterine contraction. Because it can cause bronchoconstriction, prostaglandin $F_{2\alpha}$ should not be used in asthmatics, and because it can also elicit pulmonary vasoconstriction, it is best avoided in women with severe chronic pulmonary hypertension. Prostaglandin E_2, given as a 20-mg rectal or vaginal suppository, provides another potentially safer option for these high-risk patients, without the potent side effects of severe pulmonary vasoconstriction and bronchoconstriction. Oxytocin or prostaglandin $F_{2\alpha}$ can be injected transabdominally into the myometrium. Care must be taken to avoid lacerating urinary, intestinal, and vascular tissue. An undiluted intravascular bolus of oxytocin can aggravate pre-existing hypotension or cause cardiac arrest.

Surgical Management

When excessive uterine bleeding does not respond to standard therapeutic modalities, surgical intervention is indicated. The most effective surgical procedure for controlling severe uterine bleeding is hysterectomy; however, most obstetricians prefer to use this procedure as a last resort. Other surgical procedures employed in the treatment of severe postpartum hemorrhage include (1) uterine artery ligation (Fig. 3–4), (2) uteroovarian arterial anastomosis ligation (Fig. 3–4), (3) oversewing of the placental implantation site, and (4) bilateral hypogastric (internal iliac) artery ligation (Fig. 3–5). When uterine artery ligation and uteroovarian anastomosis ligation are combined, a 95% success rate is claimed; however, bilateral hypogastric artery ligation successfully controls uterine bleeding in fewer than half who undergo the procedure. None of these techniques is associated with the same efficacy as hysterectomy; so, for an unstable patient or in the setting of torrential hemorrhage, it is advisable to proceed with the definitive therapy, hysterectomy. Transabdominal compression of the aortic bifurcation against the verte-

Uterine artery ligation

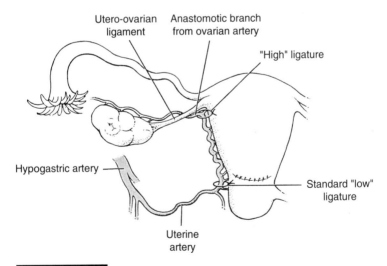

Figure 3–4

Uterine artery ligation. (From Clark SL, Phelan JP: Surgical control of obstetric hemorrhage. Contemp Obstet Gynecol 24(2):70, August 1984.)

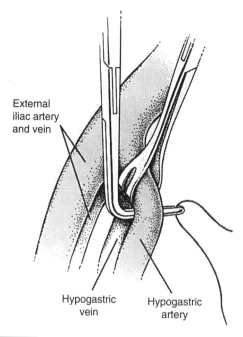

Figure 3-5

Hypogastric artery ligation. (From Clark SL, Phelan JP: Surgical control of obstetric hemorrhage. Contemp Obstet Gynecol 24(2):70, August 1984.)

brae may be used as a temporizing measure while the hemorrhaging woman is stabilized. Postoperatively, military antishock trousers (MAST) may be indicated for patients with persistent bleeding or when reexploration is best avoided. During MAST use, the circulatory well-being of the lower extremities must be closely monitored. Pressure damage to the peroneal nerve incurred during prolonged MAST suit inflation can result in foot drop (see Chapter 18).

Bibliography

Placenta Previa

Clark SL, Koonings PP, Phelan JP: Placenta previa/accreta and prior cesarean section. Obstet Gynecol 1985;66:89.

Cotton DB, Read JA, Paul RH, et al.: The conservative aggressive management of placenta previa. Am J Obstet Gynecol 1980;137:687.

Rizos N, Doran TA, Miskin M, et al.: Natural history of placenta previa ascertained by diagnostic ultrasound. Am J Obstet Gynecol 1979;133:287.

Placental Abruption

Hurd WW, Miodovnik M, Hertzberg V, et al.: Selective management of abruptio placentae: A prospective study. Obstet Gynecol 1983;61:467.
Scholl JS: Abruptio placentae: Clinical management in nonacute cases. Am J Obstet Gynecol 1987;156:40.

Postpartum Hemorrhage

Mengert WF, Burchell C, Blumstead RW, et al.: Pregnancy after bilateral ligation of the internal iliac and ovarian arteries. Obstet Gynecol 1969;34:664.
Watson P, Besch N, Bowes WA: Management of acute and subacute puerperal inversion of the uterus. Obstet Gynecol 1980;55:12.
Weis FR, MarKello R, Mo B, et al.: Cardiovascular effects of oxytocin. Obstet Gynecol 1975;46:211.

PHILIP SAMUELS

Acute Care of Thrombocytopenia and Disseminated Intravascular Coagulation Complicating Pregnancy

Life-threatening hematologic complications are rare during pregnancy. This is because obstetricians are attuned to the pathophysiology and antecedent events that may lead to these occurrences and take preventive action before the situation becomes an actual emergency. Nonetheless, despite the best possible obstetric care, such events occasionally occur. Rapid and decisive action on the part of the obstetrician averts a poor outcome in most cases. In this chapter I cover the areas of clinically significant thrombocytopenia and disseminated intravascular coagulation (DIC). Some aspects of these topics are controversial, and the purpose of this chapter is to serve as a guide for therapy. There are other acceptable approaches to treating the same clinical situations; this chapter presents general guidelines.

■ Thrombocytopenia

Etiology

Thrombocytopenia coincides with approximately 4% of all pregnancies and is the most common reason for hematology consultation during gestation. The common and rare causes of thrombocytopenia during pregnancy are listed in Table 4–1. Gestational thrombocytopenia occurs more frequently than thrombocytopenia of all other causes combined. It is generally characterized by mild, progressive thrombocytopenia detected incidentally on a routine complete blood count (CBC). It has come to attention recently because the automated blood cell counters presently used routinely measure and report platelet

Table 4–1

Causes of Thrombocytopenia During Pregnancy

Common Causes

Gestational thrombocytopenia
Severe preeclampsia
    HELLP syndrome
Immune thrombocytopenic purpura
Disseminated intravascular coagulation

Rare Causes

Lupus anticoagulant/antiphospholipid antibody syndrome
Systemic lupus erythematosus
Thrombotic thrombocytopenic purpura
Hemolytic uremic syndrome
Type IIb von Willebrand's syndrome
Folic acid deficiency
Human immunodeficiency virus infection
Hematologic malignancies
May-Hegglin syndrome (congenital thrombocytopenia)

counts, as the counters used 10 to 15 years ago did not. To make this diagnosis, the patient must have no history of a bleeding diathesis outside of pregnancy and should have a normal platelet count earlier in or prior to pregnancy (although this is not mandatory). Fewer than 1% of pregnant women have a platelet count below 100,000/mm^3, so the lower the platelet count, the more likely it is that the patient has an ongoing pathologic process. To be classified as gestational thrombocytopenia, the platelet count should be greater than 50,000/mm^3. The important fact is that this is a benign condition that poses virtually no risks to mother or fetus/neonate. The obstetrician, however, is obliged to rule out other serious causes of thrombocytopenia, including incipient preeclampsia, immune thrombocytopenic purpura (ITP), and DIC from a variety of causes. In most cases, invasive testing and therapy are more likely than the disease process to lead to misadventure for the patient. Problems arise when a patient who has had little prenatal care in the third trimester presents with a depressed platelet count. Such patients are often poor historians, and it is uncertain whether or not these patients have true ITP. The way we manage them is depicted in Figure 4–1. Occasionally, however, a patient with suspected gestational thrombocytopenia has a platelet count below 50,000/mm^3 and this requires special attention.

ITP, an autoimmune disorder that results in increased platelet destruction by the reticuloendothelial system, complicates as many as three pregnancies in every thousand. This can be an acute disorder with rapid remission and rare relapses, as in the case of childhood ITP that usually follows an acute viral illness. Conversely, it can be a chronic disorder that may eventually require constant glucocorticoid therapy. The importance and ramifications of this disorder have been a point of significant controversy among obstetricians. As this is an autoimmune phenomenon, platelet antibody testing is used to diagnose ITP. Platelet antibodies may be bound to platelets (platelet-associated, platelet-bound, or direct) or may be circulating (free, serum, indirect). Unfortunately, these antibodies cannot be used to diagnose ITP during pregnancy, as some patients with gestational thrombocytopenia and preeclampsia also demonstrate these immunoglobulins.

Some 13% to 24% of infants born to mothers with true ITP have platelet counts below 50,000/mm³. The presence of free,

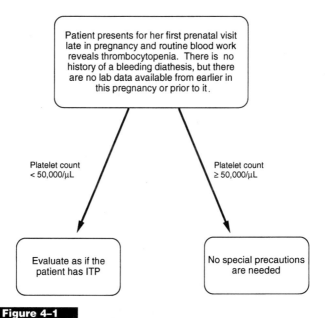

Figure 4–1

Obstetric management of the patient who presents for her first prenatal care late in pregnancy with scant information and an incidentally discovered depressed platelet count.

circulating immunoglobulin (IgG) class antibodies, when identified in a laboratory accustomed to dealing with pregnant patients, may serve as a rough indicator of women at risk for giving birth to a thrombocytopenic infant. They are only a rough predictor because their negative predictive value is excellent but their positive predictive value poor. These antibodies may serve as a screen to identify which patients might benefit from invasive testing and closer surveillance.

The controversies surrounding this disorder deal with mode of delivery and the need for cordocentesis to diagnose fetal thrombocytopenia. No prospective studies have investigated mode of delivery and fetal outcome. The problem is that all of these studies have been retrospective, and the largest have been metaanalyses. These studies have been contaminated by including many patients who have gestational thrombocytopenia, which carries negligible risk of poor outcome. In adults, a platelet count below 50,000/mm^3 is associated with increased morbidity. It is difficult to believe that a fetus, with its incompletely developed hemostatic capability, is at no risk when the platelet count is less than 50,000/mm^3. Even if the mode of delivery is not a concern in a fetus with profound thrombocytopenia, knowing the fetal platelet count may still be useful. If it is known that the fetus has a platelet count below 50,000/mm^3, the obstetrician may choose not to use a scalp electrode, not to allow a prolonged second stage, not to use forceps or vacuum delivery. These issues have not been studied. Perhaps, because of the risk of bleeding, neonates with a platelet count below 50,000/mm^3 should be delivered at a high-risk center. Our method of evaluating and managing pregnancies complicated by ITP is shown in Figure 4–2.

Thrombotic thrombocytopenic purpura (TTP) is a rare disorder but one that must be considered when a pregnant patient's platelet count is severely depressed. Pathologically, platelets aggregate, producing platelet thrombi that occlude arterioles and capillaries. This can produce ischemia and infarction in any organ system, but it frequently affects those most dependent on microcirculation, such as brain and kidneys. The cause of TTP remains elusive, but inadequate production of prostacyclin by endothelial cells, instability of produced prostacylin, or deficient plasminogen activator production by endothelial cells may play a role in the pathophysiology of this disorder.

TTP is a clinical diagnosis, and the disorder is characterized by a pentad of findings (Table 4–2). The complete pentad occurs in only about 40% of patients, but approximately 75 percent

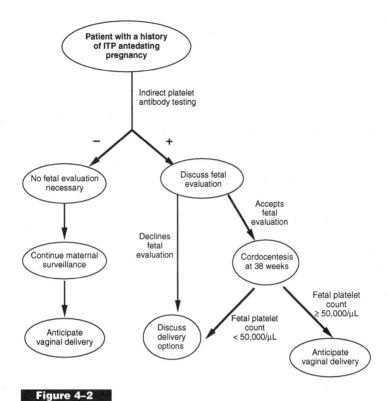

Figure 4-2

Obstetric management of the patient with ITP antedating pregnancy. This management plan, which utilizes platelet antibody testing, sharply narrows the number of patients who are offered invasive testing, with its inherent risks. This plan omits fetal scalp sampling, which we have found difficult to standardize. It may be utilized by experienced operators and would be useful to those who believe thrombocytopenic infants should be delivered by cesarean section. The management plan outlined here does not recommend a mode of delivery but leaves that decision to the obstetrician, patient, and pediatrician.

present with the triad of microangiopathic hemolytic anemia, thrombocytopenia, and neurologic changes. If TTP occurs during pregnancy, it usually occurs antepartum, and possibly during the second trimester. The disease may mimic severe preeclampsia or HELLP (hemolytic anemia, elevated liver function tests, and low platelets). Antithrombin III is frequently depressed in preeclampsia but not in TTP, so this laboratory test may help distinguish between the two serious disorders. TTP usually oc-

---

Table 4-2

Classic Findings in Thrombotic Thrombocytopenic Purpura*

Microangiopathic hemolytic anemia†
Thrombocytopenia†
Neurologic abnormalities† (confusion, headache, paresis, visual hallucinations, seizures)
Fever
Renal dysfunction

*The classic pentad is found in 40% of patients.

†This triad of findings is present in 75% of cases.

---

curs as an isolated incident with little risk of recurrence. Intermittent TTP is a rare disorder characterized by occasional episodes at irregular intervals. The rarest form of this disorder is chronic relapsing TTP that recurs at almost monthly intervals.

Treatment

When do gravidas with ITP or gestational thrombocytopenia require therapy? Previously, anyone with a platelet count below 50,000/mm³ received therapy. Spontaneous bleeding usually does not occur unless the platelet count approaches 20,000/mm³, and surgical bleeding does not occur until the platelet count falls below 50,000/mm³. Many hematologists, therefore, do not treat patients with platelet counts higher than 20,000/mm³ unless they are having spontaneous bleeding. Glucocorticoids are the first-line treatment to raise a depressed platelet count. Methylprednisolone is often used, as it has little mineralocorticoid effect. The usual dose of intravenous methylprednisolone is 1.0 to 1.5 mg/kg *total body weight*/day in divided doses. A response is usually seen in 2 days, but, rarely, it takes as long as 10 days to see a maximum rise in platelet count. After the desired response has been seen, the patient may be switched to oral prednisone. The usual starting dose is 1 mg/kg *total body weight*/day. The dose can be rapidly tapered to 40 mg/day and then slowly thereafter to maintain the mother's platelet count at approximately 100,000/mm³ for the remainder of the pregnancy. Approximately 70% of patients respond to glucocorticoids.

For those patients who fail to respond to glucocorticoids, intravenous immunoglobulin (IVIG) should be administered.

The usual dose is 0.4 gm/kg/day for 3 to 5 days, but an occasional patient requires as much as 1 gm/kg/day. The response usually begins in 2 to 3 days and usually peaks within 5 days. The duration of response is variable, so if IVIG is being administered to raise the maternal platelet count before delivery, proper timing is essential. In general, if a peak platelet count is needed for delivery, the course of therapy should be started 5 to 8 days before the planned induction or cesarean delivery. Although IVIG is a blood product, several steps in production make it extremely safe. Plasma is thawed and pooled. After the cryoprecipitate is removed, the remaining effluent undergoes several steps of cold ethanol fractionation, which inactivates viruses. Furthermore, the liquid form of IVIG is incubated for 21 days at pH 4.25, which inactivates both enveloped and nonenveloped DNA and RNA viruses, thus increasing its safety.

If there is inadequate response to IVIG, splenectomy can be performed safely during gestation. The best time is during the second trimester, before the uterus enlarges enough to interfere with surgical exposure. Splenectomy can be carried out at the time of cesarean delivery if necessary, by extending a midline skin incision cephalad after uterine closure.

Platelet transfusion is indicated for profoundly thrombocytopenic patients who have clinically significant bleeding while awaiting the effect of other therapies or before vaginal delivery, cesarean delivery, or splenectomy. Furthermore, platelets should be administered before surgery if the maternal count is below $50,000/mm^3$ or before vaginal delivery if the maternal platelet count is around $20,000/mm^3$. The viability of transfused platelets is extremely short lived because the same antibodies and reticuloendothelial cell clearance that affect the mother's endogenous platelets also destroy and sequester the transfused platelets. Transfusion at the time of skin incision should provide adequate hemostasis to complete the case. Each unit of platelets increases the maternal platelet count approximately $10,000/mm^3$. A scheme for treating maternal ITP is shown in Figure 4–3. Certain technical surgical precautions should be taken when performing cesarean delivery on patients with severe thrombocytopenia. Some of these are listed in Table 4–3.

Intensive plasma manipulation is the key to treating TTP. Therapy usually entails a combination of plasmapheresis and plasma exchange with platelet-poor normal fresh-frozen plasma (FFP, 3 to 4 L/day). Plasmapheresis removes platelet-aggregating substances, and plasma infusion provides some antiaggregating substances deficient in the patient's plasma. If exchange plasma-

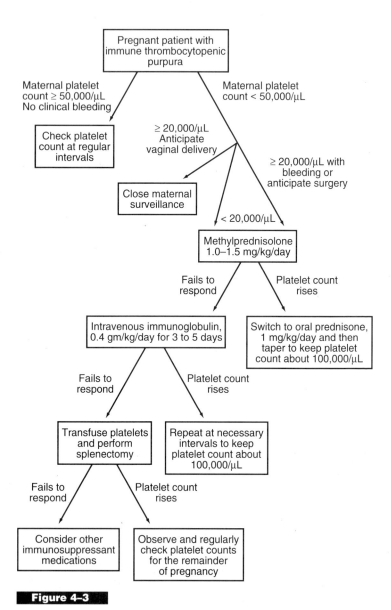

Figure 4–3

The management of maternal thrombocytopenia in the gravida with ITP antedating pregnancy.

> ### Table 4–3
>
> ### Surgical Tips for Performing a Cesarean Delivery on a Severely Thrombocytopenic Woman
>
> If the patient is experiencing clinically significant bleeding, use a midline skin incision; otherwise a Pfannenstiel incision is acceptable
>
> Use electrocautery liberally.
>
> Close the uterus in two layers.
>
> Leave the bladder flap open to prevent hematoma formation that could later lead to fever or abscess.
>
> Close the peritoneum. This prevents bleeding from vessels at the edge that often are not seen and allows a space for subfascial drains.
>
> Place subfascial drains and leave them in place until they stop draining.
>
> Use skin staples, even with a Pfannenstiel incision. This allows the obstetrician to open only part of the incision if a subcutaneous hematoma forms.
>
> Place a pressure dressing over the incision, and do not remove it for 48 hr unless signs of active bleeding are observed.

pheresis is not readily available, infusion of FFP (30 mL/kg/day) can be used as a temporizing measure. If this is done, the treating physician must be careful to observe for signs of volume overload. If a patient responds completely to plasmapheresis, this procedure should be continued for at least 5 days. In patients who exhibit a partial response without clinical deterioration, plasmapheresis and plasma exchange should be continued for 3 to 4 weeks to achieve complete remission.

Glucocorticoids should be administered to all patients with TTP immediately after diagnosis. The U.S. TTP Study Group recommends administering 0.75 mg/kg of methylprednisolone intravenously every 12 hours until the patient recovers.

If patients do not begin to respond within 5 days of therapy, or if their condition deteriorates within the first 3 days, other therapies should be considered, for example, vincristine, azathioprine, or splenectomy. Occasionally, in refractory cases cryosupernatant may be substituted for FFP in the plasma exchange protocol. Treatment of the pregnant patient with TTP is outlined in Figure 4–4.

Disseminated Intravascular Coagulation

DIC describes a widespread hematologic condition characterized by accelerated fibrin formation and lysis. It is truly a consump-

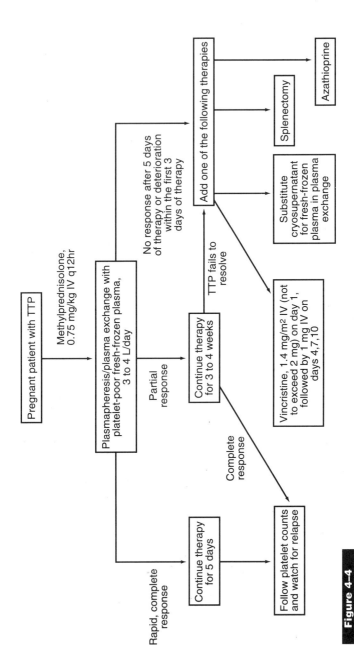

Figure 4-4

See legend on opposite page

Table 4–4
Causes of Disseminated Intravascular Coagulation in Pregnancy
Common Causes
Greater than expected blood loss with inadequate crystalloid and/or colloid replacement
Placental abruption
Severe preeclampsia/HELLP syndrome
Rare Causes
Sepsis
Acute fatty liver of pregnancy
Retained dead fetus
Septic abortion
Amniotic fluid embolus
Adult respiratory distress syndrome
Autoimmune disease
Acute hemolytic transfusion reactions
Hematologic malignancies
Solid tumors

tive coagulopathy. DIC occurs when regulatory systems that control the fine balance between the coagulation cascade and the fibrinolytic system go awry. In acute situations, the massive activation of the coagulation cascade may simply overwhelm control mechanisms. DIC may be initiated by exposure of blood to tissue factor or a host of proteolytic enzymes. Release of tissue factor may occur as a result of trauma, release from mononuclear cells after stimulation by endotoxin, or obstetric events such as placental abruption.

Etiology

The most common obstetric causes of DIC are listed in Table 4–4. The most common cause is probably underestimation of

---

Figure 4–4

The management of the gravida with TTP. Before adopting this patient care plan, the treating physician must be certain of the diagnosis. TTP is a clinical diagnosis and can mimic severe preeclampsia. The criteria for diagnosing TTP are listed in Table 4–2.

blood loss at delivery with inadequate replacement by crystalloid or colloid. In these cases, vasospasm occurs with resultant endothelial damage and initiation of DIC. Also, hypotension results in decreased perfusion leading to local hypoxia and acidosis at the tissue level, thus starting the DIC cascade. By keeping the patient's volume replete, DIC can often be avoided, even when anemia is severe.

Although every medical student is taught that a retained dead fetus can cause DIC, this is unusual. This process must continue for at least 3 weeks before DIC can occur. The exception, of course, is fetal death caused by placental abruption. In this scenario, the abruption initiates DIC. Previously, most obstetricians believed that the problems seen in a second twin after its monozygotic twin died in utero were secondary to embolization of thromboplastin from the deceased twin to the surviving one, with resultant DIC. Current evidence, however, implicates hypotension in the second twin after death of the first as the etiology of these phenomena.

Placental abruption can cause DIC. When the retroplacental blood clot forms and expands, it consumes coagulation factors and may result in consumptive coagulopathy. This takes place if delivery does not occur in timely fashion or if coagulation factors are not administered when needed. The coagulation profile in these cases usually begins as an isolated drop in fibrinogen with an increase in fibrin degradation products. It is difficult to rely solely on an isolated fibrinogen level to determine if consumptive coagulopathy is ensuing, as the fibrinogen level is often very high in pregnancy with a wide normal range. This level needs to be followed serially to determine if abruption is leading to consumptive coagulopathy. If the abruption continues to expand before delivery, DIC develops with clinically relevant bleeding.

Both gram-negative and gram-positive bacteria (especially hemolytic streptococci) can produce sepsis resulting in DIC. In these cases, endotoxin or cytokines such as interleukin 1 and tissue necrosis factor may lead to loss of normal hemostatic mechanisms controlled by the endothelium throughout the body. Therefore, DIC should be anticipated whenever a pregnant patient presents with overwhelming sepsis and has evidence of abnormal bleeding.

Severe preeclampsia and the HELLP syndrome can result in DIC if delivery is not effected promptly. Usually, however, these patients show isolated thrombocytopenia owing to increased destruction of platelets by the reticuloendothelial system. Clinically significant DIC is rare in these patients unless the disease process goes unchecked. Even though there is no evidence of overt DIC in most severely preeclamptic patients, laboratory evidence often demonstrates subclinical DIC.

Diagnosis

The diagnosis of DIC can be made preliminarily from any sensitive laboratory parameter of fibrinolysis. Fibrin degradation products are the most readily available gauge of fibrinolysis. An increase in the fibrin D-dimer also may predict fibrinolysis. It holds some advantages over the standard tests for fibrin degradation products, as either serum or plasma may be used and incomplete clotting of the serum sample does not produce spurious results. Falling levels of plasminogen or alpha-2-antiplasmin also indicate greatly increased fibrinolytic activity. As clotting factors are consumed and the disease process continues, the prothrombin time is prolonged and the fibrinogen level drops. In pregnancy, however, the normal range for fibrinogen is so broad that a single value is not useful. The physician must serially follow levels of this parameter.

A falling level of antithrombin III (AT III) usually indicates accelerated coagulation. The prothrombin time (PT) is prolonged as the levels of most clotting factors in the extrinsic pathway (especially II, V, VII, and X) fall in DIC. Conversely, factor VIII levels often rise owing to release of factor VIII/von Willebrand's complex from endothelial cells. This explains why the activated partial thromboplastin time (aPTT) is often normal or even shortened in cases of DIC. Levels of fibrinopeptide A and the prothrombin fragment 1.2 are also sensitive and specific indicators of the degree of coagulation activation.

It is very important to note that a falling platelet count is neither sensitive nor specific for DIC. The peripheral smear can show schistocytes and other findings typical of DIC. A normal peripheral smear, however, does not preclude the diagnosis of DIC.

Treatment

The basic treatment of DIC involves correcting the inciting event. In placental abruption, delivery in a timely fashion is the definitive therapy. If the fetus is stable, vaginal delivery can be accomplished as long as the mother's fluid status and hematologic parameters are monitored and therapy is initiated when appropriate. If an amniotic fluid embolus is the cause, the mother's cardiovascular status must be supported and the coagulopathy treated rapidly, as cardiovascular collapse and DIC are the most frequent causes of maternal death. In the case of a retained dead fetus, delivery should be accomplished after DIC is diagnosed. In this situation, DIC takes several weeks to develop and is related to the gestational age and size of the fetus at the time of death. In the case of DIC related to severe preeclampsia or HELLP, definitive treatment is delivery. Vaginal delivery is preferable, but if the condition of the fetus is unstable or if the mother's condition is deteriorating, cesarean delivery should be seriously considered.

Treating the patient with DIC secondary to sepsis requires rapid and special care. Broad-spectrum antibiotics should be given, and the choice of antibiotics depends on the site of the suspected underlying infection. If the infection is due to an abscess (including intrauterine infection), the site should be drained. If the infection is due to an indwelling intravascular or urethral catheter, these must be removed. Although most patients with DIC suffer most from hemorrhage, when the disorder is secondary to infection there is a concomitant risk of thrombosis. Heparin should not be administered unless there is strong evidence of thrombosis in these patients with DIC secondary to infection.

Table 4–5 summarizes the use of clotting factors in DIC. Plasma replacement therapy should be considered when the PT is approximately 1.5 times the control value. This test is a rough indicator of the extent to which the extrinsic clotting system has

---

Table 4–5

Treatment of Disseminated Intravascular Coagulation in Pregnancy

Treat underlying cause.

If the prothrombin time is greater than 1.5 times the control value, transfuse FFP. The goal is to keep PT within 2 to 3 sec of the control value.

If the fibrinogen concentration is <100 mg/dL, transfuse cryoprecipitate.
  Ten units of cryoprecipitate are usually given after every 2 to 3 units of plasma.
  Each unit of cryoprecipitate increases the fibrinogen by 10 mg/dL.

Platelets should be transfused if the platelet count is <20,000/mm^3 or if clinically significant bleeding occurs with a platelet count between 20,000 and 50,000/mm^3. The usual rate of platelet transfusion is 1 to 3 U/10 kg/d.

been activated. The goal is to keep the PT within 2 to 3 seconds of the control value. In addition to clotting factors, fresh-frozen plasma contains inhibitors of fibrinolysis and coagulation as well as other factors that promote healing of endothelial cells. When administering plasma, the physician must carefully evaluate the patient's volume status and renal function, to prevent fluid overload. If the fibrinogen is below 100 mg/dL, cryoprecipitate should be administered. Each unit of cryoprecipitate raises the fibrinogen level about 10 mg/dL. In patients with DIC and a fibrinogen level below 100 mg/dL, the usual transfusion regimen is 10 units of cryoprecipitate for every 2 to 3 U ⌄f plasma. This infuses maximal fibrinogen in a small volume. If the patient develops clinically significant anemia, red blood cells should be replaced as indicated. This depends on the patient's hemodynamic status, the rate of drop of hemoglobin concentration, and the concentration of hemoglobin before the onset of DIC. With the exception of severe preeclampsia/HELLP, profound thrombocytopenia is not usually a part of the DIC syndrome. If the platelet count falls below 20,000/mm^3 or if clinical bleeding occurs with a platelet count between 20,000 and 50,000/mm^3, platelet transfusion may be indicated. The usual rate of platelet transfusion is 1 to 3 units/10 kg/day.

Vitamin K and folate should be administered because patients with DIC are often deficient in these vitamins. There is some growing evidence that administering antithrombin III concentrate to patients with DIC may ameliorate the condition and shorten its course. It may promote healing of endothelial cells and retard overactive fibrinolysis. There is some evidence that heparin may be useful in treating DIC in a patient with a retained dead fetus. This has been reported in twin pregnancies when attempts have been made to prolong the gestation of the surviving twin. Unless the patient is at an extremely early point in gestation, the preferred treatment for this condition is delivery.

■
Bibliography

Aster RH: Gestational thrombocytopenia. A plea for conservative management. N Engl J Med 1990;323:264.

Burrows RF, Kelton JG: Low fetal risks in pregnancies associated with idiopathic thrombocytopenic purpura. Am J Obstet Gynecol 1990;163:1147.

Burrows RF, Kelton JG: Fetal thrombocytopenia and its relation to maternal thrombocytopenia. N Engl J Med 1993;329:1463.

Cines DB, Dusak B, Tomaski A, et al.: Immune thrombocytopenic purpura and pregnancy. N Engl J Med 1982;306:826.

Gabbe SG, Neibyl JR, Simpson JL (eds): Obstetrics: Normal and Problem Pregnancies, ed 2. New York: Churchill Livingstone, 1991;1137–1150.

Hoffman R, Benz EJ Jr, Shattil SJ, et al. (eds): Hematology: Basic Principles and Practice. New York: Churchill Livingstone, 1991;1394–1405.

Hoffman R, Benz EJ Jr, Shattil SJ, et al. (eds): Hematology: Basic Principles and Practice. New York: Churchill Livingstone, 1991;1495–1500.

McCrae KR, Samuels P, Schreiber AD: Pregnancy-associated thrombocytopenia: Pathogenesis and management. Blood 1992;80:2697.

Repke JT (ed): Intrapartum Obstetrics. New York: Churchill Livingstone, 1996;431–446.

Rousell RH, Good RA, Pirofsky B, et al.: Non-A non-B hepatitis and the safety of intravenous immunoglobulin pH 4.25: A retrospective survey. Vox Sang 1988;54:6.

Samuels P, Bussel JB, Braitman LE, et al.: Estimation of the risk of thrombocytopenia in the offspring of pregnant women with presumed immune thrombocytopenic purpura. N Engl J Med 1990;323:229.

Weiner CP: Thrombotic microangiopathy in pregnancy and the postpartum period. Semin Hematol 1987;24:119.

WILLIAM H. CLEWELL

Hypertensive Emergencies in Pregnancy

5

Almost all hypertensive emergencies in pregnancy are related to preeclampsia. The exceptions to this rule are rare but important causes of hypertension. The initial management is the same, regardless of the disease, so therapy can be initiated while the evaluation to determine the correct diagnosis is carried out. Preeclampsia can be either "pure" or superimposed on chronic hypertension. The incidence of this problem peaks in the late third trimester of pregnancy. When it is superimposed on chronic hypertension it may develop late in the second trimester. In the circumstance of underlying lupus anticoagulant or anticardiolipin antibody it may present as early as 20 to 25 weeks. When associated with a molar pregnancy, it may develop before 20 weeks' gestation.

Since both maternal and fetal well-being must be considered, treatment must balance the need to reduce blood pressure for the mother's benefit with the need to maintain uteroplacental perfusion for fetal oxygenation. In this chapter I deal primarily with the diagnosis and management of preeclampsia and its variants during labor and delivery.

■ Pathophysiology

Etiology

The underlying cause of preeclampsia has not been determined. Progress in this area is hampered by the fact that there is not an animal model that duplicates the human disease. The human disease can present in several different ways, and only in their fullest expression are these diverse syndromes recognized as variants of preeclampsia. A number of observations have contributed to our understanding of the underlying physiology, but they do not make a complete theory or model in that not all patients exhibit all the pathologic or laboratory abnormalities and not all patients with the abnormalities develop preeclampsia.

The earliest change noted in patients who develop preeclampsia is relative failure of trophoblastic invasion of the spiral arteries of the placental bed. In normal pregnancies there is extensive invasion of the musculoelastic layers of the spiral arteries, beginning with implantation and lasting until 8 to 10 weeks' gestation. A second wave of trophoblastic invasion takes place around 18 to 20 weeks' gestation. This process converts the muscular spiral arteries into passive, nonmuscular, low-resistance vessels that supply the intervillous space of the placenta. Patients destined to develop preeclampsia exhibit relative failure of this second wave of trophoblastic invasion. This abnormality of the spiral arteries, known as "acute atherosis," is most prominent in patients who develop severe preeclampsia. Since this event occurs at the point of contact between mother and fetus, it has been suggested that an immune-mediated process is involved. It has also been suggested that women destined to develop preeclampsia have a genetic abnormality that causes the failure of trophoblastic invasion. This placental abnormality may contribute to the increased incidence of placental abruption and antepartum hemorrhage seen with preeclampsia.

Histochemical studies of the pregnant and nonpregnant uterus have shown almost complete adrenergic denervation of the uterus in normal pregnancies. Patients with preeclampsia have less complete denervation. Patients with preeclampsia have higher uterine tissue levels of norepinephrine. The combination of retention of the musculoelastic coat of the spiral arteries, incomplete adrenergic denervation, and elevated norepinephrine concentration has the potential to cause constriction of the spiral arteries and to decrease placental perfusion.

Normal healthy pregnant women are relatively insensitive to pressor substances. It has been shown that women who later develop preeclampsia fail to develop this resistance. After 20 weeks' gestation, women who will not develop preeclampsia require progressively larger amounts of infused angiotensin to cause a 15-mm Hg rise in diastolic blood pressure. Women who will develop preeclampsia do not show this decrease in sensitivity. The physiologic mechanism of this decreased pressor sensitivity has not been determined.

It has been suggested that a relative increase in the ratio of concentrations of thromboxane and prostacyclin is present in patients who later develop preeclampsia. Small doses (81 mg per day) of aspirin have been shown to reduce the incidence of preeclampsia in high-risk patients. It is thought that this dose of aspirin selectively reduces the synthesis of thromboxane and adjusts the ratio of thromboxane to prostacyclin back toward normal.

Physiologic Changes

In preeclampsia, the patient's cardiac output can be normal, increased, or decreased. Systemic vascular resistance frequently is increased. Depending on the balance of these factors the patient may have marked hypertension or normal blood pressure. Patients with preeclampsia almost always have a smaller plasma volume than normal pregnant patients. The vasospasm and variable cardiac output changes lead to labile hypertension. Further changes in blood volume due to intravenous fluids, pharmacologic vasodilatation, or blood loss can lead to rapid— and at times dangerous—fluctuations in blood pressure.

Diffuse endothelial cell injury seems to play a role in the pathogenesis of preeclampsia. The mechanism or agent of this injury remains obscure, but the injury causes activation of intravascular coagulation and fibrin deposition. This in turn appears to be responsible for much of the organ dysfunction associated with severe disease. This includes the consumption of platelets and other clotting factors, seizures and coma, abnormal renal and liver function, fetal growth restriction, and placental abruption.

■ Management Plan

The goal of management in maternal hypertensive emergencies is delivery of a healthy infant without placing at undue risk the mother's life and health. Since the only definitive treatment of preeclampsia is delivery, the approach to this goal, especially in early-onset preeclampsia, often involves compromises between maternal and fetal considerations. Figure 5–1 reviews, in algorithm format, the management of severe preeclampsia or hypertension in obstetric patients.

■ Diagnostic Evaluation

As for all clinical diagnoses, a clear assessment of past and present medical history is essential in arriving at the correct

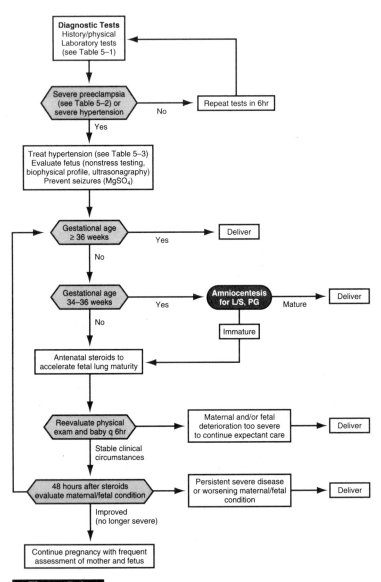

Figure 5–1

Algorithm for management of severe preeclampsia and hypertension.

diagnosis. It is important to seek underlying medical conditions that would predispose to the development of preeclampsia. Specifically, a history of chronic hypertension, renal disease, collagen vascular disorders, and diabetes should be sought. Superimposed preeclampsia tends to occur at an earlier gestational age and may be more severe than "pure" preeclampsia. Recurrent preeclampsia probably reflects an underlying predisposing condition.

Measurement of blood pressure must be accurate if the physician is to make a correct diagnosis. Indirect pressure determination with an appropriate sized sphygmomanometer cuff placed on the right arm of the seated patient correlates best with directly determined systolic, diastolic, and mean arterial pressures. It is generally agreed that blood pressure greater than 140/90 is diagnostic of hypertension in pregnancy. A rise above baseline values of more than 30 mm Hg for systolic pressure or 15 mm Hg for diastolic pressure is often used. Since a basal, nonpregnant or first trimester blood pressure often is not known, using the 140/90 definition of hypertension is most practical. A diastolic pressure greater than 110 mm Hg is considered severe hypertension. Occasional patients with severe preeclampsia or HELLP (*h*emolytic anemia, *e*levated *l*iver function tests, and *l*ow *p*latelets) syndrome do not manifest hypertension.

Edema is considered a hallmark of preeclampsia but is highly variable. Many normal pregnant patients have marked edema of the upper and lower extremities. Facial edema can be dramatic in preeclampsia but can be difficult to identify and distinguish from normal changes of pregnancy. If serial weight records on the patient are available, rapid weight gain can provide an objective assessment of excessive fluid retention.

Laboratory evaluation in this condition starts with urine testing for proteinuria. Semiquantitative assessment by "dipstick" giving a value of 1+ is considered significant. This corresponds to more than 300 mg of protein in a 24-hour urine collection. While proteinuria is not always present, it is a defining characteristic of preeclampsia. Table 5–1 lists laboratory tests that may be helpful in diagnosing preeclampsia. For almost all of these tests, the *trend* of values is more important than a single value. The interval over which they should be repeated depends on the clinical severity of the condition. Often it is necessary to follow values at intervals as short as to 4 to 6 hours to establish a trend and rate of change.

Preeclampsia is categorized as mild or severe. If one or more of the items listed in Table 5–2 is present, it is severe.

Table 5–1

Laboratory Test Findings Useful for the Diagnosis of Preeclampsia

Test	"Suspect" Value
Hemoglobin	11 mg% (rising value, hemoconcentration)
Hematocrit	35% (rising value, hemoconcentration)
Uric acid	>4.5 mg/dL
Platelet count	<150,000/mm³
Serum glutamic-oxaloacetic transaminase (SGOT)	>41 IU/L
Serum glutamic-pyruvic transaminase (SGPT)	>30 IU/L
Blood urea nitrogen	>14 mg/dL (rising value)
Creatinine	>0.8 mg/dL
Proteinuria	1+ or 300 mg/24-hr collection

Table 5–2

Diagnostic Criteria of Severe Preeclampsia

Clinical

Epigastric pain
Visual disturbances
Headache unresponsive to conventional therapy
Associated severe intrauterine growth restriction
Cyanosis or pulmonary edema
Blood pressure of ≥160 mm Hg systolic, or ≥110 mm Hg diastolic, recorded on at least two occasions at least 6 hr apart with patient at bed rest
Oliguria (<400 mL in 24 hr)

Laboratory

Thrombocytopenia (<150,000/mm³)
Proteinuria (≥5 gm in 24 hr or 3+ or 4+ on dipstick qualitative exam)
Elevated liver function test (SGOT, SGPT)

While the mother's condition is being evaluated, the fetus' condition must also be assessed. The fetus may be acutely affected and in immediate danger, may be chronically compromised with intrauterine growth restriction (IUGR) and oligohydramnios or both. The immediate well-being of the fetus can be quickly assessed with nonstress testing (NST), contraction stress testing (CST), or biophysical profile (BPP). Of these three tests, CST is most sensitive at detecting uteroplacental insufficiency. A positive CST result indicates lack of fetal reserve, but it does not mandate immediate delivery. Given a reactive NST or normal BPP and a positive CST, one can often defer delivery while awaiting maternal stabilization or acceleration of fetal lung maturation with glucocorticoids.

Fetal compromise of longer standing is generally detected by the demonstration of IUGR and oligohydramnios. It is not uncommon, however, to observe fetal growth restriction before any clinical evidence of preeclampsia appears. When preeclampsia is suspected, an ultrasound examination for IUGR and oligohydramnios is needed. If there is independent confirmation of gestational age, the finding of IUGR supports the diagnosis of severe preeclampsia and alerts the clinician to the presence of fetal compromise. The growth-restricted fetus is at high risk for acute distress before or during labor, especially if oligohydramnios is present.

■ Control of Hypertension

Since acute hypertension represents an immediate threat to the mother, measures must be taken to control and reduce arterial pressure. The first-line drug in the treatment of acute hypertension during pregnancy, hydralazine, is safe and has a long history of use in this condition. It can be given as a continuous intravenous infusion or as intermittent intravenous doses. Table 5–3 lists the dosage for this and other drugs that can be used to treat maternal hypertension. The reader is also referred to Table 8–2 for a more comprehensive table of antihypertensive agents used during pregnancy. The goal of treatment is to prevent hypertensive damage to the mother and at the same time preserve adequate uteroplacental perfusion for fetal oxygenation. In practice, this means reducing maternal diastolic pressure to between 90 and 100 mm Hg. If maternal diastolic pressure exceeds 110, specific antihypertensive therapy should be insti-

---

Table 5–3

First-Line Medications for the Treatment of Severe Hypertension in Critically Ill Gravidas*

Hydralazine
Mechanism of action: Direct smooth muscle relaxation
Half-life: 1 hr
Elimination: Liver and gut
Dosage: 5–10 mg slow IV push, repeated every 10–20 min as needed (up to a total of 30 mg)
Maternal side effects: Headaches, tachycardia, nausea, flushing, hypotension, angina, lupuslike syndrome
Fetal effects: None

Labetalol
Mechanism of action: α_1- and nonselective β-blockade (PO, balanced α and β effects; IV, primarily β effect with small α-blocking effect)
Half-life: 4–6 hr
Elimination: Hepatic
Dosage: 10–20 mg slow IV push, followed by 20–80 mg IV push every 10 min to a total dose of 300 mg
Maternal side effects: Bradycardia, postural hypotension, cold extremities, sleep disturbance, rebound hypertension; may exacerbate asthma and mask hypoglycemia
Fetal effects: May cause respiratory depression and bradycardia

Nifedipine
Mechanism of action: Calcium channel blocker
Half-life: 1.8 hr
Elimination: Hepatic
Dosage: 10 mg sublingual every 10–30 min as needed (three doses)
Maternal side effects: Postural hypotension, flushing, headache, tachycardia
Fetal effects: None in humans

---

*Table 8–2 contains additional antihypertensive drugs commonly used in the obstetric intensive care setting.

---

tuted. Magnesium sulfate, which is usually used to prevent eclamptic seizures, has little or no antihypertensive effect.

Prevention of Convulsions

Equally important to blood pressure control is prevention of convulsions. While the likelihood of their occurrence increases with increasing blood pressure, they can occur with diastolic pressures as low as 95 mm Hg. Headache and hyperreflexia with ankle clonus generally antedate seizures. The mainstay of preventive treatment is magnesium sulfate. Some authors have advocated other agents, such as benzodiazepines, but the wide experience with magnesium sulfate and its relative safety for both mother and infant have made it the drug of choice in the United States. While it can be given by deep intramuscular injection, the rate of absorption from this site and the difficulty of predicting and adjusting the systemic effect makes the intramuscular route less useful than the intravenous one. The goal of therapy is to prevent eclamptic seizures. This endeavor requires a steady-state serum magnesium level of 4 to 6 mEq/L. This can generally be achieved with an intravenous bolus infusion of 4 gm magnesium sulfate over 5 minutes followed by a continuous infusion of 1 to 2 gm per hour. In patients with impaired renal function, lower rates of infusion may be needed. In patients with an increased volume of distribution and blood volume, such as those with a multiple gestation, higher rates of infusion may be required. It is generally sufficient to follow magnesium therapy with clinical signs. At therapeutic levels hyperreflexia diminishes. At a level of 10 mEq/L there is loss of deep tendon reflexes. Respiratory arrest occurs at a level of 15 mEq/L and cardiac arrest at levels above 25 mEq/L. Since patients with preeclampsia often have decreasing renal function, serum levels can rise rapidly during constant intravenous infusion. Frequent assessment of the patient's deep tendon reflexes, respiratory rate, and mental status is important to avoid toxicity. With changes in any of these parameters determination of a serum magnesium concentration is useful for confirming therapeutic or toxic levels. If toxicity is suspected, the infusion rate should be reduced or discontinued until the level is determined. For acute toxicity calcium gluconate (10 mL of 10% solution) can be given intravenously over 3 minutes as an antidote.

■
Liver Function

Hepatic injury is a common feature of severe preeclampsia. Manifestations can range from mild elevation of serum liver enzymes to frank liver failure. Subcapsular hematoma of the liver is an unusual but life-threatening complication of preeclampsia. Patients with preeclampsia often complain of epigastric pain, which is due to swelling of the liver with stretching of the capsule. With severe epigastric or right upper quadrant pain, sudden exacerbation, or an unexplained hypotensive blood pressure trend, one must strongly consider subcapsular hepatic hematoma. Ultrasound of the liver can make the diagnosis in most cases. The only definitive treatment of the liver dysfunction is delivery. Maternal steroid treatment has been shown in small, uncontrolled trials to transiently improve hepatic function and platelet abnormalities. Rarely, in cases of expanding or ruptured subcapsular hematoma, surgery is needed to control the hemorrhage.

Renal Function

The glomerular lesion typical of preeclampsia no doubt accounts for the proteinuria. It may also contribute to decreased glomerular filtration. Most of the impairment of renal clearance, however, is caused by intravascular plasma volume constriction. Urine output must be followed hourly in these patients. Only with continuous catheter drainage can the renal output be monitored adequately. The initial treatment of oliguria is cautious expansion of the blood volume. In young healthy women without clinical evidence of heart failure or pulmonary edema, this can safely be done with intravenous crystalloid solution. Usually, 500 to 1000 mL of normal saline or lactated Ringer's solution given over 1 to 2 hours results in improved urine output. For patients who do not respond with appropriate diuresis it is necessary to use invasive hemodynamic monitoring with a pulmonary artery catheter. Accurate assessment of hemodynamic variables, including systemic vascular resistance, cardiac output, pulmonary capillary wedge pressure, and serum colloid oncotic pressure, allows optimization of physiologic functions, improving both renal function and uteroplacental perfusion. This process may entail use of vasodilator, colloid, crystalloid, or diuretic therapy (see Chapters 1 and 8).

Hematologic Alterations

The most common and often the first hematologic change noted in preeclampsia is hemoconcentration. Rising hematocrit values found on serial evaluations can signal worsening of disease. This pathophysiologic aberration reflects the overall constriction of the plasma volume. The relative hypovolemia contributes to the oliguria noted above and makes the patient very susceptible to sudden changes in blood pressure due to volume expansion, blood loss, or the sympathectomy associated with conduction anesthesia (see Chapter 20).

Thrombocytopenia commonly develops in severe pre-eclampsia, principally owing to consumption of platelets. The degree of thrombocytopenia can be mild and evident only on serial measurements or profound with peripheral counts as low as 1000 platelets/mm^3. It is rarely necessary to treat the thrombocytopenia directly. Excessive bleeding is unusual, even during surgery, unless the count falls below 50,000 platelets/mm^3. Since the problem is manifested by rapid platelet destruction, platelet transfusion provides only transient improvement. For this reason, platelet transfusion should be given only when it will provide the most timely benefit. In the case of operative delivery, platelet transfusion at the start of surgery or during the operation near the time of closing seems most prudent.

Glucocorticoid therapy has been shown in uncontrolled trials to transiently normalize both platelet count and liver enzyme values. This therapy can, in some cases, allow for significant prolongation of the pregnancy.

In addition to the antepartum benefit of glucocorticoid therapy, postpartum administration has also been shown, again in an uncontrolled trial, to be effective in shortening the postpartum recovery period in patients with severe HELLP syndrome.

Glucocorticoid therapy for HELLP syndrome:

Antepartum: Dexamethasone, 10 mg IV every 12 hours (36-hour course).
Postpartum: Dexamethasone, 10 mg IV; then 10 mg, 5 mg, 5 mg IV at 12-hour intervals (36-hour course).

Delivery as Definitive Treatment

The only definitive cure for preeclampsia is delivery. If the patient is near term, delivery by induction of labor—or by cesarean section if the fetus will not tolerate labor or if labor cannot be successfully induced—is curative. When the pregnancy is far from term, delivery is less easy to achieve and may not be in the best interest of the fetus. Management then becomes an exercise in weighing the risks for the fetus in utero versus in the nursery, and the risks for the mother of continuing the pregnancy. If the pregnancy is between 34 and 36 weeks, amniocentesis to determine fetal lung maturity is useful. Many fetuses, in pregnancies complicated by preeclampsia, have mature lung studies at this gestational age. Beyond 36 weeks, delivery is appropriate without amniocentesis.

Management of the pregnancy before 34 weeks or with immature fetal lungs is more difficult. Treatment with glucocorticoids to accelerate fetal lung maturity is safe for patients with preeclampsia as long as fetal testing is employed. Since it takes 48 hours to achieve optimal fetal benefit from this treatment, the administration should occur as early as practical in the course of management. Since there seem to be no adverse maternal or fetal effects, steroids should be administered as soon as the patient is admitted to the hospital and fetal well-being is ascertained. If further evaluation of the mother indicates that delivery cannot be delayed, then the fetus has had the maximal benefit, even if it has been only a few hours. This may be particularly important for extremely premature infants (less than 30 weeks' gestation). A very premature fetus may benefit because the risk of intracranial hemorrhage is reduced after only a few hours of steroid therapy. At 48 hours after the initial steroid injection the patient should be reevaluated for delivery. If there has been amelioration of the signs and symptoms and if the fetus is doing well, further prolongation of the pregnancy can be considered. During this expectant management period, frequent maternal and fetal assessments must be made to assess the safety of continuing the pregnancy. Delivery can be accomplished by induction of labor or by cesarean section. The choice depends on multiple fetal and maternal considerations. If the fetus is in a vertex position and the cervix is favorable or can be ripened, induction of labor is reasonable. Vaginal delivery certainly carries less risk of morbidity for the mother, and it may improve initial pulmonary function of the newborn. If the mother's condition is deteriorating rapidly and delivery is likely to take many hours, cesarean section after maternal stabilization is the best option.

Anesthesia for delivery of a hypertensive patient poses several specific problems. Chapter 20 offers a detailed discussion of anesthesia for critically ill obstetric patients. Lumbar epidural anesthesia has become the favored technique for both labor analgesia and cesarean delivery. Stabilization of the mother and adequate plasma volume expansion are required for safe conduct of any anesthesia. Conduction anesthesia is contraindicated in the presence of coagulation abnormalities or uncorrected hypovolemia. General anesthesia may be used for cesarean section when fetal distress indicates rapid delivery or when conduction anesthesia is contraindicated or inadequate. As with conduction anesthesia, adequate blood volume expansion and control of hypertension are important prerequisites to safe induction of general anesthesia.

■
Management Post Partum

Preeclampsia generally resolves shortly after delivery. The onset of spontaneous diuresis marks the beginning of resolution. Magnesium therapy should be continued until the diuresis is well-established. This often takes 24 hours or more after delivery. At times hypertension and central nervous system irritability persist longer than 24 hours and require continued magnesium therapy. The hematologic and hepatic manifestations of the disease generally begin resolving within a few days of delivery. In 80% of patients with thrombocytopenia the platelet count returns to normal by the fourth day post partum. Complete resolution of all clinical and laboratory abnormalities may take several weeks. Initially, laboratory evaluations may need to be repeated daily until values appear to be normalizing.

Once a normalizing trend is established and hematologic, renal, and hepatic functions are in a safe range, the patient can be managed as a routine post partum patient. If hypertension persists, the patient should remain on antihypertensive agents until the blood pressure has normalized and remains normal off therapy; often this takes several weeks. These patients should be evaluated for underlying predisposing conditions such as collagen vascular disease, lupus anticoagulant, anticardiolipin antibody, and renal disease. Any of these disease processes will greatly increase the patient's risk of developing preeclampsia in subsequent pregnancies and the patient should be counseled accordingly.

■
Bibliography

Cunningham FG, Lindheimer MD: Hypertension in pregnancy. N Engl J Med 1992;326:927–932.

Davies NJ: Hypertensive disorders of pregnancy for the trainee. Br J Hosp Med 1992;47:613–619.

Dildy GA, Clark SL: Recent developments in pregnancy-induced hypertension. Current Opin Obstet Gynecol 1991;3:783–791.

Kyle PM, Redman CWG: Comparative risk-benefit assessment of drugs used in the management of hypertension in pregnancy. Drug Safety 1992;7:223–234.

Lowe SA, Rubin PC: The pharmacological management of hypertension in pregnancy. J Hypertension 1992;10:201–207.

JORDAN H. PERLOW

Obesity in the Obstetric Intensive Care Patient

About one third of the female U.S. population are obese. The remarkably high prevalence of this condition and its significant negative impact on overall health make its treatment a top priority in primary care medicine. Obese women are at significantly increased risk for a variety of medical complications, cancers, and premature sudden death (Table 6–1). Obesity should be of particular interest and importance to those who provide health care to women because age-adjusted rates of obesity for females of all races significantly exceed those for

Table 6–1

Medical Complications of Obesity

Sudden death	Dermatologic diseases
	Acanthosis nigricans
Stroke	Fragilitas cutis inguinalis
Coronary artery disease	Gout
Hypertension	Osteoarthritis
Thromboembolic disease	Digestive diseases
	Cholelithiasis
Diabetes mellitus	Hiatal hernia
Hypercholesterolemia	Pulmonary function impairment
	Pickwick syndrome
	Obesity-hypoventilation
	syndrome
Carcinoma	
Colon	Hepatic steatosis
Gallbladder	
Ovary	Endocrine abnormalities
Endometrium	Menstrual disorders
Breast	Infertility
Cervix	Polycystic ovaries
Compromised obstetric outcome	

males. It has been estimated that if the U.S. population were at ideal body weight, coronary heart disease, congestive heart failure, and stroke could be reduced by 25% to 35% and life expectancy would be extended 3 years!

Obesity and its relation to the obstetric intensive care patient seem to be underemphasized. Eighteen percent of obstetric causes of maternal death and 80% of anesthesia-related maternal deaths are associated with obesity. These patients are indeed at high risk and deserving of intense efforts to minimize morbidity and mortality.

This chapter serves to inform the reader of the various aspects of critical obstetric care for the obese gravida.

■ Definition

Obesity has been defined and described in a variety of colorful ways. Terms such as "severe," "massive," "morbid," and "grotesque" appear in the literature to describe different degrees of obesity. Unfortunately, standardized definitions are lacking. In general, however, obesity is defined as "an excess of body fat, frequently resulting in impairment of health." Obesity is usually caused by an excess of caloric intake versus expenditure; however, its cause is primarily multifactorial, accounting for 99% of all patients with obesity. A small percentage may be caused by a diverse group of neurologic and endocrine disorders (Table 6–2). Frequently, the body mass index (BMI) or Quetelet's index is used to measure obesity (Table 6–3). Others have used percentage of ideal body weight (IBW), using actuarial tables. More sophisticated methods of quantifying percentage of body fat are available, but they are not utilized for everyday clinical situations.

Table 6–2

Obesity: Differential Diagnosis (<1% of cases)

Hypothyroidism	Insulinoma
Prader-Willi syndrome	Adiposogenital dystrophy
Laurence-Moon-Biedl syndrome	Partial lipodystrophy
Hypothalamic lesion	Polycystic ovaries
Craniopharyngioma	Cushing's syndrome
Hypogonadism	

<table>
<tr><td>

Table 6–3

Body Mass Index

$$\text{Calculated BMI} = \frac{\text{Weight (kg)}}{\text{Height (m}^2)}$$

</td></tr>
</table>

For women, obesity is present when the BMI is greater than 27.3 for women older than 20 years, greater than 25.7 for those aged 18 or 19, and greater than 24.8 for those aged 15 to 17. These values approximate weights in excess of 120% of IBW. Some studies, however, have shown adverse health consequences with an IBW greater than 110%. Patients twice IBW or 100 pounds heavier than their ideal body weight have been described as "morbidly obese."

Pathophysiology

Overview

Perinatal outcome is compromised when pregnancy is complicated by obesity (Tables 6–4, 6–5). The obese pregnant woman and fetus are both at risk for a variety of complications during

<table>
<tr><td>

Table 6–4

Obesity and Perinatal Outcome: Maternal Risks

Obstetric (direct) mortality
   Aspiration
   Hemorrhage
   Thromboembolism/stroke
Cesarean delivery
   Increased blood loss
   Increased endometritis
   Prolonged operative time
   Failed epidural placement
   Respiratory complications (atelectasis, pneumonia)
   Wound infection/dehiscence
Medical complications (see Table 6–1)
   Chronic hypertension
   Diabetes mellitus (pregestational and gestational)
Prolonged hospitalization

</td></tr>
</table>

> ### Table 6–5
> ## Obesity and Perinatal Outcome: Fetal/Neonatal Risks
>
> Increased perinatal mortality
> Low Apgar scores
> Intrauterine growth restriction
> Low birth weight
> Macrosomia
> Postdates
> Shoulder dystocia/birth trauma
> Intensive care nursery admission
> Neonatal/childhood obesity
> ?Anomalies–neural tube defects

pregnancy. These include increased risks for hypertension, pre-eclampsia, diabetes (insulin-dependent and gestational), labor abnormalities, and cesarean delivery with associated morbidity. The neonate born to the obese mother has also been noted to be at significantly increased risk for adverse outcome, including low Apgar scores, intrauterine growth restriction, preterm delivery, low birth weight, macrosomia, and intensive care requirement.

Physiologic Changes in Obese Pregnant Patients (Table 6–6)

Blood volume and cardiac output increase approximately 40% in pregnancy, and cardiac output increases even further during labor and delivery, reaching values 80% greater than pre-pregnancy values. Obesity accentuates these changes as blood volume and cardiac output expand in proportion to the increases in fat and tissue mass.

Obese patients have marked abnormal changes in respiratory physiology. In fact, obese gravidas have markedly diminished functional residual capacity, and, except for residual volume, all lung volumes, vital capacity, and total lung capacity are reduced in association with obesity. Obese parturients have also been shown to have diminished Po_2 and chest wall and lung compliance. Total compliance in obesity diminishes by an average of 50%, which is equivalent to placing a 50-lb weight on the chest and abdomen of a nonobese person! These respiratory

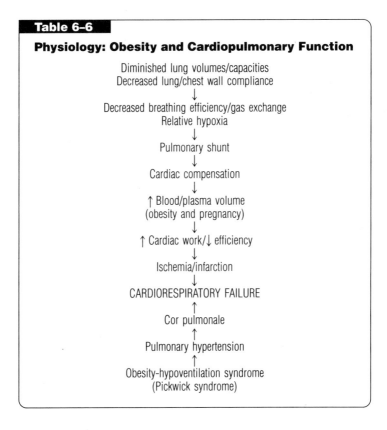

Table 6–6

Physiology: Obesity and Cardiopulmonary Function

Diminished lung volumes/capacities
Decreased lung/chest wall compliance
↓
Decreased breathing efficiency/gas exchange
Relative hypoxia
↓
Pulmonary shunt
↓
Cardiac compensation
↓
↑ Blood/plasma volume
(obesity and pregnancy)
↓
↑ Cardiac work/↓ efficiency
↓
Ischemia/infarction
↓
CARDIORESPIRATORY FAILURE
↑
Cor pulmonale
↑
Pulmonary hypertension
↑
Obesity-hypoventilation syndrome
(Pickwick syndrome)

changes in the obese parturient cause the work of breathing to be increased three times normal.

Intrapartum Management (Table 6–7)

The intrapartum management of the obese patient in labor is truly a team effort. The obstetrician, the labor and delivery nurse, and the obstetric anesthesiologist are the primary members of the team. Medical consultants who have evaluated the patient for given medical complications may be notified of the patient's admission to labor and delivery for additional management input.

Given the marked physiologic changes in the obese gravidas and the high probability of coexisting medical complications,

Table 6–7

Obesity and Pregnancy: Intrapartum and Postpartum Management Challenges

Obesity-Related Problem	Potential Solution or Adjunctive Measures
Difficult peripheral IV access	Central IV line
Inaccurate or difficult blood pressure monitoring	Arterial line
Preexisting cardiopulmonary disease	Continuous electrocardiography, arterial blood gas monitoring, chest radiography, pulse oximetry
Increased risk of general anesthesia, difficult emergent regional anesthesia placement	Prophylactic epidural catheter
Difficult intubation	Regional anesthesia
	Prophylactic epidural
	Capability for awake intubation/ fiberoptics (see Chapter 20, Failed Intubation Drill)
Aspiration risks	Prophylactic epidural
	H$_2$ antagonists (e.g., ranitidine HCl, 50 mg IV q6–8hr and 45 min before surgery)
	Sodium citrate with citric acid (30 mL of 0.3 M before anesthesia)
	Metoclopramide (10 mg IV over 1–2 min and 45 min before surgery)
	NPO status in labor
Thromboembolic risks	Low-dose heparin (5000 U SC q8–12hr)
	Elastic antithrombotic hose (thigh-high)
	Sequential pneumatic compression boots
	Early postoperative ambulation
	Minimize operative/immobilization times
Endometritis/wound infection	Prophylactic antibiotics (broad-spectrum, before incision)
	Thorough skin preparation
	Pelvic/wound irrigation (consider placing antibiotics in the irrigant)
	Surgical drains
	If Pfannenstiel's incision—maintain dry surgical site postoperatively

it is suggested that all such women have an anesthesiology consultation—preferably during the antepartum period, but certainly at the time of admission to labor and delivery. In addition to careful evaluation of the patient's cardiovascular and pulmonary status, meticulous assessment of the patient's airway is critical. This cannot be overemphasized: a recent study indicated that 80% of all anesthesia-related maternal deaths occurred among obese patients, and the inability to accomplish endotracheal intubation was the principal cause. Securing intravenous access and accurate blood pressure monitoring may also prove challenging, owing to the obese body habitus. The use of central venous access and an arterial line may be helpful in individual cases.

Particular attention should be given to the obese gravida's laboring position. The left lateral position is preferred to increase maternal oxygenation and uteroplacental blood flow and to prevent aortocaval compression. Obese patients may also benefit from elevation of the head and chest to prevent airway closure and improve oxygenation and overall comfort. Continuous pulse oximetry provides the clinician with important information about maternal oxygen saturation and allows administration of oxygen as needed.

Another important aspect of labor management includes maximizing pulmonary function and decreasing myocardial oxygen requirements. Recall that the obese gravida's respiratory work requirement is approximately three times that for the gravida of ideal body weight. Epidural anesthesia decreases respiratory work, improves oxygenation, and, by decreasing the perception of pain, can decrease the release of catecholamines, which cause increased cardiac work (output).

Operative Management

Perhaps the most important aspect of epidural anesthesia lies in the fact that, in an emergent situation, should cesarean section be required, a regional anesthetic can be administered through the catheter already in place. It has been shown that neonatal outcome is not compromised by this approach. This is critically important, as at least 90% of maternal deaths from anesthetic causes are attributed to general anesthesia, principally to complications of aspiration of gastric contents and failed endotracheal intubation.

The risks of general anesthesia for the obese parturient are intensified because of the greater difficulty in intubation secondary to anatomic barriers, a greater gastric volume with lower pH, and diminished barrier pressure (difference between lower esophageal sphincter tone and intragastric pressure). Therefore, regional anesthesia should be considered the modality of choice unless contraindications exist. Such contraindications may include maternal hypocoagulable states, hemodynamic instability, acute hemorrhage, and infection over the site of planned needle insertion. With increased utilization of regional anesthesia, one would anticipate a significant impact on the reduction of anesthesia-related maternal mortality. Therefore, "prophylactic" placement of an epidural catheter should be considered in the intrapartum management of obese laboring patients.

Other benefits of regional anesthesia include reduction in postoperative pulmonary complications. Intraspinal or epidural narcotics may be administered for postoperative analgesia, and their use reduces risks of respiratory depression from parenteral narcotics. Additionally, these patients ambulate earlier, which has the potential to decrease risk of thromboembolic complications.

Patients undergoing cesarean section should receive 30 mL of 0.3 M sodium citrate with citric acid just prior to anesthesia induction (general or regional), and the dose should be repeated each hour if surgery continues beyond 1 hour in a patient with regional anesthesia. Should general anesthesia be required, the use of H_2 antagonists (cimetidine, ranitidine) or dopamine antagonists (metoclopramide) administered intravenously during labor may help to reduce the sequelae of aspiration, should this potentially lethal complication occur. When cimetidine is given parenterally, at least 60 minutes are required to decrease gastric acidity to a "safe pH." Therefore, its use is preferred on admission and during labor rather than in the acute situation. For scheduled cases or induction of obese gravidas, ranitidine may be administered the night before surgery and then repeated on admission to the hospital and at appropriate intervals thereafter. Citric acid solutions should also be administered in addition to H_2 antagonists if cesarean section is required. These prophylactic measures raise gastric pH above 3.0 in nearly 99% of patients. The importance of these measures cannot be overemphasized, as pneumonitis and respiratory failure resulting from aspiration of gastric contents have been the most common single cause of maternal mortality related to anesthesia, accounting for 25% of 2700 maternal deaths from 1979 to 1986. In situations when evaluation of the patient's airway indicates the probability of difficult intubation, awake intubation and fiberoptic laryngos-copy should be considered. To decrease the risk of maternal morbidity and mortality associated with general anesthesia for obese parturients, regional anesthesia should be considered the anesthesia of choice for those undergoing cesarean delivery.

Recent data indicate that massively obese gravidas (>300 lb) are at significantly increased risk for perioperative morbidity associated with cesarean section. These risks include unsuccess-ful initial placement of the epidural catheter and the need for more time, as compared to controls, to deliver the fetus surgi-cally. These findings emphasize the potential benefit of the "prophylactic epidural." Other risks noted for obese gravidas undergoing cesarean section include increased blood loss, pro-longed hospitalization, and a nearly 10-fold increase in postop-erative endomyometritis.

Various adjuncts to perioperative care have been utilized to prevent morbidity associated with cesarean section in obese parturients. These include H_2 antagonists and metoclopramide to avoid the risk of aspiration with general anesthesia (discussed above), "antithromboembolic" stockings, intermittent sequential compression boots, and prophylactic doses of heparin to de-crease thromboembolic complications, and prophylactic antibi-otics to decrease the risk of postoperative infection. Unfortu-nately, these adjuncts have not been studied in the setting of randomized clinical trials. Therefore, there are few definitive data on the utility of these adjuncts, specifically in the obese population.

Nevertheless, in other populations prophylactic antibiotics have been shown to decrease the risk of infectious morbidity, and it is clear that obese patients are at significantly increased risk for postoperative infection. Thus, it would seem that the benefit of prophylactic antibiotics would outweigh the risk. Simi-larly, the use of prophylactic "minidose" heparin has not been studied in a prospective randomized fashion for this population. Given, however, that maternal obesity is a serious risk factor for maternal death and that a large portion of that mortality is related to thromboembolic complications, it would seem that a risk-benefit evaluation would favor the use of prophylactic doses of heparin perioperatively for obese parturients. One suggested protocol is 5000 U given subcutaneously every 8 to 12 hours, beginning 6 to 8 hours before surgery and continuing until the patient is fully ambulatory. Table 6–7 reviews the intrapartum and postpartum management recommendations.

Choice of Incision

The incision of choice for cesarean section in obese patients is not entirely clear. A recent study reported that 86% of massively obese patients had a transverse incision—72% Pfannenstiel's and 14% transverse periumbilical. Benefits of the transverse incision include more secure closure, less fat transection, and less post-operative pain. Perhaps the most compelling reason to utilize a transverse incision is its association with diminished risk for atelectasis and hypoxemia postoperatively and decreased pain leading to earlier ambulation and deep breathing, all critically important given the increased risk for pulmonary and thrombo-embolic complications. Drawbacks of Pfannenstiel's incision include placement of a surgical wound in the warm, moist inter-triginous area beneath the panniculus, which could increase the risk of infection and impede exploration of the upper abdomen, should that become necessary. Wolfe has shown that the type of incision was not independently related to operative morbidity.

A suggested approach includes retraction of the pannus.

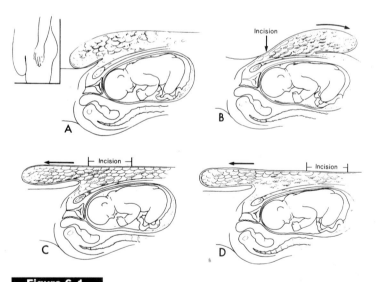

Figure 6–1

Diagram of massively obese pregnant patient showing the following: panniculus in place *(A)*; placement of a Pfannenstiel's incision following retraction of the panniculus *(B)*; location of a low midline vertical incision above the panniculus *(C)*; placement of a midline vertical incision higher in the abdomen or periumbilically *(D)*. (Gross TL: Operative considerations in the obese pregnant patient. Clin Perinatol 1983;10:411–421.)

This affords exposure of the lower abdomen, allowing the Pfannenstiel incision to be made through a minimum of adipose tissue (Fig. 6–1). At times, when the pannus is too large to be retracted, doing so may lead to marked cardiorespiratory compromise. Alternatively, a transverse periumbilical incision may be utilized. This approach affords excellent exposure without pannus retraction and the potential for cardiorespiratory compromise (Fig. 6–2). The incision circumvents the intertriginous area beneath the pannus and avoids the thick and edematous portion of the panniculus transected in "high Pfannenstiel" or vertical incisions.

Fascial wound closure requires special attention. If a vertical incision is utilized, a Smead-Jones or modified Smead-Jones closure is preferred (Fig. 6–3). Transverse fascial incisions may be closed with a permanent or delayed absorbable monofilament suture. The placement of closed surgical drains has not been studied prospectively in randomized clinical trials. Again, this option should be individualized to the clinical situation, as they may indeed be useful both subfascially and subcutaneously.

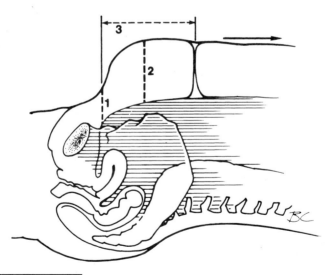

Figure 6–2

Possible sites of abdominal incisions. The panniculus retracted in the direction of the solid arrow: (1) Low suprasymphyseal transverse abdominal incision; (2) high suprasymphyseal transverse abdominal incision; (3) low midline abdominal incision. (Krebs HB, Helmkamp FB: Transverse periumbilical incision in the massively obese patient. Obstet Gynecol 1984;63:241–245.)

88   Obstetric Intensive Care: a practical manual

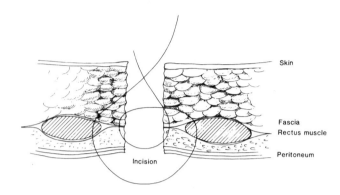

Figure 6-3

Diagram showing placement of a Smead-Jones suture. (Gross TL: Operative considerations in the obese pregnant patient. Clin Perinatol 1983;10:411–421.)

The use of subcutaneous sutures is controversial. Some investigators feel they serve as a nidus for infection in the poorly vascularized and infection-prone subcutaneous adipose tissue, potentially increasing the risk for wound dehiscence and infection. Others, however, believe in the importance of closing the "dead space" and taking tension off the skin edges to enhance skin closure. Recent work has demonstrated a decreased dehiscence rate when subcutaneous sutures were utilized in a group that included some obese patients.

Sterile skin staples may be used for skin closure; however, one should be careful not to remove them prematurely from obese patients. Since postcesarean patients are being discharged as early as the second postoperative day, some may need to return as outpatients for staple removal several days later.

Finally, these patients should be given thorough discharge instructions, including the signs and symptoms of wound infection and dehiscence, thromboembolic complications, and follow-up with respect to continued management of any existing medical complications.

In conclusion, the management and care of obese gravidas is very challenging. The course of pregnancy affords us not only the opportunity to markedly improve perinatal outcome and reduce maternal mortality but the time to develop mutual trust and rapport with the patient, permitting us to attempt some "long-term" intervention directed toward the patient's obesity. Truly, any impact made in this regard has the potential for tremendous health benefit throughout the patient's life and in subsequent pregnancies.

■
Bibliography

Epidemiology

Bray GA: Complications of obesity. Ann Intern Med 1985;103:1052–1062.

Burton BT, Foster WR, Hirsch J, et al.: Health implications of obesity: An NIH consensus development conference. Int J Obesity 1985;9:155–169.

Garfinkel L: Overweight and cancer. Ann Intern Med 1985;103:1034–1036.

Kral JG: Morbid obesity and related health risks. Ann Intern Med 1985;103:1043–1047.

Lew EA, Garfinkel L: Variations in mortality by weight among 750,000 men and women. J Chron Dis 1979;32:563–576.

McDowell A, Engel A, Massey JT, et al.: Plan and Operation of the Second National Health and Nutrition Examination Survey, 1966–1980. DHHS publication no. (PHS) 81-1317. Hyattsville, MD: National Center for Health Statistics, 1981.

National Center for Health Statistics: Anthropometric Reference Data and Prevalence of Overweight, United States, 1976–1980. DHHS publication no. (PHS) 87-1688. Hyattsville, MD: National Center for Health Statistics, 1987.

U.S. Public Health Service: The Surgeon General's Report on Nutrition and Health. DHHS publication no. (PSH) 88-50210. Washington, DC: US Department of Health and Human Services, 1988.

Obesity and Perinatal Outcome

Freedman MA, Preston LW, George WM: Grotesque obesity: A serious complication of labor and delivery. South Med J 1972;65:732–736.

Garbaciak JA Jr, Richter M, Miller S, et al.: Maternal weight and pregnancy complications. Am J Obstet Gynecol 1985;152:238–245.

Gross T, Sokol RJ, King K: Obesity in pregnancy: Risks and outcome. Obstet Gynecol 1980;56:446–450.

Johnson SR, Kolberg BH, Varner MW, et al.: Maternal obesity and pregnancy. Surg Gynecol Obstet 1987;164:431–437.

Naeye RL: Maternal body weight and pregnancy outcome. Am J Clin Nutr 1990;52:273–279.

Perlow JH: Obstetric Management of the Obese Patient. Contemp Ob/Gyn 1995;40:15–18.

Perlow JH, Morgan MA, Montgomery DM, et al.: Perinatal outcome in pregnancy complicated by massive obesity. Am J Obstet Gynecol 1992;167:958–962.

Wolfe HM, Zador IE, Gross TL, et al.: The clinical utility of maternal body mass index in pregnancy. Am J Obstet Gynecol 1991;164:1306–1310.

Obesity and Surgical Risks, Cesarean Section

Ahern JK, Gooklin RC: Cesarean section in the massively obese. Obstet Gynecol 1977;51:509–510.

Del Valle GO, Combs P, Qualls C, et al.: Does closure of Camper fascia reduce the incidence of post-cesarean superficial wound disruption? Obstet Gynecol 1992;80:1013–1016.

Gallup DG: Modifications of celiotomy techniques to decrease morbidity in obese gynecologic patients. Am J Obstet Gynecol 1984;150:171–178.

Gross TL: Operative considerations in the obese pregnant patient. Clin Perinatol 1983;10:411–421.

Krebs HB, Helmkamp FB: Transverse periumbilical incision in the massively obese patient. Obstet Gynecol 1984;63:241–245.

Nielsen TF, Hokegard KH: Postoperative cesarean section morbidity: A prospective study. Am J Obstet Gynecol 1983;146:911–916.

Pelle H, Jepsen OB, Larsen SO, et al.: Wound infection after cesarean section. Infect Control 1986;7:456–461.

Perlow JH, Morgan MA: Massive obesity and perioperative cesarean morbidity. Am J Obstet Gynecol 1994;170:560–565.

Sicuranza BJ, Tisdall LH: Cesarean section in the massively obese. J Reprod Med 1975;14:10–11.

Wolfe HM, Gross TL, Sokol RJ, et al.: Determinants of morbidity in obese women delivered by cesarean. Obstet Gynecol 1988;71:691–696.

Obesity, Pregnancy, and Anesthetic Morbidity and Mortality

Conklin KA: Can anesthetic-related maternal mortality be reduced? [Letter] Am J Obstet Gynecol 1990;163:253–254.

Endler GC: The risk of anesthesia in obese parturients. J Perinatol 1990;10:175–179.

Endler GC, Mariona FG, Sokol RJ, et al.: Anesthesia-related maternal mortality in Michigan, 1972 to 1984. Am J Obstet Gynecol 1988;159:187–193.

Maeder EC, Barno A, Mecklenburg F: Obesity: A maternal high risk factor. Obstet Gynecol 1975;45:669–672.

May JW, Greiss FC Jr: Maternal mortality in North Carolina: A forty-year experience. Am J Obstet Gynecol 1989;161:555–561.

ROBERT L. JOHNSON

Thromboembolic Disease Complicating Pregnancy

Thromboembolic disease (TED) in pregnancy has since 1989 been the leading cause of maternal mortality and morbidity. The complex changes in maternal coagulation leading to the diagnosis and treatment of TED require a basic understanding of the pathophysiology, sensitivity, and specificity of diagnostic tests and the myriad treatment options available to clinicians. The major classifications of TED in pregnancy are outlined in Table 7–1.

Maternal mortality may exceed 10% to 15% in untreated deep venous thrombosis (DVT) from pulmonary embolus (PE). Proper treatment reduces this risk to less than 1%. In this chapter I focus on specific risk factors, coagulation changes during pregnancy, and the diagnosis and treatment of TED.

■ Pathophysiology

Numerous changes in pregnancy contribute to the relatively hypercoagulable state:

- All procoagulant factors increase except factors XI and XIII.
- Procoagulant factors II, V and XII are relatively unchanged.
- Fibrinogen nearly doubles.
- Cofactor protein C and C-46-binding protein increase.
- Cofactor protein S decreases.
- Antithrombin III (AT-III) and pregnancy-specific protein-neutralizing AT-III (PAPP-A) are unchanged.
- Cellular components such as platelets and red blood cells generally increase during pregnancy.

Table 7–1

Thromboembolic Diseases*

TED	Incidence (%)
Superficial thrombophlebitis	0.15–1.35
Deep vein thrombophlebitis	0.36–3.0
Thrombosis (arterial, venous)	Exact incidence unclear
Pulmonary embolism	0.04–1.2
Septic pelvic thrombophlebitis	0.1

*Overall incidence for pregnancy is 5 times higher than in the nonpregnant state.

Table 7–2 outlines the normal values for coagulation factors during pregnancy. The normal components of the coagulation system are intact in normal pregnancy, as is the fibrinolytic pathway (see Figs. 7–1, 7–2). Proteins C and S exhibit anticoagulant and fibrinolytic activity (Fig. 7–3). The delicate balance of the coagulation system during pregnancy provides effective maternal hemostasis at the time of placental separation. The

Table 7–2

Normal Values for Coagulation Factors

Factor	Nonpregnant	Pregnant
I (fibrinogen)	200–400 mg%	350–650 mg%
II (prothrombin)	75–125 mg%	100–125 mg%
III (thromboplastin)	———	———
IV (calcium ions)	4.7–5.5 mg%	4.7–5.5 mg%
V (proaccelerin)	75–125 mg%	100–150 mg%
VII (proconvertin)	75–125 mg%	150–250 mg%
VIII (antihemophilic globulin)	75–150 mg%	200–500 mg%
IX (plasma thrombin component)	75–125 mg%	100–150 mg%
X (Stuart-Power factor)	75–125 mg%	150–250 mg%
XI (plasma thromboplastin antecedent)	75–125 mg%	50–100 mg%
XII (Hageman factor)	75–125 mg%	100–200 mg%
XIII (fibrin-stabilizing factor)	75–125 mg%	35–75 mg%
Antithrombin III/PAPP-A	0.8–1.2 U/mL	0.8–1.2 U/mL

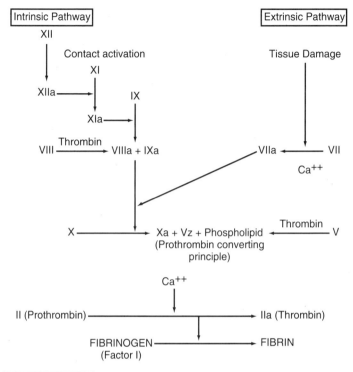

Figure 7–1

The normal components of the coagulation system.

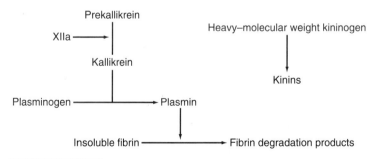

Figure 7–2

The components of the fibrinolytic pathway in pregnancy.

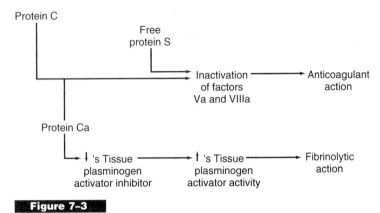

The role in the fibrinolytic pathway of cofactors proteins C and S.

following additional physiologic changes, however, may impose increased risk for thromboembolic disease:

- Low-grade chronic disseminated intravascular coagulation (DIC) within the placental bed with deposition of fibrin in the spiral arteries
- Venous stasis secondary to uterine enlargement
- Placental inhibition of fibrinolysis
- Placental separation with subsequent tissue thromboplastin release
- Endothelial damage to vessels during operative or vaginal delivery increases maternal thrombotic risk.

The anticoagulant system is best represented by the cofactors protein C, protein S, heparin, and AT-III. AT-III serves as the most important endogenous factor for inhibition and limitation of thrombus formation and acts synergistically with exogenous heparin during therapy for TED. Proteins C and S exhibit physiologic anticoagulant and fibrinolytic activity (see Fig. 7–3). Deficiency of these important vitamin K–dependent anticoagulant cofactors is associated with profound thrombogenic morbidity and mortality.

Additional clinical risk factors important for the clinician to recognize include the following:

- Previous TED, recent or remote to pregnancy
- Primary hypercoagulable disorders—AT-III, protein C, protein S deficiencies
- Concurrent malignant disease

- Preeclampsia or eclampsia
- Previous TED associated with hyperestrogenic state (oral contraceptive drugs)
- The presence of lupus anticoagulant or anticardiolipin antibody
- Advanced age, multiparity, obesity, blood type other than O, sickle cell disease

■
Diagnosis of Specific Thromboembolic Diseases

The diagnosis of any thromboembolic event requires careful contemplation for both diagnostic accuracy and consideration of the implications this diagnosis may have for life-long therapy. The fact that a patient has on her record "history of thromboembolic disease" may seriously impede psychosocial, lifestyle, and occupational goals and insurance coverage. Therefore, ensuring the accuracy of the diagnosis is crucial. Table 7–3 conceptualizes the diagnosis of thromboembolic disease from non–life-threatening superficial thrombophlebitis to pulmonary embolus. Universally, DVT and PE are not likely to be confirmed by clinical diagnosis alone. Extensive (and expensive) diagnostic evaluations are generally indicated. Patient concerns about the invasive nature of the tests and potential fetal risks should be discussed thoroughly.

CLOT (*c*linical findings, *l*aboratory, *o*bjective data, *t*reatment) is an easy mnemonic that can guide the clinician through the steps of patient care, addressing each specific disease.

Table 7–3 (Objective Data) reviews the methods and the positive predictive values for the testing associated with the diagnosis of DVT/PE. Increasingly sophisticated and invasive tests are used to diagnose the various disease entities. Clinicians must be aware that the gold standards for diagnosis of DVT and PE are venography and pulmonary angiography, respectively. The algorithm for diagnosis of DVT is shown in Figure 7–4. *Any* clinical suspicion of DVT should be pursued with at least one confirmatory test to rule out the diagnosis. Extended observation of suspected clinical disease is not prudent during pregnancy. Prompt treatment may avert major complications.

Figure 7–5 is an algorithm for pulmonary embolus. The high degree of clinical suspicion associated with the findings in Table 7–3 requires a definitive diagnostic investigation. The ventilation-perfusion scan is a relatively low-risk procedure. Simple first-pass kinetics prevent excessive fetal radiation exposure. No

Table 7-3
Approach to Thromboembolic Disease

	Superficial Thrombophlebitis	PPV for Deep Vein Thrombosis* (%)	PPV for Pulmonary Embolism* (%)
Clinical findings	Painful, warm, erythematous, localized vein, varicosity, ± febrile	Pain, tenderness, and swelling: 50 Homan's sign‡: 30 Lowenberg test‡: 50 Calf tenderness: 60–90 Unilateral edema: 40–75 Superficial venous dilatation: 30	Dyspnea, hemoptysis, pleuritic pain: 50 Tachypnea: 97 Hemoptysis: 30 Diaphoresis: 40 Shock: 14 Syncope: 15
Laboratory investigation	None	AT III Protein S Protein C Activated protein C resistance (factor 5 mutation) PT, PTT, fibrin split products Lupus anticoagulant Anticardiolipin } None	Electrocardiogram Chest film Lactate dehydrogenase } None Arterial blood gas Labs same as for DVT }

Table continued on opposite page

		*		*
Objective data (testing)	Recurrence related to history of venous stasis (varicosities) No untoward maternal-fetal risks *Clinical diagnosis only*		Invasive Pulmonary angiography: (morbidity 4–5%; mortality 0.2–0.3%)	99
	Invasive Venography (gold standard): Fibrinogen ^{125}I (contraindicated):	99 78		
	Noninvasive Impedance plethysmography: Color flow Doppler:	92 90+	Noninvasive Ventilation-perfusion scan:	97
Treatment	Symptomatic Heat Elevation Prevent stasis Nonsteroidal antiinflammatory drugs <32 wk		O₂, pressor support IV heparin (see Table 7–6) Continued therapy throughout pregnancy and postpartum Rare use of thrombolytic agents	None
	IV heparin See Raschke's protocol (Fig. 7–6) Warfarin—rarely antepartum, routinely postpartum for 6 wk Low molecular weight heparin (consider) Long-term therapeutic heparin See Table 7–5	None		

*Positive predictive value of clinical tests.
†Pain in calf elicited on dorsiflexion of the foot.
‡Pain occurring distal to a blood pressure cuff rapidly inflated to 180 mm Hg.

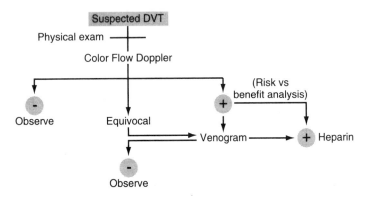

Figure 7-4

Algorithm for suspected deep venous thrombosis (DVT).

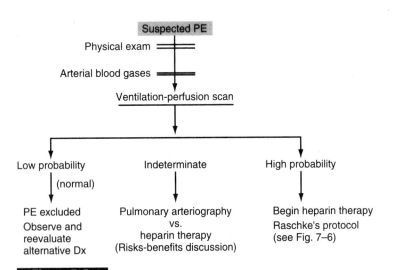

Figure 7-5

Algorithm for suspected pulmonary embolus (PE).

fetal side effects have been reported from this procedure. Patients in the "indeterminate"-result group require additional consideration of the risks and benefits of empiric therapy versus pulmonary angiography for confirmation.

■
"Acute" Anticoagulation for DVT/PE

The decision to begin anticoagulation must not be made without reliable objective data. Since the treatment and diagnosis of these disorders may affect the patient's future health care considerations, the risk-benefit discussions with patient and family must be completed before therapy is instituted.

Three types of therapeutic agents are generally available for anticoagulation: (1) agents that interfere with platelet adhesion and aggregation (dextran); (2) agents that interfere with fibrin formation (heparin, coumadin); and (3) agents that facilitate clot lysis (streptokinase, urokinase, ancrod). Generally, heparin and coumadin are used most frequently and will be discussed in detail here.

Heparin is a glycosaminoglycan with a molecular weight of 5 to 30 kd. It can be unfractionated, or fractionated (e.g., low–molecular weight heparin [LMWH]). The most experience to date has been with the use of unfractionated heparin, but recent data concerning the advantages of LMWH may dramatically increase its use (Table 7–4 compares the two forms of heparin available for use in pregnancy).

Both heparin types exert similar pharmacologic effects by catalyzing the inactivation of thrombin by AT-III. A conformational change in AT-III induced by heparin markedly accelerates its ability to inactivate the coagulation enzymes thrombin (factor IIa), factor Xa, and factor IXa. Heparin, with fewer than 18 saccharides, cannot bind thrombin and AT-III simultaneously and, therefore, cannot accelerate inactivation of thrombin by AT-III. The therapeutic basis for using LMWH is that it produces the needed pharmacologic effects without the side effects of unfractionated heparin. The biologic half-life of both types is not linear but increases disproportionately both in intensity and duration with increasing dose. Neither form has been shown to traverse the placenta.

Table 7–5 lists the usual dosage, route of administration, recommended laboratory evaluations, and complications associated with unfractionated heparin. Acutely, particular attention should be given to the Raschke's protocol for heparin dosing (Fig. 7–6). This easy-to-follow dosing regimen allows rapid anti-

Table 7-4
Unfractionated Heparin and Low Molecular Weight Heparin (LMWH) Compared

	Dosage	Frequency	Route	Advantages	Disadvantages
Unfractionated heparin	5000–10,000 IU 750–1400 IU/hr	b.i.d.–t.i.d.	SC IV	Largest body of medical literature Most clinical trials	Frequent monitoring Heparin-induced thrombocytopenia Osteoporosis
LMWH	20–40 mg	b.i.d.	SC	Increased patient compliance Decreased dosing interval Decreased heparin-induced thrombocytopenia No reports of osteoporosis to date Fewer painful skin reactions Fewer bleeding complications	New form (limited clinical trials) More expensive Dosage ill-defined Multiple LMWH products

Table 7-5

Heparin and Warfarin Anticoagulation Compared

Drug	Dosage	Route	Laboratory Tests	Complications and Risks
Heparin	Prophylaxis 5000–10,000 IU b.i.d.	SC	Baseline PT, PTT	Rare; no need for laboratory follow-up
	Adjusted (intermittent) dose 5000–10,000 IU t.i.d.	SC	Platelet count 5–14 d after starting therapy	Overall 3% risk for adverse outcome; bleeding 2%
	Continuous SC (heparin pump) 750–1400 IU/hr	SC	Heparin concentration (0.2–0.4 IU/mL)	Osteoporosis, 2% risk >20,000 IU/d for >20 wk
	Continuous IV (heparin pump) 750–1400 IU/hr (use Raschke's protocol; see Fig. 7–6)	IV	Heparin concentration (0.2–0.4 IU/mL)	Thrombocytopenia 2.4%; may be related to pharmaceutical lot and type; heparin activity reversed by protamine sulfate (1 mg/100 IU; maximum single dose 50 mg in 30 min); side effect is profound hypotension.
Warfarin	2.5–10 mg	PO	PT (1½–2 times baseline) INR (2.5–4.9)	Overall 14% adverse outcome, warfarin embryopathy 4%; CNS fetal hemorrhage 10% 2nd and 3rd trimesters. Useful in certain mechanical heart valve patients. Reversal by fresh-frozen plasma and vitamin K. American Academy of Pediatrics approves while breast feeding.

1. Make calculations using total body weight: _____ kg. (see chart)

2. BOLUS HEPARIN, 80 U/kg = _____ U IV.

3. IV HEPARIN infusion, 18 U/kg/hr = _____ U/hr.
   (25,000 U heparin in 250 mL D_5W)

4. WARFARIN _____ mg PO qd; give first dose as soon as APTT $\geq$ 50
   (nonpregnant or postpartum)

5. LABORATORY: APTT, PT, CBC now
                      CBC with platelet count q3d
                      <u>STAT</u> APTT 6 hr after heparin bolus
                      PT qd (start on third day of heparin)

6. ADJUST heparin infusion based on sliding scale below:
PTT < 35	80 U/kg bolus, increase drip by 4 U/kg/hr
PTT 35–49	40 U/kg bolus, increase drip by 2 U/kg/hr
PTT 50–70	No change
PTT 71–90	Reduce drip by 2 U/kg/hr
PTT > 90	Hold heparin for 1 hr, reduce drip by 3 U/kg/hr

2 U/kg/hr		3 U/kg/hr		4 U/kg/hr	
Weight (kg)	Dose change (U/hr)	Weight (kg)	Dose change (U/hr)	Weight (kg)	Dose change (U/hr)
40–74	100	40–50	100	40–60	200
75–124	200	51–80	200	61–87	300
125–170	300	81–115	300	88–112	400
		116–150	400	113–137	500
		151–170	500	138–162	600
				163–175	700

7. Order PTT 6 hr after any dosage change, adjusting heparin infusion by the sliding scale until PTT is therapeutic (50–70 sec). When two PTTs in a row are therapeutic, order PTT (and readjust heparin drip as needed) q24hr.

<u>Please make changes as promptly as possible</u>, and round off doses to the nearest mL/hr (nearest 100 U).

Signed _____ Date _____/_____/_____

Note: This protocol provides management guidelines for full therapeutic anticoagulation. **It should not be used for prophylactic anticoagulation or after thrombolytic agents.**

Figure 7-6

Raschke's protocol orders. APTT, activated partial thromboplastin time; CBC, complete blood count; PT, prothrombin time; PTT, partial thromboplastin time; PO, by mouth; qd, every day, STAT, immediately.

The following chart gives the initial heparin bolus dose and infusion rates (bolus of 80 U/kg, infusion of 18 U/kg/hr) rounded off.

Weight (kg)	IV bolus (U)	Infusion (U/hr)
42–47	3500	800
48–52	4000	900
53–58	4500	1000
59–63	5000	1100
64–69	5300	1200
70–75	5700	1300
76–80	6300	1400
81–86	6700	1500
87–91	7100	1600
92–97	7500	1700
98–102	8000	1800
103–108	8400	1900
109–113	8900	2000
114–119	9300	2100
120–124	9800	2200
125–130	10,200	2300
131–136	10,600	2400
137–141	11,100	2500
148–152	12,000	2700

Figure 7-6 *Continued*

coagulation safely and efficiently. Follow-up recommended laboratory evaluation and dosage adjustments are outlined in the protocol. For the acute event, intravenous treatment for 10 to 14 days is recommended.

After the acute treatment, long-term heparinization should be considered for the remainder of the gestation and approximately 6 weeks post partum, depending on the diagnosis. Those with cofactor deficiencies will require lifelong anticoagulation. Postpartum warfarin is frequently used to anticoagulate patients who require prolonged therapy and is accepted by the American Academy of Pediatrics for use during breastfeeding.

Patients with mechanical heart valves or recurrent thrombi, despite full heparinization, may be candidates for warfarin during pregnancy. Table 7–5 contains the most useful information on warfarin use in pregnancy. Post partum, warfarin is given by oral dosing during heparin treatment. Heparin is discontinued after adequate change in the prothrombin time. Usual dosage regimen is 5–10 mg on each of days 1, 2, and 3; on day 4 prothrombin time is measured prior to dosing. A prothrombin time of 1½ to 2 times the baseline value is desirable. An international normalized ratio (INR) equivalent of 2.5 to 4.9 is also of value in assessing adequate anticoagulation. Discontinuation of heparin therapy should be considered when these values have been achieved. Warfarin is avoided during pregnancy because it so readily crosses the placenta, placing the fetus at high risk for congenital malformation.

Acute intervention for thromboembolic disease includes thrombolytic therapy. This is generally reserved for the unusual clinical circumstance when conventional therapy is failing and the patient shows signs of continued deterioration. Streptokinase and urokinase are the primary thrombolytic drugs used in these circumstances. In most cases, however, these drugs are contraindicated during the acute puerperium, secondary to reports of excessive blood loss from the placental implantation site. Ancrod, another thrombolytic agent, has been associated with high fetal loss rates and hemorrhage. These treatments should be considered experimental at present, pending further clinical investigation.

Intrapartum anticoagulation is another concern for clinicians. Therapeutic anticoagulation potentially increases the risk of hemorrhage during the labor and delivery process. Three clinical choices exist: (1) Discontinue heparin therapy approximately 4 hours before delivery or withhold the last subcutaneous injection. (This is difficult since rarely can the clinician predict delivery time). (2) Decrease all dosing to prophylaxis levels (5,000 to 10,000 U subcutaneously every 12 hours). After delivery, reinstitute therapeutic heparinization. (3) Continue the heparin therapy and switch to intravenous dosing during labor. Desirable levels can be attained such as low therapeutic levels (heparin concentration 0.1 to 0.2 IU/mL or a partial thromboplastin time that is approximately 1.5 times the baseline value). If the mother is fully anticoagulated, increased blood loss should be anticipated at cesarean section, but with vaginal delivery blood loss is similar to that for patients not receiving anticoagulation therapy. Additional complications, such as vaginal vault and episiotomy hematomas, have been reported.

Reversal of heparin can be accomplished with protamine sulfate. One milligram of protamine sulfate neutralizes 100 U of circulating heparin. It is imperative to calculate the appropriate amount of protamine sulfate and to underestimate rather than overestimate the dose, since excessive dosing has been associated with an irreversible anticoagulant effect.

Circulating heparin = Plasma volume =
    (50 ml/kg body weight) × Plasma heparin concentration

Generally, small doses of protamine sulfate (5 to 10 mg) are preferable. Profound hypotension has been reported with rapid administration of the drug. Profound hypotension has occurred when large doses are given rapidly. Reversal of warfarin anticoagulation is accomplished by giving fresh-frozen plasma and vitamin K to replenish and stimulate factor production.

■
Summary

Thromboembolic disease continues to be an important cause of maternal mortality in pregnancy. Prompt recognition and diagnosis of DVT/PE can prevent maternal death. Logical care pathways have been presented to inform decision making and the therapeutic process. As for any condition, individualization of patient care is appropriate. New methods of diagnosis and treatment are being developed to decrease morbidity and enhance patient compliance in this serious disorder complicating pregnancy.

■
Bibliography

Barbour L, Pickard J: Controversies in thromboembolic disease during pregnancy: A critical review. Obstet Gynecol 1995;86:621–633.

Clark SL, Cotton DB, Harkins GDV, et al.: Critical care obstetrics. 2nd ed. New York: Blackwell Scientific Publications, 1991, pp 150–177.

Dulitzki M, et al.: Low–molecular weight heparin during pregnancy and delivery: Preliminary experience with 41 pregnancies. Obstet Gynecol 1996;87:380–383.

Ginsberg J, Hirsh J: Use of antithrombotic agents during pregnancy. Chest 1995;108:305–315.

Hirsh J, et al.: Heparin: Mechanism of action, pharmacokinetics, dosing, considerations, monitoring, efficacy, and safety. Chest 1995;108:258–275.

Raschke RA, Reilly BM, Guidry JR, et al.: The weight-based heparin dosing nomogram. Ann Int Med 1993;119:874–881.

MICHAEL F. KOSZALKA, JR.

Cardiac Disease in Pregnancy

Concern for significant cardiac instability arises when the heart is unable to adjust to the dynamic physiologic changes of pregnancy, parturition, and the puerperium. Changes in the structure of the heart due to acquired or congenital anomalies may result in abnormal channeling or flow rates. Depending on the specific

---

Table 8–1

Maternal Mortality Associated with Pregnancy

Group 1—Mortality <1%
- Atrial septal defect
- Patent ductus arteriosus
- Pulmonic/tricuspid disease
- Tetralogy of Fallot, corrected
- Bioprosthetic valve
- Mitral stenosis, NYHA class I and II

Group 2—Mortality 5–15%
- 2A
  - Mitral stenosis, NYHA class III and IV
  - Aortic stenosis
  - Coarctation of aorta, without valvular involvement
  - Uncorrected tetralogy of Fallot
  - Previous myocardial infarction
  - Marfan syndrome with normal aorta
- 2B
  - Mitral stenosis with atrial fibrillation
  - Artificial valve

Group 3—Mortality 25–50%
- Pulmonary hypertension
- Coarctation of aorta, with valvular involvement
- Marfan syndrome with aortic involvement

From Clark SL, Phelan JP, Cotton DB (eds): Critical Care Obstetrics: Structural Cardiac Disease in Pregnancy. Oradell, NJ: Medical Economics Company, Inc., 1987.

abnormality, the risk of maternal mortality may approach 50% (Table 8–1). The effective management of cardiac disease during pregnancy requires a basic knowledge of how congenital or acquired lesions may modify cardiac function during pregnancy and how commonly used cardiovascular drugs may affect the developing fetus and uterine blood flow (Table 8–2).

■ Physiology

The Most Important Cardiac Changes in Pregnancy

General
- Blood volume increases approximately 50%.
- Systemic vascular resistance falls approximately 20%.
- Blood is hypercoagulable.
- Cardiac output increases 30% to 45% (Fig. 8–1).
- Stroke volume increases early in pregnancy (Fig. 8–1).
- Heart rate increases (10 to 15 bpm), peaking in the third trimester (Fig. 8–1).

Intrapartum
- Cardiac output increases by an additional 15% with each contraction.
- Hemodynamic changes associated with contractions are less pronounced and baseline cardiac output higher with lateral supine positioning.
- Hemodynamic variables are less labile with conduction anesthesia blocking the pain-stress cascade.
- Blood pressure increases 10 to 20 mm Hg.
- Baseline cardiac output increases 60% immediately following vaginal delivery (Fig. 8–1).

Electrocardiographic (ECG) changes
- QRS axis shifts 15 degrees to left.
- Low-voltage complexes may be present.
- T-wave negativity may be present in lead III.
- "Positional" Q waves may be seen in lead III and AVF.
- Ectopic beats (ventricular and supraventricular) are common.
- Bouts of supraventricular tachycardia are more frequent.

■ Specific Congenital Cardiac Lesions (Table 8–3)

Atrial Septal Defect (ASD). Although ASDs are frequently asymptomatic, specific concerns related to this diagnosis include arrhythmias (especially atrial fibrillation) and left ventricular failure secondary to increased shunting. In patients with large

Text continued on page 113

Table 8-2

Cardiovascular Drugs Commonly Used in the Obstetric Intensive Care Setting and Their Effects on Uterine Blood Flow and the Fetus

Drug	Dose	Uterine Blood Flow	Fetal Effect
Inotropic agents			
Digoxin	Loading dose of 1.0 mg IV over 5 min	No change	Placental transfer; higher than usual maternal maintenance dose required
Dopamine	Initiate with 1.0 µg/kg/min and titrate to effect (up to 10 µg/kg/min)	Direct effect ↓ UBF. Improved maternal hemodynamics may ↑ UBF.	No adequate assessment of effects on fetus
Dobutamine	Initiate with 1.0 µg/kg/min and titrate to effect (up to 15 µg/kg/min)	Direct effect ↓ UBF. Improved maternal hemodynamics may ↑ UBF.	No adequate assessment of effects on fetus
Epinephrine	Endotracheal, 0.5 to 1.0 mg every 5 min; IV-initiate with 0.5-mg bolus and follow with infusion of 2–10 µg/kg/min	Direct effect ↓ UBF. Improved maternal hemodynamics may ↑ UBF.	No adequate assessment of effects on fetus
Vasodilators			
Nitroprusside	Start at 0.5 µg/kg/min and titrate to effect (up to 10 µg/kg/min)	↑ unless significant reduction in maternal BP	Optimal drug because of ease of titration for optimal effects. Fetal effect unknown. Concern exists for fetal cyanide toxicity with prolonged use. *Table continued on opposite page*

Hydralazine	5–10 mg IV dose given at 15–30 min intervals, total dose 30 mg	Large experience without adverse fetal effects
Nitroglycerin	0.4–0.8 mg sublingual *or* 1–2 inches of dermal paste *or* IV infusion of 0.5 μg/min up to 40 μg/min	With volume depletion, hypotension and a fall in uterine blood flow more likely

β-Blockers (Intravenous preparations)

Propranolol	0.1 mg/kg IV over 5 min	May ↓ by ↑ uterine tone and/or ↓ maternal BP	Potential for premature labor and smaller than average birth weight. If taken at the time of delivery the newborn may have bradycardia and hypovolemia.
Labetalol	10–20 mg IV followed by 20–80 mg IV every 10 min to total dose of 300 mg	↑ unless significant reduction in maternal BP	
Atenolol	25 mg IV over 5 min	↑ unless significant reduction in maternal BP	
Metoprolol	15 mg IV over 1 min; repeat dose in 10 min		
Esmolol	500 μg/kg IV with infusion rate of 50–300 μg/kg/min		Rapid metabolism of esmolol (11-min half-life) by mother also occurs in the fetus

Calcium channel blockers

Verapamil	5–10 mg IV bolus, repeat p.r.n. in 5 min, then every 30 min p.r.n.	Mild decrease	No evidence for teratogenicity or adverse fetal effects
Nifedipine	10 mg sublingual, repeat every 10–30 min p.r.n. × 3	Mild decrease	
Diltiazem	20 mg IV bolus over 2 min, repeat with 25 mg in 15 min	Few data available	

Table continued on following page

Table 8-2

Cardiovascular Drugs Commonly Used in the Obstetric Intensive Care Setting and Their Effects on Uterine Blood Flow and the Fetus *Continued*

Drug	Dose	Uterine Blood Flow	Fetal Effect
Vasoconstrictors			
Ephedrine sulfate	5–15 mg IV bolus, repeat every ½ min p.r.n. × 3	No effect on UBF	Because it does not decrease UBF, from this group, ephedrine is the agent of choice.
Metaraminol	Initiate with 0.1 mg/min and titrate to effect up to 2.0 mg/min	Mild ↓ in UBF	If improved ventricular function is desired along with vasoconstriction, then dopamine is preferable (see Inotropic agents).
Antiarrhythmic agents			
Lidocaine	Initial bolus of 1.0 mg/kg; repeat ½ bolus at 10 min and drip at 0.05 mg/kg/min (total dose 3 mg/kg)	None of these agents has a significant effect on uterine blood flow.	Each agent crosses the placenta. Experience greatest with lidocaine, procainamide, and quinidine with no clear adverse fetal effects
Procainamide	15 mg/kg over 30 min, then drip at 0.08 mg/kg/min (total dose 17 mg/kg)		

Table continued on opposite page

Quinidine	15 mg/kg over 60 min, then drip at 0.02 mg/kg/min
Bretylium	IV bolus of 5 mg/kg then drip at 1–2 mg/min
Phenytoin	300 mg IV in central line, then 100 mg every 5 min to total of 1000 mg
Amiodarone	5 mg/kg IV over 3 min, then 10 mg/kg/d

AV node-blocking agent

Adenosine	6 mg IV bolus over 1–3 sec, may repeat at 12 mg in 1–2 min × 2 doses	Transient ↓ Mild ↑
Verapamil	As stated above	No adequate assessment of effects on fetus
β-Blocking agent	As stated above	
Digoxin	As stated above	

Adapted from McAnulty JH: Heart and other circulatory diseases. In Bonica JJ, McDonald JS (eds): Principles and Practice of Obstetric Analgesia and Anesthesia, ed 2. Baltimore: Williams & Wilkins, 1995, pp 1019–1020.

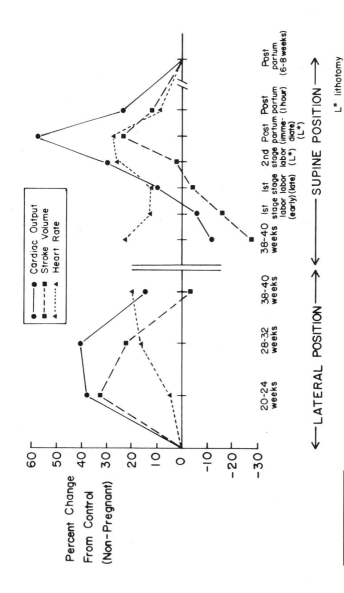

Figure 8-1

See legend on opposite page

> ### Box 8–1
>
> **"Avoids" for ASD**
>
> 1. Avoid increases in systemic vascular resistance (may increase left-right shunt).
> 2. Avoid decreases in pulmonary vascular resistance (may increase left-right shunt).
> 3. Avoid supraventricular dysrhythmias (may increase left-right shunt).
> 4. If pulmonary hypertension is present, avoid circumstances that may worsen pulmonary vascular resistance: Metabolic acidosis, excess catecholamines, hypoxemia, nitrous oxide, hypercarbia, pharmacologic vasoconstrictors, lung hyperinflation.

shunts corrected nonsurgically, pulmonary hypertension may develop and lead to shunt reversal; however, in the absence of Eisenmenger's syndrome (see below), increased cardiac demands in pregnancy are usually tolerated well.

Management. Avoiding fluid overload is important. The left lateral recumbent position is optimal for labor. Endocarditis prophylaxis is *not* generally recommended. Supplemental oxygen should be administered. Epidural anesthesia is optional but useful for pain management (Box 8–1).

Ventricular Septal Defect (VSD). Small VSDs are generally tolerated well. Larger ones, however, are more often associated with arrhythmias, pulmonary hypertension, and congestive heart failure. Pulmonary hypertension carries the risk of shunt reversal during hypotensive episodes. Large VSDs may also be associated with aortic regurgitation that can add to the risk of congestive failure.

Figure 8–1

Maternal cardiovascular changes during pregnancy and labor from studies on patients in the lateral and supine positions. (Data from Ueland K, Hansen J: Maternal cardiovascular dynamics. II. Posture and uterine contractions. Am J Obstet Gynecol 1969;103:1; Ueland K, Hansen J: Maternal cardiovascular dynamics. III. Labor and delivery under local and caudal analgesia. Am J Obstet Gynecol 1969;103:8; and Ueland K, Novy M, Peterson E, et al.: Maternal cardiovascular dynamics. IV. The influence of gestational age on the maternal cardiovascular response to posture and exercise. Am J Obstet Gynecol 1969;104:156.)

Table 8-3

Considerations for the Management of Cardiac Disease During Pregnancy

Problem	Maternal Mortality (%)	SBE Prophylaxis (see Table 8–1)	Labor Anesthesia*	Central Monitoring	Special Concerns§
Septal Defects					
Atrial	<1	No	Regional†	No	1,3,7,8
Ventricular	<1	Yes	Regional†	No	1,5,8†
Valvular					
Aorta					
Coarctation	5–15 (25–50 if valvular involvement)	Yes	Narcotic epidural	No	3,4,10
Stenosis	5–15	Yes	Narcotic epidural	Yes	3,4,10
Insufficiency	<1	Yes	Regional	No	8,9,10
Mitral					
Stenosis	5–15	Yes	Regional	Yes/No	1,3,4,5,6
Insufficiency	<1	Yes	Regional	No	1,8,9,10
Pulmonary					
Stenosis	<1	Yes	Regional	No	1,3,4,9,10
Insufficiency	<1	Yes	Regional	No	1,6,10
Tetralogy of Fallot (uncorrected)	≤15 (<1% if corrected)	Yes	Narcotic epidural	Yes	3,9
Tricuspid					
Stenosis	<1	Yes	Epidural	No	1,5
Insufficiency	<1	Yes	Epidural	No	1,6

Table continued on opposite page

Other					
Eisenmenger's	25–50	Yes	Narcotic epidural	Yes	2,3,4,6,9
IHSS	<1	Yes	Narcotic epidural	No	3,4,5
Marfan's with aortic root >4 cm	25–50 (5–15 with normal aorta)	No‡	Regional	No	1,4,5
Cardiomyopathy	25–50	No	Regional	Yes	1,2,8
PDA	<1	Yes	Regional†	No	1,8†

*A regional anesthetic may be utilized for a C-section delivery. In cases when a narcotic epidural is recommended, C-sections should be managed with general anesthesia.

†In the absence of pulmonary hypertension.

‡In the absence of significant valvular insufficiency.

Note:

All cardiac patients should be labored in the left lateral uterine tilt position and oxygen should be given.

§Special concerns:

1. Avoid fluid overload.
2. Heparinization.
3. Avoid hypotension/decreases in systemic vascular resistance.
4. Forceps-assisted delivery to shorten second stage of labor.
5. Avoid tachycardia.
6. Avoid increases in pulmonary vascular resistance: metabolic acidosis, excess catecholamines, hypoxemia, nitrous oxide, hypercarbia.
7. Avoid decreases in pulmonary vascular resistance.
8. Avoid increases in systemic vascular resistance.
9. Avoid myocardial depressant drugs.
10. Avoid bradycardia.

From Dajani AS, Bisno AL, Chung KJ, et al: Prevention of bacterial endocarditis: recommendations of the American Heart Association. JAMA 1990;264:2919–2922. Reprinted with permission. Copyright 1990, American Medical Association.

Management. Avoid fluid overload. The left lateral recumbent position during labor optimizes cardiac function. Endocarditis prophylaxis is advisable (Table 8–4). In the absence of Eisenmenger's syndrome (Fig. 8–2 and Box 8–2), epidural anesthesia is a reasonable option.

Patent Ductus Arteriosus (PDA). PDA is uncommon during pregnancy. In most circumstances patients are relatively asymptomatic. If PDA is uncorrected, however, large volumes of aortic blood are shunted at high pressure through the patent ductus into the pulmonary circulation and can lead to pulmonary hypertension. What in effect occurs is a left heart–to–right heart shunt with secondary left and right ventricular and atrial hypertrophy.

Table 8–4	
Prevention of Bacterial Endocarditis	
Drug	**Dosage**
Standard Regimen	
Ampicillin, gentamicin, and amoxicillin	Ampicillin, 2 gm, IV or IM plus gentamicin, 1.5 mg/kg IV or IM (not to exceed 80 mg), 30 min before procedure; followed by amoxicillin, 1.5 gm PO 6 hr after initial dose; alternatively, the parenteral regimen may be repeated once 8 hr after initial dose
Regimen for Those Allergic to Ampicillin/Amoxicillin/Penicillin	
Vancomycin and gentamicin	Vancomycin, 1 gm IV over 1 hr, plus gentamicin, 1.5 mg/kg IV or IM (not to exceed 80 mg), 1 hr before procedure; may be repeated once 8 hr after initial dose
Alternate Low-Risk Patient Regimen	
Amoxicillin	3 gm PO 1 hr before procedure; then 1.5 gm 6 hr after initial dose

From Dajani AS, Bisno AL, Chung KJ, et al.: Prevention of bacterial endocarditis: Recommendations of the American Heart Association. JAMA 1990;264:2919–2922. Reprinted with permission. Copyright 1990, American Medical Association.

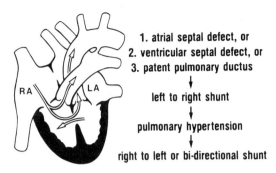

1. atrial septal defect, or
2. ventricular septal defect, or
3. patent pulmonary ductus
   ↓
left to right shunt
   ↓
pulmonary hypertension
   ↓
right to left or bi-directional shunt

Figure 8-2

Pathophysiology of Eisenmenger's syndrome. RA, right atrium; LA, left atrium. (Adapted from Mangano DT: Anesthesia for the pregnant cardiac patient. *In* Shnider SM, Levinson G (eds): Anesthesia for Obstetrics, ed 3. Baltimore: Williams & Wilkins, 1992.)

Management. Endocarditis prophylaxis is recommended (see Table 8–4). Epidural anesthesia is reasonable in the absence of pulmonary hypertension. Management of PDA is similar to that for Eisenmenger's syndrome (Box 8–3).

Pulmonary Hypertension and Eisenmenger's Syndrome. Left-to-right shunting may occur with PDA, ASD, or VSD. The high-pressure blood in the left side of the heart passes into the low-pressure right heart, eventually producing pulmonary hypertension, which in a pregnant woman has a grave prognosis. During the antepartum period, declining systemic vascular resistance associated with pregnancy causes some degree of right-to-left ("reverse") shunting. With progressively more shunt reversal, pulmonary perfusion declines and hypoxia increases (Eisenmenger's syndrome; see Fig. 8–2). Systemic hypotension

Box 8-2

"Avoids" for VSD

1. Avoid marked increases in heart rate (may increase left-right shunt).
2. Avoid increases in systemic vascular resistance (may increase left-right shunt).
3. With pulmonary hypertension avoid marked decreases in systemic vascular resistance and marked increases in pulmonary vascular resistance (see #4 Avoids for ASD) (may increase right-left shunt).

Box 8–3

"Avoids" for PDA

1. Avoid increase in systemic vascular resistance.
2. Avoid fluid overload (increases in blood volume).
3. With pulmonary hypertension avoid increases in pulmonary vascular resistance (see #4 Avoids for ASD) and decreases in systemic vascular resistance (may increase left-right shunt).

---

in these patients can further decrease right ventricular filling. In the presence of severe pulmonary hypertension, right heart pressures may be insufficient to perfuse the hypertensive, vasoconstricted pulmonary arterial bed and severe, rapid hemodynamic deterioration may ensue. Therefore, avoidance of hypotension is the principal clinical concern in the management of patients with pulmonary hypertension of any cause. Owing to the high risk of maternal mortality associated with Eisenmenger's syndrome and pulmonary hypertension, consideration of pregnancy termination in the first or early second trimester may be warranted. The prognosis for the mother is poor if maternal hematocrit exceeds 65%. Fetal wastage in the setting of Eisenmenger's syndrome can approach 75%. Maternal Pao_2 should be maintained at no lower than 60 to 70 mm Hg (see Chapter 22). Third trimester fetal surveillance is advised.

Management. (See also primary pulmonary hypertension) Intrapartum management should include placement of a pulmonary artery catheter to monitor the effects of filling pressure on cardiac output. Continual monitoring of the mixed venous oxygen saturation is recommended as a reliable technique for assessing cardiopulmonary function. Decreasing preload or systemic vascular resistance can result in inadequate pulmonary vascular perfusion. Epidural anesthesia (with local anesthetic) is contraindicated owing to the associated risk of systemic hypotension (secondary to induced sympathectomy). Epidural or intrathecal morphine, a technique devoid of adverse effects on systemic vascular resistance, may be the best type of anesthetic for these difficult cases. Additional problems include a propensity for thromboembolic phenomena owing to the hypercoagulability of pregnancy and the associated polycythemia of this disease. Prophylactic heparin during gestation and full heparinization for 10 days after delivery have been proposed. Endocarditis prophylaxis is also advised (see Table 8–4 and Box 8–4).

Box 8–4

"Avoids" for Pulmonary Hypertension and Eisenmenger's Syndrome

1. Avoid decreases in systemic vascular resistance.
2. Avoid increases in pulmonary vascular resistance (see #4 Avoids for ASD).
3. Avoid decreases in venous return.
4. Avoid myocardial depressant drugs.

Coarctation of the Aorta. In most circumstances, severe coarctation of the aorta has been surgically corrected early in infancy. The most common site of aortic coarctation is at the origin of the left subclavian artery. Although most patients are asymptomatic, resting cardiac output may be decreased. Aortic dissection or rupture, congestive heart failure, cerebral vascular accidents, or bacterial endocarditis may complicate the clinical picture and may increase maternal mortality to as high as 17%.

Management. Endeavor to avoid systemic hypotension. Narcotic epidural anesthesia is therefore a reasonable option during labor. Shortening of the second stage with forceps is suggested. Endocarditis prophylaxis is recommended (see Table 8–4 and Box 8–5).

Pulmonic Stenosis. Although the exact site of the pulmonary artery obstruction varies, it is the degree of obstruction that is the principal prognostic factor. A valvular pressure gradient exceeding 80 mm Hg is considered severe, and surgical correction should be considered. Otherwise, no additional measures are suggested other than avoidance of iatrogenic fluid overload and endocarditis prophylaxis (see Table 8–4 and Box 8–6).

Tetralogy of Fallot. The features of this cardiac anomaly include VSD with an overriding aorta, right ventricular hypertrophy, and pulmonary stenosis. The decline in the systemic vascular

---

Box 8–5

"Avoids" for Coarctation of Aorta

1. Avoid decreases in left ventricular filling.
2. Avoid decreases in systemic vascular resistance.
3. Avoid bradycardia.

Box 8–6

"Avoids" for Pulmonic Stenosis

1. Avoid bradycardia.
2. Avoid myocardial depressant drugs.
3. Avoid decreases in systemic vascular resistance.
4. Avoid fluid overload.
5. Avoid significant decreases in venous return.

---

resistance that accompanies pregnancy can result in right-to-left (i.e., "reverse") shunting, as discussed earlier. Prognosis is more likely to be poor in the presence of a hematocrit exceeding 65%, syncope, congestive failure, ECG evidence of right ventricular strain, cardiomegaly, right ventricular pressures in excess of 120 mm Hg, or peripheral oxygen saturation below 80%. Cyanosis may increase during pregnancy owing to decreasing peripheral vascular resistance and right-to-left shunting through the VSD. Cyanosis can also be increased by hypotension or a decrease in venous return.

Management. Left lateral recumbency is recommended. A narcotic epidural anesthetic is acceptable. If significant blood loss occurs at delivery, immediate replacement is recommended. Endocarditis prophylaxis is advised (see Table 8–4). Intrapartum use of support hose is warranted to minimize positional effects on preload (Box 8–7).

Acquired Cardiac Lesions (see Table 8–3). Rheumatic heart disease still accounts for 90% of cardiac disorders of pregnant women worldwide. Mitral stenosis is the most common rheumatic lesion. Endocarditis secondary to intravenous drug abuse is an increasingly common cause of acquired valvular disease, especially in the right side of the heart. Maternal morbidity and mortality in this setting generally result from congestive failure, arrhythmias, or thromboembolism.

Box 8–7

"Avoids" for Tetralogy of Fallot

1. Avoid decreases in blood volume and venous return.
2. Avoid significant decreases in systemic vascular resistance.
3. Avoid myocardial depressant drugs.

Memory Aid. The cardiac valves most often affected, in order of prevalence, are *m*itral, *a*ortic, *t*ricuspid, and *p*ulmonic ("*M*ary *a*nd *T*im *P*lay").

Pulmonic and Tricuspid Lesions. Isolated right-sided valvular lesions are uncommon but among intravenous drug abusers are seen with increasing frequency secondary to bacterial endocarditis. Pregnancy-associated hypervolemia is less likely to be problematic with these cardiac lesions, owing to the lower pressures found in the right heart. Invasive monitoring is not usually required.

Mitral Stenosis. Mitral stenosis impedes the flow of blood from the left atrium to the left ventricle. A relatively fixed cardiac output results. Pulmonary hypertension may occur from chronic untreated disease (Fig. 8–3).

Management. These patients often require relatively elevated left atrial pressures (and thus pulmonary capillary wedge pressures of 14 to 16 mm Hg) to maintain adequate left ventricular filling. Gravidas unable to accommodate the increasing volume status and heart rate associated with pregnancy may decompensate, with resultant pulmonary edema. Careful modulation of the preload with venodilators or diuretics may help decrease pulmo-

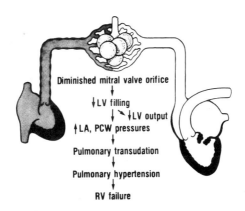

Figure 8–3

Pathophysiology of mitral stenosis. LV, left ventricle; LA, left atrium; PCW, pulmonary capillary wedge; RV, right ventricle. (Adapted from Mangano DT: Anesthesia for the pregnant cardiac patient. *In* Shnider SM, Levinson G (eds): Anesthesia for Obstetrics, ed 3. Baltimore: Williams & Wilkins, 1992.)

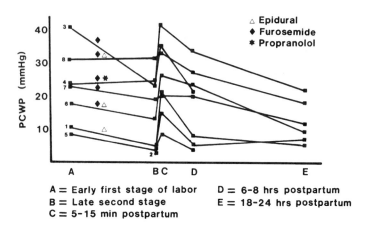

A = Early first stage of labor   D = 6-8 hrs postpartum
B = Late second stage   E = 18-24 hrs postpartum
C = 5-15 min postpartum

Figure 8-4

Intrapartum alterations in PCWP in eight patients with mitral stenosis. (From Clark SL, Phelan JP, Greenspoon J, et al.: Labor and delivery in the presence of mitral stenosis: Central hemodynamic observations. Am J Obstet Gynecol 1985; 152:984.)

nary congestion. Afterload reduction may be accomplished by use of a vasodilator (see Table 8–2). Since blood flows across a fixed mitral orifice, tachycardia can diminish diastolic filling time and further reduce cardiac output. To avoid hazardous tachycardia, beta-blockade should be utilized in any parturient with severe mitral stenosis and a pulse rate exceeding 90 bpm. Intrapartum fluctuations of cardiac output may be minimized by use of epidural anesthesia. The most hazardous time for these patients is immediately post partum, owing to the increased cardiac output and large volume shifts (increased preload) that follow delivery. Post partum, large increases (up to 16 mm Hg) in the wedge pressure can be expected (Fig. 8–4). The additional pressure in the left atrium and pulmonary vasculature can result in pulmonary edema. Postpartum dosing of the epidural local anesthetic may help to increase blood vessel capacity, which may help to accommodate the large postpartum fluid shifts. Historically, recommendations for delivery have included liberal forceps assistance during vaginal delivery. Endocarditis prophylaxis is advised (see Table 8–4 and Box 8–8).

Mitral Insufficiency. Mitral insufficiency of rheumatic origin often occurs in conjunction with other valvular lesions. It is generally tolerated well during pregnancy. In severe cases, mitral insuffi-

> **Box 8–8**
>
> ### "Avoids" for Mitral Stenosis
>
> 1. Avoid tachycardia, which decreases ventricular filling.
> 2. Avoid fluid overload, as it can result in right ventricular failure, pulmonary edema, or atrial fibrillation.
> 3. Avoid decreases in systemic vascular resistance.
> 4. Avoid increases in pulmonary vascular resistance (see #4 Avoids for ASD), which can precipitate right ventricular failure.

ciency can be associated with the development of atrial enlargement and fibrillation (Fig. 8–5). Since pregnancy itself increases the risk of atrial fibrillation, consideration of prophylactic digitalization has been recommended for patients with significant mitral insufficiency. Endocarditis prophylaxis before delivery is recommended (see Table 8–4 and Box 8–9).

Aortic Stenosis. Aortic stenosis is most frequently of rheumatic origin and occurs in conjunction with other valvular lesions. With severe disease, cardiac output may be fixed (Fig. 8–6).

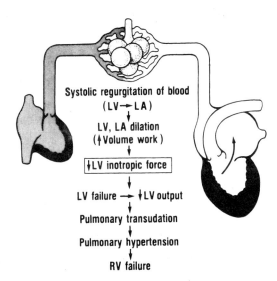

Figure 8–5

Pathophysiology of mitral insufficiency. LV, left ventricle; LA, left atrium; RV, right ventricle. (Adapted from Mangano DT: Anesthesia for the pregnant cardiac patient. *In* Shnider SM, Levinson G (eds): Anesthesia for Obstetrics, ed 3. Baltimore: Williams & Wilkins, 1992.)

Box 8-9

"Avoids" for Mitral Insufficiency

1. Avoid severe increases in systemic vascular resistance (they increase regurgitant flow).
2. Avoid bradycardia; keep the heart rate normal to slightly tachycardiac to reduce time for regurgitant backflow.
3. Avoid atrial fibrillation (treat immediately if it occurs).
4. Avoid myocardial depressant drugs.

During exertion or in the setting of hypotension, cardiac output may be insufficient to maintain coronary arterial and cerebral perfusion. This can result in angina, syncope, and sudden death. Limitation of physical activity is vital for patients with severe disease. Delivery is the time of greatest risk for those with severe aortic stenosis. Patients with pressure gradients exceeding 100 mm Hg are at greatest risk. Pulmonary artery catheterization allows more exact hemodynamic assessment during labor and delivery.

Management. Management is similar to that for pulmonary hypertension. Hypotension is avoided by maintaining adequate preload. Acute hypotensive events can reduce coronary artery

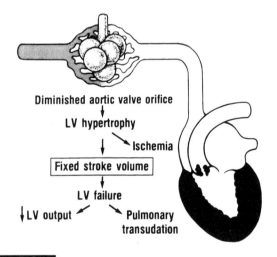

Figure 8-6

Pathophysiology of aortic stenosis. LV, left ventricle. (Adapted from Mangano DT: Anesthesia for the pregnant cardiac patient. *In* Shnider SM, Levinson G (eds): Anesthesia for Obstetrics, ed 3. Baltimore: Williams & Wilkins, 1992.)

Box 8-10

"Avoids" for Aortic Stenosis

1. Avoid bradycardia.
2. Avoid significant decreases in systemic vascular resistance.
3. Avoid decreases in venous return and left ventricular filling.

---

perfusion and result in sudden death. Epidural anesthesia is contraindicated unless a narcotic epidural is utilized. As with mitral stenosis, managing these patients in the left lateral recumbent position and maintaining a wedge pressure of 14 to 16 mm Hg is optimal for maintaining adequate left ventricular preload. Forceps-assisted delivery should be considered. Continuous invasive monitoring is generally utilized during labor and delivery and post partum. Endocarditis prophylaxis is advised (see Table 8–4 and Box 8–10).

Aortic Insufficiency. Aortic insufficiency is also commonly of rheumatic origin. Pregnancy and delivery are usually tolerated well. Concern arises when diastolic regurgitation of blood from the aorta to the left ventricle results in left ventricular dilatation (Fig. 8–7). Chronic problems lead to a decrease in left ventricular inotropic force, which may result in left ventricular failure.

Management. Maintenance of adequate venous return and avoidance of hypertension are mainstays of therapy. Elastic support stockings facilitate maintenance of venous return. Endocarditis prophylaxis is recommended during labor and delivery (see Table 8–4 and Box 8–11).

Other Categories

Primary Pulmonary Hypertension. Pulmonary hypertension is associated with mortality rates of 50%. The principal hemodynamic defect is elevated pulmonary vascular resistance. The

---

Box 8-11

"Avoids" for Aortic Insufficiency

1. Avoid marked increases in systemic vascular resistance.
2. Avoid myocardial depressant drugs.
3. Avoid bradycardia.

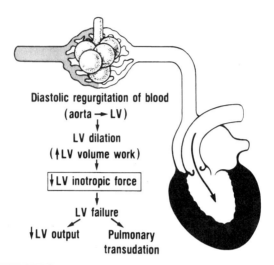

Figure 8-7

Pathophysiology of aortic insufficiency. LV, left ventricle. (Adapted from Mangano DT: Anesthesia for the pregnant cardiac patient. *In* Shnider SM, Levinson G (eds): Anesthesia for Obstetrics, ed 3. Baltimore: Williams & Wilkins, 1992.)

increased cardiac output and blood volume are poorly tolerated as is decreased venous return late in pregnancy and during delivery.

Management (see also Eisenmenger's Syndrome). Management includes the avoidance of hypotension and the maintenance of venous return to the heart. Left lateral positioning and elastic support stockings should be utilized. A narcotic epidural is recommended to avoid hypotension. Immediate fluid replacement is vital if losses are excessive. Endocarditis prophylaxis is indicated (see Table 8–4). Ambulation with elastic support socks is recommended post partum. Additionally, prophylactic heparin is suggested during the antepartum period.

Marfan's Syndrome. Marfan's syndrome is transmitted in an autosomal-dominant pattern of inheritance. Cystic medial necrosis of the aorta can result in aortic regurgitation or dissecting aortic aneurysm. Increasing aortic regurgitation and aortic root dilation increase the risk of rupture from dissecting aneurysms. Echocardiographic measurements of aortic root diameters may be of benefit. Risks are substantially increased with root diameters in excess of 4 cm.

Management. Prevention of tachycardia and excessive pulsatile pressures on the aortic wall appears to reduce the risk of dissecting aneurysms. Empiric beta-blockade for hypertension or maternal heart rate in excess of 90 bpm is recommended and should be considered for all patients. Labor in the left lateral recumbent position and epidural anesthesia are beneficial. Forceps-assisted delivery is warranted. Cesarean delivery may be preferred to prevent the potentially deleterious effects of bearing down. Caution, however, should be exercised during surgery on patients with Marfan's syndrome, owing to friable tissue and poor healing.

Idiopathic Hypertrophic Subaortic Stenosis (IHSS). IHSS is an inherited autosomal-dominant cardiac anomaly. Outflow of blood from the left ventricle is impeded by an abnormal outflow tract (asymmetric septal hypertrophy—ASH). The hemodynamic effects of this lesion and the management principles are very similar to those for valvular aortic stenosis. Outflow obstruction can be decreased by increasing venous return. In pregnancy, cardiac demands are generally well tolerated.

Management. Caution is advised when utilizing conduction anesthesia. Conduction anesthesia may decrease venous return, thereby increasing outflow obstruction. Endocarditis prophylaxis is recommended (see Table 8–4 and Box 8–12).

Cardiomyopathy of Pregnancy. Biventricular myocardial failure and secondary pulmonary congestion may occur in the third trimester or the postpartum period in a previously healthy patient without underlying cardiac disease. The mortality rate is 5% to 60%; of the survivors approximately 50% will completely

---

Box 8–12

"Avoids" for IHSS

1. Avoid decreases in systemic vascular resistance.
2. Avoid decreases in venous return.
3. Avoid increases in myocardial contractility.
4. Avoid tachycardia.

recover cardiac function but bear increased risk of recurrence during a subsequent pregnancy.

Management. Fluid restriction, appropriate diuretic therapy, a low-sodium diet, and bed rest have been described as cornerstones of therapy. Digitalis preparations are helpful but must be utilized cautiously because these patients are quite sensitive to this medication and may rapidly develop evidence of digitalis toxicity. Prophylactic heparinization is advised. Full heparinization for 10 days post partum should be considered because of the increased risk of thromboembolism.

■
Bibliography

Burlew BS: Managing the pregnant patient with heart disease. Clin Cardiol 1990;13:757–762.

Clark SL, Phelan JP, Cotton DB (eds): Critical Care Obstetrics: Structural Cardiac Disease in Pregnancy. Medical Economics Company, Inc., Oradell, NJ: 1987.

Mangano DT: Anesthesia for the pregnant cardiac patient. *In* Shnider SM (ed): Anesthesia for Obstetrics, ed 3. Baltimore: Williams & Wilkins, 1993.

McAnulty JH: Heart and other circulating diseases. In Bonica JJ, McDonald JS (eds): Principles and Practice of Obstetric Analgesia and Anesthesia, ed 2. Baltimore: Williams & Wilkins, 1995.

Pitkin RM: Pregnancy and congenital heart disease. Ann Internal Med 1990;112:445–454.

MICHAEL C. GORDON

Maternal Sepsis

Sepsis is the systemic response to infection and, despite the improvement in antibiotics, remains a serious problem in obstetrics. In the general U. S. population, sepsis and septic shock have been increasing over the past 30 years and are now the thirteenth most common cause of death. Terminology has been confusing owing to the use of imprecise terms with varying definitions and has resulted in confusion in the medical literature. Recent attempts have been made to standardize the terminology for infection, bacteremia, sepsis, and septic shock in order to enhance our ability to diagnose, treat, and formulate the prognosis for these infections. In this new terminology, "sepsis" represents a subgroup of what is termed the "systemic inflammatory response syndrome" (SIRS; Fig. 9–1).

SIRS is a systemic response caused by activation of the host's own inflammatory system that results in a wide variety of insults and is seen in association with many clinical conditions. In addition to infection, other causes of SIRS include pancreatitis, ischemia, hemorrhage, shock, immune-mediated organ injury, and burns. Sepsis is the systemic inflammatory response caused by a number of infectious organisms: gram-negative bacteria, gram-positive bacteria, fungi, parasites, and possibly viruses. Obviously, not all persons with infection develop sepsis, and there is a continuum in the severity of infection from a localized process to bacteremia to sepsis to septic shock. The following definitions are suggested by a consensus conference of the American College of Chest Physicians and the Society of Critical Care Medicine for these various manifestations of infection:

> Infection: Microbial phenomenon characterized by an inflammatory response to the presence of microorganisms or the invasion of normally sterile host tissue by these organisms.
> Bacteremia: The presence of viable bacteria in the blood.
> Sepsis (Simple): The systemic response to infection, manifested by two or more of the following conditions

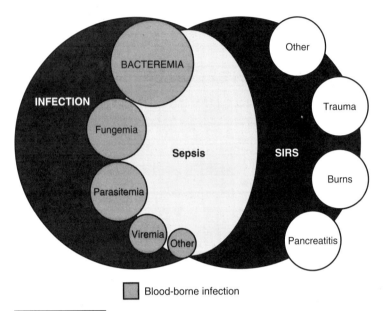

Blood-borne infection

Figure 9–1

The relationship among systemic inflammatory response syndrome (SIRS), sepsis, and infection. (From Bone RC, Balk RA, Cerra FB, et al.: Definitions for sepsis and organ failure and guidelines for the use of innovative therapies in sepsis. Chest 1992;101:1644.)

as a result of infection: (1) a temperature greater than 38°C or less than 36°C; (2) an elevated heart rate greater than 90 beats per minute; (3) tachypnea, manifested by a respiratory rate greater than 20 breaths per minute *or* a $Paco_2$ of less than 32 mm Hg; and (4) an alteration in the white blood cell count, such as a WBC greater than 12,000/mm^3 or less than 4000/mm^3, or the presence of more than 10% immature neutrophils.

Sepsis (Severe): Sepsis associated with organ dysfunction, hypoperfusion, or hypotension. Hypoperfusion and perfusion abnormalities that may include, but are not limited to, lactic acidosis, oliguria, or an acute alteration in mental status.

Septic Shock: Sepsis-induced hypotension despite adequate fluid resuscitation, along with the presence of perfusion abnormalities that may include, but are not limited to, lactic acidosis, oliguria, or an acute alteration in mental

status. Patients who are receiving inotropic or
vasopressor agents may not be hypotensive at the time
that the perfusion abnormalities are measured. This is a
subset of severe sepsis.

Sepsis-Induced Hypotension: A systolic blood pressure
<90 mm Hg or a reduction of ≥40 mm Hg from baseline
in the absence of other causes for hypotension.

The terms "septicemia" and "septic syndrome" have been
used so variously in the medical literature that these terms have
become confusing and ambiguous, and it has been recommended they be dropped entirely. Sepsis is the third most
common cause of shock in the United States, and shock occurs
when the patient's functional intravascular blood volume does
not meet the needs of the body's vascular capacity, which
results in lowering of the blood pressure and decreased tissue
perfusion.

■
Maternal Concerns

The prevalence of bacteremia in the obstetric-gynecologic patient population has been reported to be 0.2% to 0.7% of all
women admitted to an OB-GYN ward. Bacteremia occurs in
approximately 5% to 10% of women with acute chorioamnionitis, pyelonephritis, or postpartum endometritis. Of these
women with bacteremia, 4% to 5% develop sepsis or septic
shock and as many as 3% of them die. The mortality of septic
shock in the nonpregnant population is much higher. The mortality of septic shock in this population is 20% to 50% and
depends on the patient's underlying medical conditions. The
reasons for the better prognosis for pregnant women is multifactorial and includes (1) younger age, (2) transient nature of the
bacteremia in obstetric infections, (3) less toxic organisms, (4)
primary site of infection more amenable to treatment, and (5)
previously healthy patients without underlying chronic medical
conditions. Although pregnant patients in septic shock have a
more optimistic outcome than do the general medical population, animal studies indicate that pregnant animals are less tolerant of septic shock than are similar nonpregnant animals. The
pregnant animals died more rapidly of gram-negative sepsis
(3.5 hours versus 14 hours) with more pronounced metabolic
acidosis. Therefore, although the pregnant patient's prognosis is
better than that for the general medical population, pregnancy

places a woman at higher risk for developing septic shock and she is more intolerant to its consequences than if she were not pregnant.

The most frequent cause of bacteremia (70% to 85%) in the obstetric patient is the development of endometritis after a cesarean delivery; therefore, not surprisingly, the majority of sepsis (80%) in obstetrics occurs in the postpartum period (Table 9–1). Cesarean delivery is associated with a higher incidence of bacteremia than vaginal delivery (3% versus 0.1% in one study); thus, cesarean delivery is one of the greatest risk factors for the development of bacteremia and sepsis. Other risk factors for sepsis whose frequency is increasing in the obstetric population include immunosuppressive or cytotoxic drugs, parenteral hyperalimentation, immune deficiency, and chronic debilitating diseases.

As in the nonobstetric population, gram-negative, endotoxin-producing, aerobic bacilli (mainly Enterobacteriaceae) are the isolates found most frequently in obstetric patients with bacteremia or sepsis. The majority of these organisms are endogenous from the vaginal flora and are not acquired nosocomially. Although these bacteria cause as much as 60% to 80% of all sepsis in pregnancy, any organism may cause sepsis; and in 20% of obstetric cases the sepsis is polymicrobial (Table 9–2). In addition to bacteria, sepsis is (rarely) caused by fungi, viruses, and parasites; and in as many as 10% of cases the infectious cause is unknown.

Table 9–1	
Prevalence of Infectious Causes of Septic Shock in Pregnancy	
Infection	Prevalence (%)
Endometritis after cesarean delivery	70–85
Pyelonephritis	1–4
Septic abortion	1–2
Endometritis after vaginal delivery	1–4
Wound infections	1–2
Chorioamnionitis	0.5–1
Pneumonia	2
Toxic shock syndrome	<1

Table 9-2	
Bacterial Causes of Sepsis in Obstetric Patients	
Pathogen(s)	Prevalence (%)
Gram-negative bacilli (Enterobacteriaceae)	
Escherichia coli	50
Klebsiella spp	
Serratia spp	30
Enterobacter spp	
Gram-positive cocci	
Streptococcus pyogenes (group A)	
Streptococcus agalactiae (group B)	
Streptococcus faecalis (group D Enterococcus)	
Staphylococcus aureus	
Obligate anaerobes	20
Bacteroides fragilis	
Provotella spp (formerly *Bacteroides* spp)	
Peptostreptococci spp	
Clostridium perfringens	
Fusobacterium spp	

■
Pathophysiology

Sepsis is the result of multiple normal body defense mechanisms responding too aggressively in an attempt to eradicate an overwhelming infection, which results in the body's own defense mechanisms' causing systemic side effects (simple sepsis), organ damage (severe sepsis), or cardiovascular instability (septic shock). It is the activation of the body's defense mechanisms by bacterial endotoxins, exotoxins, proteases, or cellular debris—not the actual bacteremic infection—that is responsible for most of the serious clinical manifestations of sepsis and septic shock. Sepsis is usually the result of a gram-negative bacillary bacteremia. Endotoxin, a lipopolysaccharide component of the outer membrane gram-negative cell wall, is released at the time of the organism's death and has been implicated as the most common initiator of the cascade of events leading to septic shock (Fig. 9–2).

Endotoxin is composed of an oligosaccharide side chain, a core polysaccharide, and lipid A, which is thought to be the major toxic component of the endotoxin molecule. After release

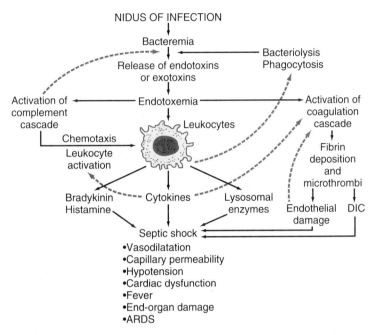

NIDUS OF INFECTION
↓
Bacteremia
↓
Release of endotoxins
or exotoxins

Bacteriolysis
Phagocytosis

Activation of
complement
cascade ← Endotoxemia → Activation of
coagulation
cascade

Leukocytes

Chemotaxis
Leukocyte
activation

Fibrin
deposition
and
microthrombi

Bradykinin
Histamine   Cytokines   Lysosomal
enzymes   Endothelial   DIC
damage

Septic shock
• Vasodilatation
• Capillary permeability
• Hypotension
• Cardiac dysfunction
• Fever
• End-organ damage
• ARDS

Figure 9–2

The sequence of events seen in the development of septic shock caused by endotoxin.

from the gram-negative cell wall, endotoxins cause activation of at least three separate body defense mechanisms: release of macrophage-derived cytokines, activation of complement pathway, and activation of the coagulation cascade. Initiated by the endotoxin, the release of cytokines appears early in the sequence of events and plays a central role in amplifying the subsequent release of additional mediators of the body's host defense system. Key cytokines in the development of septic shock appear to be tumor necrosis factor and interleukins. The activation of the complement pathway, along with the recruitment of leukocytes by cytokines, leads to systemic activation of the body's defense mechanisms. This is aimed at eradicating the infection but results in the paradoxic release of further bacteria-derived endotoxin secondary to bacteriolysis of the cell wall and release of leukocyte-derived intracellular toxins such as superoxide free radicals, lysosomal enzymes, and hydrogen peroxide. These intracellular toxins then cause local tissue injury.

In addition, histamine and bradykinin are released by the leuko-cytes, which causes increased capillary permeability, endothelial damage, and peripheral vasodilatation. Activation of the coagu-lation cascade can lead to fibrin deposition and multiple mi-crothrombi within an organ. This results in impaired organ per-fusion and eventually leads to disseminated intravascular coagulopathy (DIC) due to consumption of the coagulation fac-tors.

Although the most comprehensive research on the causes of sepsis has focused on gram-negative derived endotoxin, it is also apparent that septic shock can be caused by exotoxins and hemolysins from gram-positive organisms, anaerobes, and fungi. In addition, during septic shock endotoxemia can occur in the absence of bacteremia.

■
Clinical Manifestations

Shock occurs when tissue perfusion is inadequate, and it results in cell dysfunction and eventually cell death, if prolonged. The organ systems most commonly affected include the heart, kid-neys, lungs, liver, central nervous system, and coagulation sys-tem. In addition, in pregnancy the uterus and the fetus can be affected. The prognosis for survival worsens as the number of affected organ systems increases. Death usually is a result of one or more organ systems failing completely or from refractory hypotension.

Cardiovascular Effects

The hemodynamic changes observed in septic shock differ from the other causes of shock: cardiogenic, vascular obstructive, and hypovolemic. In these forms of shock the systemic vascular resistance is elevated as a compensatory mechanism to maintain blood pressure and the arteriovenous oxygen difference is ele-vated, reflecting enhanced systemic extraction of oxygen by hypoperfused tissues. The hemodynamic changes that result from sepsis or septic shock are more complex and classically have been divided into three distinct phases (1) early (warm) shock, (2) late (cold) shock, and (3) secondary (irreversible) shock. The first phase represents a hyperdynamic shock syn-drome with decreased systemic vascular resistance (SVR) and an elevated cardiac output (warm shock). The onset of sepsis is accompanied by hypovolemia, owing to the combination of arterial and venous dilatation and leakage of plasma into the extravascular space due to endothelial damage. If this hypovolemia is treated, the patient will be found to have a low SVR (as low as 400 dyne/s/cm/^{5}; normal pregnancy value is 1210 $\pm$ 266 dyne/s/cm/^{5}), increased cardiac output, tachycardia, and decreased arteriovenous oxygen difference. The vasodilatation results from the release of cytokines, bradykinin, histamine, and prostaglandins. Although there is an overall increase in the cardiac output, owing mainly to an increase in the heart rate, ventricular function is depressed by a circulating myocardial depressant factor. This results in a depressed ejection fraction and ventricular dilatation. Finally, the decreased arteriovenous oxygen difference is due to decreased peripheral oxygen use. This is a result of maldistribution of blood flow (oxygen) to tissues with the development of lactic acidosis.

The late ("cold") stage of septic shock is classically characterized by a decrease of cardiac output as a consequence of increasing SVR (afterload) and worsening of the myocardial dysfunction. The SVR increases owing to severe vasoconstriction caused by circulating catecholamines and vasoactive prostaglandins (thromboxane) and may occur only in a minority of patients with cold shock. However, it appears that the majority of patients maintain a decrease in the SVR; and the clinical signs of cold shock are due to the depressed cardiac output, accumulation of lactic acid, persistent hypovolemia, and microvascular insufficiency. In this stage, tissue perfusion is inadequate and does not respond to fluid boluses; therefore, inotropic and vasoactive agents are necessary to maintain adequate blood pressure.

The final stage of shock represents the period of worsening hypotension that is unresponsive to conventional therapy with fluids and inotropic or vasoactive agents. The development of irreversible end organ damage occurs during this period.

Clinical Signs and Symptoms

The clinical signs of septic shock begin with bacteremia, which is usually intermittent and typically precedes the onset of temperature elevation and chills. The earliest clinical signs of sepsis (preshock) are tachypnea and respiratory alkalosis. During this period, the first signs of a hyperdynamic state appear, with mildly increased cardiac output and decreased SVR without a change in blood pressure. Early shock is characterized by a hyperdynamic state with hypotension (systolic blood pressure <60 to 90 mm Hg or a reduction of ≥40 mm Hg from baseline). The earliest clinical symptoms are often anxiety, combativeness, confusion, and disorientation. Other clinical signs during this stage of early septic shock include temperature instability, flushing, and peripheral vasodilatation. With the development of late shock there is profound hypotension, cold and clammy skin, hypoxemia, oliguria, and worsening of the mental status changes. During the period of early shock, signs of end organ damage can be seen, and these typically worsen with the development of late shock.

Organs Often Affected by Septic Shock
(Table 9–3)

End organ damage is caused by the combined effects of tissue hypoxia and the body's inflammatory response. In the general medical population, mortality is greatly influenced by the type and number of injured organ systems. If more than three organ systems are involved the mortality rate is 80% to 100%. Adult respiratory distress syndrome (ARDS) occurs in 25% of persons with septic shock and leads to hypoxemia with a mortality rate of 50%. Thrombocytopenia occurs in as many as 50% of patients, but only 5% develop DIC. DIC is thought to be more common with gram-negative sepsis. Rarely, extensive fibrin deposition leads to organ necrosis and death (the Shwartzman reaction). Hepatic dysfunction is not uncommon, and elevations in liver function tests are modest. If there is severe ischemia, more serious liver damage can occur—"shock liver"—and the patient's liver function tests will be markedly elevated. In addition, hypoglycemia can result from impaired gluconeogenesis.

Fetal Effect

Although a pregnant woman appears more susceptible to the effects of sepsis, the fetus is also at increased risk. The fetal risks do not appear to be due to the direct effects of the infection or the endotoxin, as the fetus has greater resistance to the endotoxin than the mother. However, the endotoxin causes a decrease in the uteroplacental blood supply and results in an increase in uterine contractions. The overall result is diminished fetal blood supply, which carries the risk of fetal hypoxia, acidosis, and preterm labor. If severe enough, this can lead to fetal distress and death; however, attempts at delivering the fetus may

Table 9–3

Organ Systems Affected by Septic Shock

Organ System	Clinical Findings	Mechanism
Pulmonary—ARDS	Bilateral diffuse infiltrates on chest film Hypoxemia Normal PCWP (<18 mm Hg)	Increased vascular permeability Direct endothelial damage
Renal Oliguria	<30 mL/hr	Hypotension and renal vasoconstriction
Acute tubular necrosis	Fractional excretion of filtered sodium ≥2, urine sodium >40 mEq/L	Prolonged cortical hypoxia secondary to decreased renal blood flow
Interstitial nephritis Hematologic		Immune mediated
DIC	Elevated fibrin degradation products, prothrombin time, partial thromboplastin time Decreased platelets and fibrinogen Spontaneous bleeding (uncommon)	Endotoxin activation of Hageman factor
Leukocytosis	>20,000 cells/μL	Demargination Neutrophil-releasing substance
Neurologic—mental status changes	Somnolence, coma, combativeness (uncommon, usually due to hypoxia)	Decreased cerebral blood flow Hypoxia

Adapted from Pearlman MD, Faro S: Obstetrical septic shock: A pathophysiologic basis for management. Clin Obstet Gynecol 1990;33:485.

worsen the maternal/fetal status and usually are not indicated unless the septic shock is due to chorioamnionitis. Otherwise, the best treatment for the fetus is to improve the mother's condition.

■
Diagnosis (Table 9–4)

The early diagnosis of sepsis or septic shock depends on the clinician maintaining a high index of suspicion and vigilance when caring for a patient with a febrile illness and early nonspecific signs: tachypnea, dyspnea, tachycardia with a hyperdynamic state, peripheral vasodilatation, temperature instability, and mental status changes. This is particularly important in women at higher risk for septic shock—women with pyelonephritis, chorioamnionitis, endometritis, septic abortion, or recent surgical procedures, for example. Early diagnosis and initiation of appropriate therapy has been shown to improve survival.

The actual presenting symptoms depend on the stage (warm versus cold) of the septic shock when the patient presents and the type of end organ damage present, although hypotension is a constant finding and usually is obvious. The majority of patients have an elevated temperature and an elevated white blood cell count with a shift to the left; however, some women's temperature and white blood count are below normal ($<36°C$ and <4000 per microliter, respectively). As a result of the hyperdynamic cardiac state, some women present with cardiac symptoms due to ischemia, left ventricular failure, or arrhythmia. The clinical consequences of DIC include hemorrhage, thrombosis, and microangiopathic hemolysis. In addition, because of the potential for renal dysfunction and hypovolemia, other possible

Table 9–4
Differential Diagnosis of Septic Shock
Hypovolemic shock Acute pulmonary embolism Cardiogenic shock Cardiac tamponade Thyroid storm Hemorrhagic pancreatitis Diabetic ketoacidosis

clinical manifestations include oliguria, anuria, hematuria, and proteinuria.

Owing to the 25% risk to the mother of developing ARDS with respiratory failure, the clinician needs to watch for signs of respiratory distress, hypoxemia, and worsening acidosis. In early sepsis the patient may present with respiratory alkalosis due to hyperventilation; but as the sepsis worsens severe metabolic and respiratory acidosis develops that is the result of accumulation of lactic acid from cellular anaerobic metabolism. The level of lactate corresponds with the severity of the organ hypoxia, and rising levels correlate directly with worsening prognosis and can be used as a treatment parameter.

To help in diagnosing septic shock and treating affected organ systems, certain laboratory studies should be performed (Table 9–5). In addition, a physical examination, cultures, and radiographic studies need to be done to help determine the origin of the infection responsible for the sepsis and decide on appropriate treatment. Physical examination of the obstetric patient should initially focus on the genitourinary, gastrointestinal, and respiratory systems and wounds (episiotomy and skin incisions); but if findings appear normal, more atypical sites of infection need to be considered. Possible foci of infection in a woman post partum include retained products of conception, uterine microabscesses, pelvic abscesses, wound infections, and septic pelvic thrombosis. At least two separate sets of blood

---

Table 9–5

Laboratory Evaluation of Sepsis

Complete blood count with differential and platelet count
Electrolytes, glucose, blood urea nitrogen, and creatinine
Liver function tests
DIC panel: fibrinogen, prothrombin time, partial thromboplastin time, and fibrin degradation products
Urinalysis
Arterial blood gas
Serum lactate
Cultures (aerobic, anaerobic, fungi) and Gram stains of (1) urine, (2) blood, *and if suspected* (3) wound, abscess, or episiotomy, (4) amniotic fluid (amniocentesis), and (5) sputum
Chest film
Consider other imaging studies if clinically indicated: abdominal series, computed tomography, or ultrasound of abdomen and pelvis.

cultures should be obtained. The sensitivity of a single culture for bacteremia is 80%, of two cultures 89%, and of three cultures 99% in patients with soft tissue infections.

Two uncommon agents of postpartum septic shock deserve mention owing to their extreme virulence and high mortality rates: *Streptococcus pyogenes* (group A streptococcus) and *Clostridium sordellii*. Group A streptococcal puerperal infection was a very common lethal infection before the advent of antibiotics, but since the 1960s has been an uncommon cause of maternal septic shock. Within the last 5 years, however, there appears to be a small resurgence of this infection, with a mortality of 30%, even though the majority of affected persons are young and previously healthy. This infection causes profound septic shock with hematologic, renal, and pulmonary involvement within a few hours of delivery and is believed to be caused by a type A exotoxin. On physical examination there is usually no obvious pelvic disease, but inspection of the pelvic organs at the time of surgery reveals edematous tissues with foci of gangrenous and hemorrhagic necrosis without purulence. Similarly, *C. sordellii* infection is due to an exotoxin that presents on the second to sixth postpartum day owing to a limited soft tissue infection. The type of septic shock has a distinctive clinical course characterized by sudden onset of severe and unrelenting hypotension associated with marked generalized tissue edema and third spacing of fluid, resulting in high hematocrits ($>50\%$) and very low serum albumin levels (1 to 2 mg/dL). In addition, a marked leukemoid reaction develops with a total neutrophil count of 60,000 to 90,000/mm^3 and absence of fever. This type of septic shock has been reported to be nearly uniformly fatal.

■
Treatment

As many as 70% of maternal deaths from infection are thought possibly to be preventable. To accomplish this goal, septic shock needs to be diagnosed early and the correct treatment initiated early. The goals of treatment are to maintain normal cardiac output, improve end organ perfusion and oxygenation, treat the infectious source of the bacteremia, maintain adequate ventilation, and treat the end organ damage or support of the patient until that damage resolves.

Fluid Resuscitation

The initial treatment needs to be directed at improving cardiac output and ensuring adequate oxygenation. Before transferring

> ### Table 9-6
> #### The "7–3 Rule" for Fluid Challenges with Swan-Ganz Catheter
>
> Infuse 200 mL of crystalloid over 10 min. Then,
> If PCWP rises <3 repeat fluid challenge.
> If PCWP rises 3–7, wait 10 min and repeat measurements. If <3 repeat fluid challenge. If 3–7 stop.
> If PCWP rises >7 stop fluid challenges.

the patient to a monitored setting, intravenous access with a large-gauge catheter needs to be established and vigorous and rapid fluid resuscitation must be started. The patient should be transferred to a monitored setting as soon as possible after the initial resuscitation has occurred. A peripheral vein usually provides access fastest to give the initial dose of fluid, and central access can be established later if needed. The initial fluid resuscitation is usually done with 1 to 2 L of lactated Ringer's solution or normal saline over 15 to 20 minutes without the need for central monitoring. If additional fluid administration is needed, a flow-directed pulmonary artery (Swan-Ganz) catheter should be placed to help to determine the correct amount of fluid, because of the risk of pulmonary edema, ARDS, and myocardial dysfunction. The "7–3 rule," as reviewed in Table 9–6, is one possible guide to fluid management. The use of central venous pressure (CVP) monitoring in place of PCWP determinations has been shown to be inadequate. Additional intravenous fluid should be given targeting an optimal pulmonary capillary wedge pressure (PCWP) of 12 to 17 mm Hg. If there is acute blood loss or the starting hematocrit is below 30%, the most appropriate fluid is packed red blood cells. Whether colloid solutions should be used in place of crystalloid solutions in all patients remains a matter of debate. Some authorities believe that colloid (5% albumin or 6% hetastarch) may reduce the incidence of pulmonary and systemic edema, but others believe it may increase the risk. To help monitor fluid requirements a Foley catheter and an arterial line should also be placed.

Oxygenation and Ventilation

Because of the risk of ARDS, women in septic shock need to be followed closely for development of hypoxemia and respiratory failure. A continuous pulse oximeter should be used to monitor arterial oxygen saturation in addition to occasional arterial blood gases. Oxygen treatment is indicated if pulse oximetry is <90%, the arterial oxygen saturation is <92%, or the Pao_2 is <60 mm Hg. The goal of oxygen therapy is to maintain, at minimum, these values so as to maintain adequate oxygen delivery to the tissues. This may require intubation and ventilatory support with positive end-expiratory pressure (PEEP).

Use of Vasoactive or Inotropic Drugs

If after appropriate fluid resuscitation (PCWP 12–17 mm Hg) the cardiovascular function remains suboptimal as reflected by persistent hypotension (mean arterial pressure <60 mm Hg or systolic pressure <90 mm Hg), inadequate urine output (<0.5 mL/kg/hr), inadequate cardiac output, or worsening lactic acidosis, then pharmacologic intervention is indicated. The choice of drugs is a complicated matter and must be individualized for each clinical situation and at times requires a combination of agents. Pressure support is best obtained with α-agonist and inotropic support with β_1-agonist (Table 9–7). Experimental observations indicate that in septic shock the response to these agents is blunted; and therefore, large doses are often required to achieve the desired effects.

Dopamine is the initial drug of choice if hypotension persists after volume administration. In small doses (<2 μg/kg/min), dopamine selectively dilates the renal and mesenteric vascular beds through specific dopaminergic receptors. This results in

Table 9-7

Cardiovascular Adrenergic Agents Used to Treat Septic Shock

Drug	Usual IV Dosage	Adrenergic Effect			Mixture (mg/amp)
		α	β	Dopamine	
Dopamine	1–2 μg/kg/min	+		+ +	400
	2–10 μg/kg/min	+ +	+	+	
	10–30 μg/kg/min	+ + +	+ +		
Dobutamine	2–30 μg/kg/min	+	+ + +		250
Norepinephrine	1–80 μg/kg/min	+ + +	+ +		4
Epinephrine	2–10 μg/min	+ +	+ + +		

increased urine output without affecting heart rate or increasing blood pressure. As the dose increases there is less dopaminergic and β_1-adrenergic effect and more α-adrenergic effect. At doses of 5 to 10 μg/kg/min the α-adrenergic effect results in increases in SVR and PCWP without decreasing cardiac output, owing to a persistent β_1-adrenergic effect. At doses above 10 μg/kg/min cardiac output can be decreased, and at doses above 20 μg/kg/min dopamine has effects similar to those of norepinephrine. Therefore, the initial dose should start at 5 μg/kg/min and be increased, as needed, up to 20 μg/kg/min. If doses above 20 μg/kg/min are needed, then a second agent, either dobutamine or norepinephrine, should be added. Dobutamine (or epinephrine) is added if the myocardium is depressed and SVR is normal. It is a direct myocardial β_1-receptor stimulant that increases cardiac output with minimal increases in heart rate. Norepinephrine (or phenylephrine) is added if there is refractory hypotension due to persistent low SVR (starting dose, 1 to 2 μg/min; average dose, 2 to 12 μg/min).

Treatment of Infection

Treatment of the infection is of primary importance in the treatment of septic shock. Early antibiotic therapy can decrease the complication rate by 50%. Treatment of infection involves the use of appropriate broad-spectrum antibiotics and surgical removal of the infected tissue when clinically indicated. The antibiotic coverage needs to be broad, owing to the polymicrobial nature of pelvic infections (Table 9–8). At times, when the mother's status is deteriorating, surgery will be necessary to remove the nidus of infection. Delay can be fatal in the presence

---

Table 9–8

Appropriate Antibiotic Coverage for Obstetric Septic Shock

Ampicillin + gentamicin + clindamycin
Imipenem-cilastatin + vancomycin or clindamycin
Extended-spectrum penicillin (ticarcillin or piperacillin) + gentamicin or tobramycin
Cefoxitin or ceftizoxime + gentamicin
Add amikacin if *Pseudomonas* is a possible pathogen.
Add nafcillin or vancomycin for evidence of toxic shock syndrome or a wound infection.

of necrotizing fasciitis, a severe wound infection, retained products of conception, or uterine necrosis. Intraabdominal abscesses usually require drainage and potentially, if persistent, will require exploratory laparotomy.

Potential Future Therapy

Recently attempts have been made to improve patient outcome through hemodynamic therapy aimed at achieving supranormal values for the cardiac index, peripheral oxygen consumption (Vo_2), and oxygen delivery (Do_2). The determinants of Do_2 are the oxygen-carrying capacity of blood [Cao_2 = hemoglobin $\times$ 1.36 $\times$ arterial oxygen saturation (%)] and the cardiac output (Do_2 = Cao_2 $\times$ CO). The Do_2 is maximized by maintaining hemoglobin at 10 to 12 g/dL, arterial oxygen saturation >90%, and a high cardiac output; however, a recent large, randomized study of critically ill patients did not find that outcome improved in patients so treated as compared with the group of patients whose therapy aimed only at restoring hemodynamic parameters to normal.

Finally, attempts have been made to develop new therapies for septic shock that are designed to inhibit the bacterial toxins or the endogenous mediators of the inflammatory system. Large doses of corticosteroids have been shown in two large, recent studies to not be beneficial. Likewise, the use of anti–interleukin 1, anti–tumor necrosis factor, and antiendotoxin antibodies have failed to show improvement in patients in septic shock.

■ Bibliography

Beller FK, Schmidt EH, Holzgreve W, et al.: Septicemia during pregnancy: A study in different species of experimental animals. Am J Obstet Gynecol 1985;151:967–975.

Blanco JD, Gibbs RS, Castaneda YS: Bacteremia in obstetrics: Clinical course. Obstet Gynecol 1981;58:621–625.

Bone RC, Balk RA, Cerra FB, et al.: Definitions for sepsis and organ failure and guidelines for the use of innovative therapies in sepsis. Chest 1992;101:1644–1655.

Gonik B: Septic shock in obstetrics. In Clark SL, Cotton DB, Hankins GDV, et al. (eds): Critical Care Obstetrics, ed 2. Boston: Blackwell Scientific, 1991.

Lee W, Clark SL, Cotton DB, et al.: Septic shock during pregnancy. Am J Obstet Gynecol 1988;159:410–416.

Nathan L, Peters MT, Ahmed AM, et al.: The return of life-threatening puerperal sepsis caused by group A streptococci. Am J Obstet Gynecol 1993;169:571–572.

Parrillo JE: Pathogenetic mechanisms of septic shock. N Engl J Med 1993;328:1471–1477.

Pearlman M, Faro S: Obstetric septic shock: A pathophysiologic basis for management. Clin Obstet Gynecol 1990;33:482–492.

Rackow EC, Astiz ME: Pathophysiology and treatment of septic shock. JAMA 1991;266:548–554.

Septic shock. The American College of Obstetricians and Gynecologists. Technical Bulletin Number 204. pp 1–8, 1995.

ALVIN H. PERELMAN

Management of Hyperthyroidism and Thyroid Storm During Pregnancy

Hyperthyroidism is uncommon during pregnancy (0.2% of pregnancies) and thyroid storm is considered rare. Hyperthyroidism and its treatment nevertheless have many implications for mother and fetus.

■ Physiology

Thyroxine (T_4) is the major secretory product of the thyroid. The majority of circulating T_4 is converted in peripheral tissues to triiodothyronine (T_3), the biologically active form of this hormone. T_4 secretion is under direct control from pituitary thyroid-stimulating hormone (TSH). The cell surface receptor for TSH is similar to the receptors for luteinizing hormone (LH) and human chorionic gonadotropin (hCG). T_4 and T_3 are transported in the peripheral circulation bound to thyroxine-binding globulin (TBG), transthyretin (formerly called "prealbumin"), and albumin. Less than 0.05% of plasma T_4 and less than 0.5% of plasma T_3 is unbound and able to interact with target tissues. Routine T_4 measurements reflect total serum concentration and may be factitiously altered by increases or decreases in concentrations of circulating proteins. Plasma concentrations of TBG increase 2.5-fold by 20 weeks' gestation, owing to an estrogen-induced change in the structure of TBG that prolongs the serum half-life. The result is a 25% to 45% increase in serum total T_4 from a pregravid level of 5 to 12 mg% to 9 to 16 mg%. Total T_3 increases by about 30% in the first trimester and by 50% to 65% later. The increase in available protein binding induced by pregnancy causes a transient decrease in free T_4 and a compensatory increase in TSH. Increased concentrations of TSH stimulate restoration of the free serum T_4 level. Pregnancy affects other changes

147

Table 10–1
Thyroid Function Changes During Pregnancy
Normal hypothalamic-pituitary-thyroid axis
First trimester TSH depression due to hCG, normalizes thereafter
Increased renal iodide clearance (increased glomerular filtration rate)
Goiter—minimal in regions of iodine sufficiency; 30% increase in size in regions with dietary iodine deficiency
Increased serum TBG; decreased T_3 resin uptake
Increased total serum T_4 and total serum T_3
Normal serum free T_4 and free T_3

in the thyroid system and ultimately the interpretation of thyroid function tests (Table 10–1).

The fetal hypothalamic-pituitary-thyroid axis develops independently of maternal thyroid function. Fetal thyroid hormone synthesis has been demonstrated by 10 weeks' gestation. Although the human placenta acts as a significant barrier to circulating T_4, T_3, and TSH, Immunoglobulin G (IgG) autoantibodies, iodine, thyrotropin-releasing hormone (TRH), and antithyroid medications can readily cross the placenta and interfere with fetal thyroid activity.

■
Key Thyroid Function Tests

Serum total T_4 and T_3 measurements in euthyroid mothers tend to be high owing to elevated TBG during gestation. By contrast, free T_4 and free T_3 levels are unchanged and are more useful for the diagnosis of thyroid abnormality. The T_3 resin uptake (T_3RU) test is a measure that indirectly quantitates the binding sites on TBG. It is *not* a test of thyroid function. The patient's serum is incubated with a tracer (radioiodine-labeled T_3) and an ion exchange resin. The resin competes with the patient's serum TBG for the tracer T_3. The amount of tracer T_3 taken up by the resin dictates whether the T_3 resin uptake test result is interpreted as low, normal, or elevated. During pregnancy, the resultant increase in TBG allows more of the added tracer T_3, used during the test, to be bound. The T_3 resin uptake, therefore, is low because there is less tracer T_3 to be taken up by the resin used during the test. The free thyroxine index (FT$_4$I), also reported as T_7, is an *estimation* of unbound T_4 and represents the product of the serum total T_4 and T_3 resin uptake or is expressed as the serum total T_4 multiplied by a correction factor. (The serum free T_4 can also be estimated by the ratio of total serum T_4 to serum TBG.)

$$FT_4I = \text{Total } T_4 \times \frac{\text{Patient } T_3 \, R_U}{\text{Normal } T_3 \, R_U}$$

All laboratory methods of measuring *actual* circulating free T_4 have broad normal ranges, and a value for a given patient may drop 50% yet still fall within the normal range. Currently, TSH measurements are the most sensitive tests of thyroid function. Newer (supersensitive) assays have improved sensitivity and can detect TSH levels of 0.1 μU/mL or less.

■ Etiology and Diagnosis

The causes of hyperthyroidism in pregnancy are listed in Table 10–2. Graves' disease accounts for more than 80% of hyperthyroidism during pregnancy. Autoantibodies (thyroid-stimulating antibody [TSAb]—formerly known as LATS [long-acting thyroid stimulator]) against TSH receptors act as TSH agonists, thereby stimulating increased production of thyroid hormone. The clinical presentation of hyperthyroidism is similar to the symptoms of normal pregnancy (fatigue, increased appetite, vomiting, palpitations, tachycardia, heat intolerance, increased urinary frequency, insomnia, emotional lability) and may confound the diagnosis. More specific symptoms include tremor, brisk reflexes, muscle weakness, goiter, and weight loss. Graves' ophthalmopathy (stare, lid lag, exophthalmos) is diagnostic. The disease usually gets worse in the first trimester but moderates

---

Table 10–2

Causes of Hyperthyroidism During Pregnancy

Graves' disease
Toxic multinodular goiter (rare in the reproductive age group)
Toxic adenoma
Hyperemesis gravidarum
Trophoblastic disease
Thyroiditis (chronic, subacute, viral)
Exogenous thyroid hormone

later in pregnancy. Untreated hyperthyroidism poses considerable maternal and fetal risks (Table 10–3).

Laboratory diagnosis of hyperthyroidism is confirmed with a suppressed serum TSH in the setting of elevated free T_4 estimations. In rare circumstances, the serum total T_3 may demonstrate greater elevation than T_4 (T_3 toxicosis). Graves' disease must be differentiated from thyroiditis, which usually resolves spontaneously within a few weeks and commonly requires no treatment. The diagnosis of Graves' disease should be based on specific clinical findings combined with laboratory evidence of suppressed TSH and an elevated TSAb concentration.

Hyperthyroidism may also result from elevated serum levels of hCG, as seen with trophoblastic diseases and hyperemesis gravidarum. In these circumstances, treatment is seldom needed, since the disease spontaneously resolves after trophoblastic tissue is evacuated or vomiting resolves.

■ Cardiac Dysfunction

Cardiac decompensation in pregnancy usually occurs in poorly controlled hyperthyroid patients with anemia, infection, or hypertension. The hemodynamic changes associated with hyperthyroidism during pregnancy are outlined in Table 10–4. Clinical signs of decompensation are suggested by a diastolic murmur, an apical systolic murmur, and a displaced pulse of maximal impulse. Beta-adrenergic blockade is theoretically contraindicated with congestive heart failure, since adrenergic stimulation of the heart is the major compensating mechanism against cardiac failure. The negative inotropic effect imposed by β-adrenergic blockade may depress myocardial contractility. These drugs,

Table 10–3

Fetal and Maternal Risks with Untreated Hyperthyroidism

Fetal	Maternal
Spontaneous abortion	Preeclampsia
Prematurity	Maternal heart failure
Stillbirth	Low maternal weight gain
Low birth weight	Infection
Fetal/neonatal thyrotoxicosis	Anemia
	Thyroid storm

Table 10–4

Hemodynamic Changes with Hyperthyroidism

Increased stroke volume and cardiac output
Increased pulse rate
Reduced peripheral vascular resistance
Increased blood volume
Impaired myocardial contractility

Electrocardiographic changes
Left ventricular hypertrophy (15%)
Atrial fibrillation (21%)
Wolff-Parkinson-White syndrome

---

however, are very effective for treating atrial fibrillation and supraventricular tachycardia that may accompany hyperthyroidism. Thus, cautious use of β-blocker therapy is recommended, since congestive heart failure during pregnancy is often rate related. Utilization of a pulmonary artery catheter is an important adjunct to the effective and safe use of β-blocker therapy in these critical situations. Other helpful therapeutic modalities include a low-salt diet, diuretic therapy, digoxin, and bed rest. Cardiac dysfunction may linger for months after restoration of normal thyroid function.

■ Treatment of Hyperthyroidism During Pregnancy

The primary objective of treatment is to effectively control thyroid dysfunction until after delivery. Protecting the fetus from the effects of the disease and the side effects of the medical regimen is a secondary yet important objective. Basic treatment options are outlined in Table 10–5.

Observation alone may be a reasonable treatment plan for

Table 10–5

Treatment Options for Hyperthyroidism

Observation
Antithyroid medications
Beta-adrenergic blocking agents
Thyroid surgery

---

mild clinical disease without cardiovascular compromise. For overt disease antithyroid medications are the mainstay of treatment. Propylthiouracil (PTU) and methimazole (Tapazole) are the two thioamide agents currently available. Both drugs effectively block intrathyroidal hormone synthesis, but PTU also blocks extrathyroidal conversion of T_4 to T_3. Both agents readily cross the placenta and may inhibit fetal thyroid function. Maternal side effects include skin rash, a lupuslike syndrome, arthralgias, agranulocytosis, and hepatic necrosis. Methimazole is four times more bioavailable to fetal tissue than PTU and may be associated with aplasia cutis in infancy. Thus, PTU is the preferred medication for treating hyperthyroidism in pregnancy. Twice daily doses of 150 to 200 mg may control hyperthyroidism within 4 to 8 weeks. Lack of response is usually due to noncompliance and may require hospitalization. The goal of treatment is to use the smallest dose that maintains maternal free T_4 levels at or just above the upper limit of normal. Clinical and laboratory follow-up (TSH, free T_4, free T_3) should occur every 2 to 4 weeks. Rapid improvement necessitates a decrease in dosage. Improvement commonly occurs in the second trimester, and as many as 40% of mothers may discontinue therapy. It may, however, be reasonable to continue giving small doses to ameliorate the risks of fetal thyrotoxicosis imposed by transplacental passage of TSAb and to reduce the general overall incidence of thyroid storm during labor and delivery.

Baseline white blood cell (WBC) and liver function tests should be obtained before initiating antithyroid therapy, since hyperthyroidism itself may also cause liver enzyme elevations and leukopenia. Antithyroid medications should be discontinued if liver function values become extremely abnormal or if the WBC analysis reveals severe leukopenia. These medications may be restarted during the postpartum period as disease activity dictates. Breast feeding is permissible while taking PTU because little is passed into breast milk with standard doses.

Beta-adrenergic blockers may be used as adjunctive therapy for tremor and palpitations. Relative contraindications to the use of β-adrenergic blockers include obstructive lung disease, heart block, heart failure, and insulin use. Although unusual, there may be adverse fetal effects such as bradycardia, growth retardation, and neonatal hypoglycemia. It is advisable to minimize the duration of β-adrenergic blocker therapy during gestation.

Subtotal thyroidectomy is reserved for patients with severe antithyroid drug side effects or failed medical suppression of thyroid function. To minimize pregnancy complications, surgery is usually performed during the second trimester. Preoperatively, hyperthyroidism should be controlled with antithyroid medication for 7 to 10 days, a β-adrenergic blocker (propranolol, 20 mg four times daily), and inorganic iodide (Lugol solution, 3 drops twice daily) for 4 to 5 days. The latter two can be discontinued 48 hours postoperatively. Iodine must be used cautiously to minimize the risk for severe fetal hypothyroidism and goiter. Radioactive iodine administration generally is not warranted during pregnancy. This agent readily crosses the placenta and may cause permanent damage to the fetal thyroid.

■
Thyroid Storm

Thyroid storm is a rare but potentially fatal complication of hyperthyroidism characterized by cardiovascular compromise, hyperpyrexia, and central nervous system changes (Table 10–6). It is estimated to occur in 2% of pregnancies complicated by

---

Table 10–6

Diagnosis of Thyroid Storm

Hypermetabolism
  Fever above 100°F
  Perspiration
  Warm, flushed skin
Cardiovascular
  Tachycardia
  Atrial fibrillation
  Congestive heart failure
Central nervous system
  Irritability
  Agitation
  Tremor
  Mental status change (delirium, psychosis, coma)
Gastrointestinal
  Nausea, vomiting
  Diarrhea
  Jaundice
Supporting laboratory evidence
  Leukocytosis
  Elevated liver function values
  Hypercalcemia
  Low TSH, high free T_4 and/or T_3

Table 10–7

Common Precipitants of Thyroid Storm

Acute surgical emergency
Induction of anesthesia
Diabetic ketoacidosis
Pulmonary embolism
Noncompliance with antithyroid medications
Myocardial infarction
Infection
Hypertension/preeclampsia
Labor and delivery
Severe anemia

---

hyperthyroidism. This rare but devastating disease is usually seen in patients with poorly controlled hyperthyroidism complicated by additional physiologic stressors such as toxemia and parturition. Additional precipitating events for thyroid storm are presented in Table 10–7.

The laboratory profile of the mother with thyroid storm reveals leukocytosis, elevated hepatic enzymes, and occasionally hypercalcemia. Thyroid function test results are consistent with hyperthyroidism but do not consistently correlate with the severity of the thyroid storm.

Management is best accomplished in an obstetric intensive care unit. Table 10–8 reviews basic supportive adjunctive care for patients in thyroid storm.

Table 10–8

Supportive Adjunctive Care for the Patient in Thyroid Storm

Intravenous fluids and electrolytes
Cardiac monitoring
Consideration of pulmonary artery catheterization
  (central hemodynamic monitoring to guide beta-
  blocker therapy during hyperdynamic cardiac failure)
Cooling measures: blanket, sponge bath, acetaminophen
Oxygen therapy
  (consider arterial line to follow serial blood gases)
No salicylates (increase free T_4)
Nasogastric tube if patient is unable to swallow
  (may be only avenue for PTU administration)

Admit patient to an Obstetric Intensive Care Unit
(consult Endocrinology, Maternal-Fetal Medicine and Neonatology)

↓

Initiate supportive measures: send CBC, electrolytes, liver functions, glucose and renal functions; do not intervene on behalf of the fetus until maternal stabilization is accomplished. Use position changes, cooling measures, fluids and oxygen therapy to help improve oxygen delivery to the fetus.

1) Start electronic fetal monitoring if the fetus is potentially viable
2) Intravenous fluids/electrolyte replacement
3) Cardiac monitoring (continuous ECG [obtain 12-lead at onset])
4) Cooling measures (cooling blanket, sponge bath, acetaminophen)
5) Oxygen therapy (pulse oximetry, obtain maternal blood gas at onset)
6) Nasogastric tube if patient unable to swallow

Give agents to reduce synthesis of the thyroid hormones: PTU (propylthiouracil) followed by iodides to block T_4 release (IV sodium iodide or oral Lugols):

1) PTU orally or via nasogstric tube, 300–600 mg loading dose followed by 150–300 mg q6hr
2) 1 hour after instituting PTU give:
   A) Sodium iodide, 500 mg q8–12hr **or**
   B) Oral Lugol's solution, 30–60 drops daily in divided doses
   C) Iodides may be discontinued after initial improvement.

Give agents to control maternal tachycardia:

1) Propranolol, 1–2 mg/min IV or dose sufficient to slow heart rate to ≤ 90 bpm; or 40–80 mg PO q4–6hr.
2) Consider a pulmonary artery catheter to help guide.

Give adrenal glucocorticoids to inhibit peripheral conversion of T_4 to T_3. Consider any of the following options as appropriate:

1) Hydrocortisone, 100 mg IV q8hr **or**
2) Prednisone, 60 mg PO every day **or**
3) Dexamethasone, 8 mg PO every day
4) Glucocorticoids may be discontinued after initial improvement.

Plasmapheresis or pertioneal dialysis (to remove circulating thyroid hormones) should be considered when patient fails to respond to conventional management.

↓

If conventional therapy unsuccessful:

1) Consider subtotal thyroidectomy (during 2nd trimester pregnancy) or radioactive iodine (postpartum)

Figure 10-1

Management algorithm for thyroid storm.

Specific medical therapy includes PTU by nasogastric tube (300 to 600 mg loading dose followed by 150 to 300 mg every 6 hours) and iodides to block T_4 release (oral Lugol solution, 30 to 60 drops daily in divided doses or intravenous [IV] sodium iodide, 500 mg every 8 to 12 hours, 1 hour after initiating PTU). Propranolol (40 to 80 mg orally or by nasogastric tube every 4 to 6 hours or 1 mg per minute IV) is effective for controlling tachycardia. Adrenal glucocorticoids (hydrocortisone, 300 mg per day; prednisone, 60 mg per day; or dexamethasone, 8 mg per day) have been used to inhibit peripheral conversion of T_4 to T_3. Iodides and glucocorticoids may be discontinued after initial clinical improvement. Plasmapheresis or peritoneal dialysis to remove circulating thyroid hormone is an extreme measure reserved for patients who do not respond to conventional therapy. An algorithm for the management of thyroid storm is presented in Figure 10–1.

■
Fetal and Neonatal Implications

Fetal and neonatal hyperthyroidism is thought to be due to transplacental passage of TSAb in roughly 1% of gravidas with a current or remote history of Graves' disease. Fetal hyperthyroidism is suggested by fetal tachycardia, growth retardation, and ultrasound demonstration of goiter. To confound matters, a hypothyroid goiter may also be observed as a fetal complication of maternal PTU administration. Direct fetal blood sampling (cordocentesis) may define the fetal diagnosis and management. This test may be especially helpful in clinical situations when maternal and fetal thyroid function are dissimilar and the fetus may benefit from alternative therapy. Because of the persistent effects of maternally administered PTU on the neonate for several days following birth, neonatal hyperthyroidism may not present until later in the neonatal period. Judicious follow-up care by the pediatrician, therefore, is recommended to evaluate late-presenting neonatal hyperthyroidism in these circumstances.

■
Bibliography

Braverman LE, Utiger RD (eds): Werner and Ingbar's The Thyroid, ed 6. Philadelphia: J.B. Lippincott, 1991, pp. 1263–1279.
Clark SL, Cotton DB, Hankins GH, et al.: Critical Care Obstetrics, ed 2. New York: Blackwell Scientific Publications, 1991.

Hamburger JI: Diagnosis and management of Graves' disease in pregnancy. Thyroid 1992;2:219–223.

Kaplan MM: Assessment of thyroid function during pregnancy. Thyroid 1992; 2:57–60.

Kaplan MM: The Maternal Thyroid and Parathyroid Glands. *In* Tulchinsky D, Little AB (eds): Maternal-Fetal Endocrinology, ed 2. Philadelphia: W.B. Saunders, 1994, pp. 132–141.

Polk DH: Diagnosis and management of altered fetal thyroid status. Clin Perinatol 1994;21:647–662.

Mestman JH, Goodwin M, Montoro MM: Thyroid disorders of pregnancy. Endocrinol Metabol Clinics N America 1995;24:41–71.

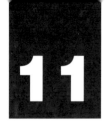

MICHAEL R. FOLEY

Diabetic Ketoacidosis in Pregnancy

Despite recent advances in the evaluation and medical treatment of diabetes in pregnancy, diabetic ketoacidosis (DKA) remains a significant concern. The fetal loss rate in most series has been estimated to range from 50% to 90%. Fortunately, since the advent and implementation of insulin therapy, the maternal mortality rate has declined to 1% or less. To favorably influence the outcome for these high-risk patients, it is imperative that obstetricians and caregivers be familiar with the basics of the pathophysiology, diagnosis, and treatment of DKA in pregnancy.

■ Pathophysiology

Simply stated, DKA is characterized by hyperglycemia and accelerated ketogenesis. Both a lack of insulin and an excess of glucagon and other counterregulatory hormones contribute significantly to these problems and their resultant clinical manifestations. In a nutshell, glucose normally enters the cells secondary to the presence of insulin. Glucose then may be utilized by the cells for nutrition and energy production. When insulin is lacking, glucose fails to enter the cells. The cells respond to this "starvation" by facilitating the release of counterregulatory hormones, including glucagon, catecholamines, and cortisol. These counterregulatory hormones are responsible for providing the cell with an alternative substrate for nutrition and energy production. By the process of gluconeogenesis, fatty acids from adipose tissue are broken down by hepatocytes to ketones (acetone, acetoacetate, and beta-hydroxybutyrate), which are then utilized by the cells of the body for nutrition and energy production (Fig. 11–1). The lack of insulin also contributes to increased lipolysis and decreased reutilization of free fatty acids, thus providing more substrate for hepatic ketogenesis. A basic review of the biochemistry of DKA is presented in Figure 11–1.

158

"In a Nutshell"

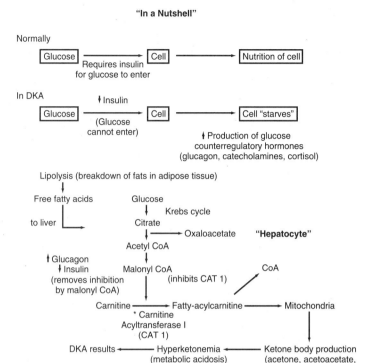

Figure 11–1

Basic biochemistry of diabetic ketoacidosis. (Adapted from Berkowitz RL (ed): Critical Care of the Obstetric Patient. New York: Churchill Livingstone, 1983, p. 416.)

Maternal Concerns

Now that we have an understanding of "how" and "why" ketone bodies are produced during DKA, what are the consequences to the gravida of excessive ketogenesis? In general, ketone bodies are considered to be moderately strong acids. In the physiologic response to the fall in pH in most body fluids created by accumulation of these acids is an attempt to correct the resultant "metabolic" acidosis. The respiratory rate and depth increase (Kussmaul respirations) in an attempt to "blow off" carbon dioxide, initiating a corrective trend toward compensatory respiratory alkalosis. Serum bicarbonate levels decline and as a result the anion gap becomes abnormally elevated. In addition to increasing fatty acid production, poor glucose utilization results in severe hyperglycemia. Untreated hyperglycemia leads to marked glycosuria, initiating significant osmotic diuresis. As a result, dehydration and electrolyte depletion may follow, and if left untreated, cardiac failure and death.

A vicious cycle is created by an increase in dehydration-mediated serum hyperosmolarity and catabolism, propagated by Kussmaul respiration, leading to further production of glucose counterregulatory hormones, lipolysis, and subsequent hyper-ketonemia. An algorithm for this clinical pathophysiologic response is presented in Figure 11–2.

Fetal Concerns

The fetus appears to be at significant risk for sudden intrauterine death during an episode of maternal DKA. The mechanism for this "sudden death" is not completely understood; however, it appears to be related to a combination of factors. Alterations in fetal fluid and electrolyte balance, poor uterine perfusion resulting from maternal hypovolemia, and increased "acid load" in the form of fatty acids and lactate all favor a reduction in fetal oxygenation and metabolic acid clearance. When caring for a patient in DKA who is carrying a potentially viable fetus, careful fetal monitoring should be judiciously utilized. Often, signs of fetal stress become apparent, reflecting the degree of maternal metabolic derangement. Delivery of a compromised baby should be prudently delayed until the mother is metabolically stable. Correction of maternal metabolic abnormalities generally rapidly improves the fetus' condition. Therefore, efforts should be directed at improving maternal deficits; emergency operative intervention is reserved for unresponsive persistent fetal compromise.

Making the Diagnosis

In pregnancy, DKA may be associated with lower plasma glucose values compared with nonpregnant patients. DKA has been observed at plasma glucose levels as low as 180 mg/dL. It appears that the relative insulin resistance of pregnancy, combined with a greater tendency toward ketosis, reduces the

Clinical Algorithm of DKA Pathophysiology

Relative Insulin Deficiency

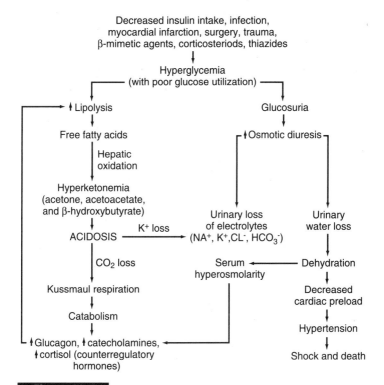

Figure 11–2

Metabolic alterations in diabetic ketoacidosis. (Modified from Hagay ZJ, Reece EA: Diabetes mellitus in pregnancy. *In* Reece EA, Hubbins JC, Mahoney MJ, et al. (eds): Medicine of the Fetus and the Mother. Philadelphia, J.B. Lippincott, 1992, pp. 982–1020.)

threshold for DKA during pregnancy. The insulin resistance during pregnancy is related to an increased production of placental hormones, insulinase, and cortisol (Fig. 11–3).

The maternal and fetal concerns resulting from DKA emphasize the importance of a rapid and reliable diagnosis. Following the axiom that laboratory tests should be utilized only to "verify or nullify" a clinical suspicion, the diagnosis of DKA should be based on clinical examination and supported by an evaluation

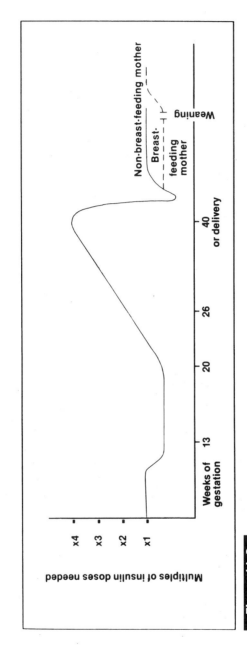

Figure 11-3

Changing insulin needs during pregnancy caused by properties of placental hormones and enzyme (insulinase) and cortisol. (From Bobak IM, Jensen MD, Zalar MK: Maternity and Gynecologic Care: The Nurse and the Family, ed 4. St. Louis, C.V. Mosby, 1989, p. 783.)

Table 11–1

Diagnostic and Biochemical Parameters of DKA

Clinical Features

General	Neurologic
Malaise	Lethargy
Drowsiness	Coma
Weakness	Respiratory
Dehydration	Kussmaul respirations
Polyuria	Tachypnea
Polydipsia	Cardiovascular
Fruity breath	Tachycardia
Gastrointestinal	Hypotension
Nausea	
Vomiting	
Abdominal pain	
Ileus	

Biochemical Definition (Memory Aid)

Diabetic $\longrightarrow$ Glucose $\geq$ 180 mg%

Keto $\longrightarrow$ Serum acetone 1:2 or greater

Acidosis $\longrightarrow$ Arterial pH $\leq$ 7.3, HCO_3^- $\leq$ 15 and anion gap $[Na^+ - (Cl^- + HCO_3^-)] > 12$

Additional Laboratory Findings

Glycosuria	Leukocytosis
Ketonuria	Elevated CPK
Metabolic acidosis	Elevated amylase
Hyperosmolality	Elevated transaminase
Hypokalemia	Elevated BUN
Hypomagnesemia	Elevated creatinine
Hypophosphatemia	

---

of biochemical parameters. Table 11–1 summarizes the clinical presentation, the biochemical definition, and additional laboratory findings associated with DKA.

■ Treatment of DKA

During pregnancy DKA is a medical emergency. The patient should be admitted to an intensive care facility and consultations obtained from maternal-fetal medicine specialists, endocrinologists, and neonatologists.

A detailed history and physical examination should be performed to seek underlying precipitating factors for DKA such as noncompliance with insulin administration or infection (urine, skin, lungs, dental or amniotic cavity). Fetal monitoring should be initiated if the fetus is potentially viable (see Chapter 26). Intervention on behalf of the fetus should be withheld until the maternal metabolic condition is stabilized. Oxygen therapy and maternal position changes, however, should be initiated to help improve fetal perfusion while correcting maternal biochemical and plasma volume abnormalities (see Chapter 22). A detailed flow sheet, including a comprehensive recording of serial laboratory values, should be started at bedside to facilitate patient assessment following therapy. Invasive hemodynamic monitoring should be reserved for patients with severe renal compromise, in an effort to properly guide rehydration while avoiding iatrogenic pulmonary edema. Other less invasive measures such as the placement of an arterial line to follow serial arterial blood gases, a Foley catheter to monitor strict urine output, and continuous peripheral pulse oximetry should be initiated as an early adjunct to beginning therapy. The basic premise for the treatment of DKA in the pregnant patient is simultaneous correction of fluid and electrolyte imbalance and treatment of hyperglycemia and acidosis (Fig. 11–4).

Treatment of Hypovolemia

Hypovolemia during DKA results principally from hyperglycemia-induced osmotic diuresis (see Fig. 11–2). Since the restoration of intravascular volume improves perfusion and augments systemic insulin delivery to peripheral tissues, repletion of the circulating intravascular volume is the number one treatment priority. The estimated total water deficit is calculated to be 100 mL/kg of actual body weight (4- to 10-L deficit). Once renal competence is established (urine output at least 0.5 mL/kg/hr), fluid replacement may be initiated. Keeping in mind that many of the patients encountered with DKA during pregnancy may have preexisting renal compromise (class F diabetes mellitus), a baseline evaluation of serum blood urea nitrogen (BUN) and creatinine would be prudent to avoid fluid overload in a patient with markedly reduced creatinine clearance. Most authorities recommend urinary isotonic normal saline as the intravenous fluid of choice for volume replacement instead of lactated Ringer's solution. The reasoning behind this recommendation is that hypotonic solutions (0.45% normal saline or lactated

Admit to OB intensive care unit or equivalent
(consult Maternal Fetal Medicine, Endocrinology, Neonatology, and Obstetric Anesthesiology)

Detailed physical exam, obtain IV access (two IV lines)

Initiate adequate monitoring. Start a flow sheet at bedside
(Hemodynamics if appropriate, vital signs, serum glucose, I/O, serum ketones,
arterial blood gas (A-line), anion gap, serum electrolytes, HCO_3, pulse oximetry)

Evaluate baby

Fetal monitoring if fetus potentially viable. Withhold intervention toward delivery on behalf of the fetus until maternal metabolic disturbances corrected. Consider O_2 therapy and maternal position changes while correcting maternal biochemical abnormalities.

Treat symptoms/signs

Acid/base
(Monitor arterial blood gas (q2hr), pH, anion gap)

If arterial pH < 7.1 or HCO_3^- < 5 mEq/L, give 44 mEq sodium bicarbonate in 1 L 0.45 NS (repeat as needed). Avoid rapid correction of acidosis, which can precipitate paradoxical fall in cerebrospinal fluid pH and hypokalemia.

Insulin Therapy

Give 0.1 U/kg IV bolus followed by 0.1 U/kg/hr IV infusion. Mix 50 U regular insulin in 500 mL NS (10 mL = 1 U). Monitor serum glucose every 1–2 hr, if serum glucose not decreased by ~ 20% within first 2 hr, double insulin infusion rate.

Glucose level should be decreased at a rate ≤ 60–75 mg%/hr to avoid rapid change in osmolarity which may precipitate cerebral edema: when the BG approaches 250 mg% add D5 to IV fluids and reduce infusion by half.

Monitor serum ketones (every 2 hr until stable)

Be aware of the failure of the ketotest to measure β-hydroxybutyrate. The ketotest primarily measures acetone. Measured serum ketones may initially appear to increase after insulin therapy, representing a shift of ketone production from β-hydroxybutyrate to acetone (oxidation) and acetoacetate.

Continue IV insulin therapy until HCO_3^- and anion gap normalized: HCO_3^- (18–31 mEq/L) anion gap (< 12).

Give SC insulin before discontinuing IV drip, to prevent rebound hyperglycemia.

Search for underlying cause of DKA
Rule out infection (urine, skin, lungs, dental, amniotic cavity). Consider urinalysis, CBC, CXR, and amniocentesis

Electrolyte abnormalities
(monitor serum electrolytes every 2–4 hr)

K^+ ——— Phosphate

If < 2.0 mg %, give K_2PO_4 instead of KCL for K^+.

Anticipate K^+ deficit of 5–10 mEq/kg even with initially normal serum K^+.

Establish and monitor for adequate urine output (at ≥ 0.5 mL/kg/hr) and wait for the serum K^+ to fall below 5 mEq/L

Replace K^+ with KCL IV, 40–60 mEq/L normal saline. If plasma K is ≥ 4 mEq/L, give 10–20 mEq/hr. If plasma K is < 4 mEq/L, give 30–40 mEq/hr. Maintain serum K^+ at 4.5–5.0 mEq/L. (Initial replacement usually is initiated after the first 2–4 hr of patient's treatment.) Monitor serum K^+ every 2–4 hr.

Hypovolemia

Evaluate renal function: Check strict I/O (consider Foley catheter), BUN/creatinine

Anticipate significant fluid deficit (~ 100 mL/kg body weight)

Correct 75% of the estimated fluid deficit over the first 24 hr (use isotonic saline)
1st hour = give 1000 mL
2nd hour = give 500 mL
3rd hour = give 500 mL
thereafter = give 250 mL/hour (use lactated Ringers or 0.45 NS) until 75% of the fluid deficit is corrected over the first 24 hr. Continue hydration over the subsequent 24–48 hr until entire deficit corrected.
If serum NA+ increases above 150–155 mEq/L, switch to hypotonic fluids (0.45 NS)

Figure 11-4   Treatment algorithm for diabetic ketoacidosis.

165

Ringer's), as initial treatment, can lead to a rapid decline in plasma osmolarity, which may lead to cellular swelling and resultant cerebral edema. Therefore, the recommended approach is to utilize isotonic normal saline and replace 75% of the total calculated fluid deficit within the first 24 hours of therapy. The remaining 25% of the deficit is replaced over the remainder of the patient's hospitalization. At our institution, 1 liter of isotonic normal saline is given over the first hour and 500 mL normal saline per hour over hours two and three. Isotonic normal saline, therefore, is used for the first 3 hours of therapy. Thereafter, however, lactated Ringer's or 0.45 normal saline is given at a rate of 250 mL/hr until 75% of the total deficit is replaced over the first 24 hours. Lactated Ringer's solution is utilized to avoid further iatrogenic contributions to the drop in serum pH, since the pH of lactated Ringer's is 6.5, as compared with 5.0 for isotonic normal saline. In addition, the sodium load with isotonic saline may create hypernatremia; this fact is behind recommendations to switch from isotonic saline to a more hypotonic solution (lactated Ringer's or 0.45% normal saline) when the patient's serum sodium increases above 150 to 155 mEq/L (Table 11–2).

Insulin Therapy

Intravenous insulin administration is the mainstay treatment for pregnant patients in DKA. An initial intravenous loading dose of 0.1 U/kg followed by a constant infusion of 0.1 U/kg/hr effectively inhibits lipolysis and ketogenesis, leading to suppression of hepatic glucose output with resultant lower serum glucose levels. The insulin infusion is prepared by adding 50 U of regular insulin to 500 mL of normal saline (1 mL = 0.1 U; 10 mL = 1

Table 11–2
Common Intravenous Fluids

1 L	gm Glu	Na	Cl	K	Ca	Lactate	pH
5% Dextrose/water	50	0	0	0	0	0	3.5–6.5
0.9% NaCl (normal saline)	0	154	154	0	0	0	5.0
Lactated Ringer's	0	130	109	4	3	28	6.5

> **Table 11–3**
>
> ## General Principles of Intravenous Insulin Infusion
>
> Use *regular* insulin when mixing the infusion.
> Pump monitor the infusion rate.
> Clearly label the insulin infusion line with units of insulin per volume.
> Intravenous insulin is compatible with both magnesium sulfate and pitocin.
> To compensate for insulin binding to the plastic tubing gently mix the insulin in the bag and thoroughly flush the tubing with insulin before beginning administration.
> Obtain blood samples from the patient's arm opposite the infusion.
> Monitor the patient's blood glucose hourly during labor.
> Have injectable dextrose 50% and dextrose 10% (500 mL) available at bedside for treatment of hypoglycemia.
> *Do not* preload with glucose containing solutions before conduction anesthesia or as a bolus infusion to improve a nonreassuring fetal heart rate tracing.
> Before discontinuing intravenous infusion give subcutaneous or intramuscular insulin to prevent rebound hyperglycemia. Remember these:
>
> *Regular Insulin Half-Lives*
>
> | |
> |---|
> | Intravenous regular insulin: 5 minute half-life |
> | Intramuscular regular insulin: 2 hour half-life |
> | Subcutaneous regular insulin: 4 hour half-life |

U). General principles of intravenous insulin infusion are listed in Table 11–3.

The intravenous insulin infusion should be titrated to reduce the serum glucose level at a rate no faster than 60% to 75 mg% per hour to avoid rapid changes in serum osmolarity that could precipitate cerebral edema. A good rule of thumb is that, if the plasma glucose level does not decrease by 10% in the first hour or by 20% by the second hour of therapy, repeat the intravenous loading dose or double the current continuous infusion rate. As the patient's blood glucose value approaches 250 mg% add 5% dextrose to the infusion and reduce the hourly insulin infusion by half. Be aware that, while monitoring serum ketones in response to insulin administration a paradoxical increase in serum acetone should be anticipated. The ketotest primarily measures serum acetone. During insulin therapy while overall

production of ketones clearly diminishes, a shift of ketone production from hydroxybutyrate to acetone (oxidation) and acetoacetate is observed. This phenomenon results in the apparent
paradoxical exacerbation of ketoacidemia at the onset of insulin
therapy. The intravenous insulin infusion should be continued
until the serum bicarbonate value and anion gap normalize.
Table 11–4 summarizes the mechanics of changing from an
intravenous insulin infusion to subcutaneous insulin.

Table 11–4

Managing the Conversion: Intravenous to Subcutaneous Insulin After Resolution of DKA

1. The patient should be tolerant of a full diet.
2. Calculate the total number of insulin units administered over 24 hours
   following stabilization.

	Before Breakfast	*Distribution*
Total units/day ⟶	2/3 of total units/day ⟶	2/3 neutral protamine Hagedorn (NPH) 1/3 regular
	Before Dinner	
	1/3 of total units/day ⟶	1/2 neutral protamine Hagedorn (NPH) 1/2 regular

(NPH may be given at bedtime instead of at
dinner if hypoglycemia occurs at 3 A.M.)

Example: Insulin infusion 2 units/hr × 24 hr (stabilized)
Total insulin/24 hr = 48 units

A.M. 2/3 × 48 = 32	2/3 as NPH = 21 units NPH 1/3 as regular = 11 units regular
P.M. 1/3 × 48 = 16	1/2 as NPH = 8 units NPH 1/2 as regular = 8 units regular

3. Remember actions of insulin in pregnancy when timing subsequent
   insulin adjustments.

Insulin	Onset	Peak (maximum effect)	Duration
Regular	1 hr	2–3 hr	4–5 hr
NPH	2 hr	8 hr	24 hr

Table 11-5

Correcting Potassium Deficit

1. Mix 40–60 mEq KCl/Liter NS
2. If plasma K^+ is:
   $\geq$ 4 mEq/L, give 10–20 mEq/hr
   < 4 mEq/L, give 30–40 mEq/hr
3. Replace K^+ cautiously, watching urinary output and serum K^+ frequently.
4. Replace entire K^+ deficit over the span of the patient's entire hospitalization.
5. Alternatively, in the face of DKA-induced maternal phosphate deficiency, K_2PO_4 (K-Phos) may be given as potassium replacement instead of KCl. Phosphate deficiency leads to depletion of red blood cell 2,3-diphosphoglycerate, which may result in impaired red cell oxygen delivery to the fetus.

Potassium Administration

The anticipated potassium deficit in a pregnant patient with DKA is 5 to 10 mEq/kg. Potassium replacement, however, is most often delayed for the first 2 to 4 hours of therapy, since the initial serum potassium value is usually normal to mildly elevated and adequate diuresis has yet to be established. Once fluid and insulin therapy have been instituted and correction of the metabolic acidosis is under way, serum potassium may fall precipitously as a result of urine loss and intracellular shift. When the patient's plasma potassium value has fallen below 5 mEq/L and adequate diuresis has been established (at least 0.5 mL/kg/hr), potassium administration should be instituted. The usual method of potassium replacement is summarized in Table 11–5.

Bicarbonate Therapy

In patients with DKA, sodium bicarbonate therapy is usually reserved for those whose arterial pH is $\leq$7.1 and/or whose HCO_3^- is <5 mEq/L. Rapid undiluted correction of metabolic acidosis with sodium bicarbonate is unwarranted and may lead to severe hypokalemia, hypernatremia, impaired oxygen delivery, and a paradoxical fall in cerebrospinal fluid pH. The contents of 1 ampule (44 mEq sodium bicarbonate) is diluted in 1000 mL of 0.45 normal saline. The total deficit of bicarbonate can be calculated (obtain base deficit on arterial blood gas) thus:

Bicarbonate (mEq) regained to fully correct metabolic acidosis

$$= \frac{\text{Base deficit (mEq/L)} \times \text{Patient weight (kg)}}{4}$$

Since oxygen-hemoglobin affinity is augmented in the presence of an alkalotic shift to the left of the oxygen-hemoglobin dissociation curve, it is prudent not to fully correct the patient's metabolic acidosis, ensuring better oxygen delivery to the fetus. Table 11–4 is an algorithm for treatment of DKA in pregnancy.

■ Bibliography

Coustan DR: Diabetic ketoacidosis. *In* Berkowitz RL (Ed): Critical Care of the Obstetric Patient. New York: Churchill Livingstone, 1983.

Demling RH, Wilson RF (eds): Decision Making in Surgical Critical Care. B.C. Decker, Inc. Burlington, Ontario: 1988, p. 216.

Golde SH: Diabetic ketoacidosis in pregnancy. In Clark SL, Cotton DB, Hankins GDV, et al. (eds): Critical Care Obstetrics, ed 2. Boston: Blackwell Scientific, 1991.

Hagay ZJ: Diabetic ketoacidosis in pregnancy: etiology, pathophysiology, and management. Clin Obstet Gynecol 37:39–49, 1994.

Landon MB: Diabetes mellitus and other endocrine diseases. In Gabbe SG, Neibyl JR, Simpson JL (eds): Obstetrics: Normal and Problem Pregnancies, ed 2. New York: Churchill Livingstone, 1991.

Plovie B: Diabetes in Pregnancy. March of Dimes, White Plains, New York, 1991.

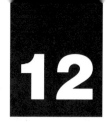

HOWARD S. SMITH

Respiratory Emergencies During Pregnancy

■ The Basics

Oxygenation is unavoidably related to ventilation of carbon dioxide. There are, however, characteristics of respiratory physiology that are unique to the oxygenation process and that merit discussion.

Terminology

Functional residual capacity (FRC) is perhaps the most important pulmonary parameter for the clinician. It is the volume of the lungs at the end of a normal exhalation during tidal breathing. FRC is affected by many variables (Table 12–1).

Vital capacity (VC) is the volume of air expired with maximal expiration following maximal inspiration (Table 12–2). The amount of air remaining in the lungs after the vital capacity has

---

Table 12–1

Factors that Decrease Functional Residual Capacity

Supine position
Obesity
Pregnancy
Impaired chest wall mechanics
Thoracoabdominal pain (splinting)
Ascent of diaphragm (abdominal distention)
Increased airway resistance
Atelectasis (pulmonary process absorption)
Decreased removal of secretions (i.e., ↓ mucociliary flow, ↓ cough)
General anesthesia
Pulmonary edema

```
Table 12-2
```

Vital Capacity

The "effective" or "working" volume of the lungs.
The volume expired with a maximal forced expiration starting from total lung capacity (50–60 mL/kg).
Correlates well with: deep breathing, effective coughing.
Decreases in patients with restrictive lung disease, massive ascites, pneumothorax, pleural effusion, or pregnancy.
If VC <15 mL/kg, consider intubation/mechanical ventilation.

been expired is called *residual volume.* Good vital capacity permits deep breathing and effective coughing.

Tidal volume (TV) is the volume of gas that moves in and out of the lungs during one normal, quiet breathing cycle (Table 12–3).

Closing capacity (CC) is the volume of the lungs at which small airways collapse (Table 12–4).

Dead space refers to those parts of the lungs and airways that act as conduits but do not participate in actual gas exchange (Table 12–5).

Intrapulmonary shunting describes a phenomenon in which a small fraction of blood goes through the lungs without being oxygenated or ventilated; it occurs when blood bypasses the alveoli (Table 12–6). The hypoxemia caused by shunting cannot be improved with supplemental oxygen.

The alveolocapillary membrane offers little resistance to the diffusion of carbon dioxide, even in disease states, as long as there is ventilation of the alveoli. Thus, carbon dioxide is considered a *ventilation-limited gas:* the more alveoli are ventilated, the more carbon dioxide is eliminated. On the other hand, the alveolocapillary membrane may present a considerable barrier

```
Table 12-3
```

Tidal Volume

Volume of gas that moves in and out of the lungs during normal quiet breathing (6–8 mL/kg)
Decreases with ↓ lung compliance, ↓ respiratory muscle strength, anesthesia
Increases with pregnancy

Table 12–4

Closing Capacity

The lung volume at which small airways begin to close.
Normally → FRC > CC
PEEP may improve FRC (thereby restoring a more normal FRC–CC
relationship).
As the FRC falls below the CC, atelectasis occurs, followed by
intrapulmonary shunting during tidal breathing. This may result in
shortness of breath.

Table 12–5

Dead Space

Anatomic
Areas of lungs where gas exchange does not occur
Trachea and conduction airways (~2 mL/kg)
Physiologic
Areas that are ventilated but not perfused (i.e., pulmonary embolism)

Table 12–6

Causes of Hypoxemia

Decreased F_{IO_2} (e.g., altitude)
Hypoventilation (e.g., decreased respiratory drive secondary to central
nervous system depressants)
Diffusion impairment (e.g., severe pulmonary fibrosis with thickened
alveolar capacity membrane)
Ventilation-perfusion (V/Q) mismatch
Shunt: alveoli that are perfused but not ventilated (e.g., intracardiac shunt;
intrapulmonary fistula); alveoli collapsed or filled with blood, pus,
edema

Box 12-1

Bedside Assessment of A-a P_{O_2} Gradient

$(7 \times F_{IO_2}) - \dfrac{P_{CO_2}}{0.8} =$ Alveolar oxygen

$(7 \times 40\%) - \dfrac{40}{0.8}$

$(280) - 50 = 230$ mm Hg (alveolar oxygen on 40% F_{IO_2} with a P_{CO_2} of 40 mm Hg)

$230 - P_{aO_2} =$ Gradient $(P_{AO_2} - P_{aO_2})$

Normal < 50 mm Hg on 100% F_{IO_2}
< 30 mm Hg on room air

---

to entry of oxygen into the blood. The *alveolar-arterial (A-a) gradient* is a clinically useful concept that reflects resistance to diffusion of oxygen across the alveolocapillary membrane. Hypoxemia in the setting of a normal A-a gradient is invariably due to low fraction of inspired oxygen (F_{IO_2}) or hypoventilation. Treatment generally entails administration of higher F_{IO_2} levels, positive end-expiratory breathing, or a different mode of ventilation (e.g., inverse ratio breathing, high-frequency jet ventilation). When a significant amount of intrapulmonary shunting occurs, for whatever reason, the A-a gradient is high. In this clinical circumstance there is nothing wrong with the alveolocapillary membrane: simply, the blood is not going through the lungs.

Compliance, defined as the change in lung volume for a given change in lung pressure, varies with the degree of elasticity (i.e., the ease of lung distention). Monitoring lung compliance may alert us to impending improvement or deterioration, sometimes well in advance of changes in other parameters.

■ Carbon Dioxide Physiology and Blood Gas Interpretation

Cellular processes generate carbon dioxide and certain metabolic acids (Table 12–7). Indeed, sufficient carbon dioxide is generated to create partial pressure in the blood. The mother's buffer systems (e.g., bicarbonate, phosphate) possess an enormous capacity to neutralize metabolic acids, thus minimizing substantial changes in the body's acid concentration (Table 12–8). In the blood, carbon dioxide is carried as dissolved

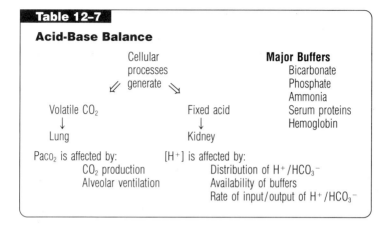

Table 12-7

Acid-Base Balance

	Cellular		**Major Buffers**
	processes		Bicarbonate
	⤢ generate ⤡		Phosphate
			Ammonia
Volatile CO_2		Fixed acid	Serum proteins
↓		↓	Hemoglobin
Lung		Kidney	

$Paco_2$ is affected by: $[H^+]$ is affected by:
          CO_2 production   Distribution of H^+/HCO_3^-
          Alveolar ventilation   Availability of buffers
                              Rate of input/output of H^+/HCO_3^-

carbon dioxide and bicarbonate in a state of equilibrium between its gaseous (dissolved) and ionized components:

$$CO_2 + H_2O \rightleftarrows H^+ + HCO_3^-$$

Normally, pH is kept within a range of 7.35 to 7.45. A pH <7.35 represents acidemia, whereas a pH value >7.45 reflects alkalemia.

Interpretation of arterial blood gas results should occur in a systematic fashion (Fig. 12–1). If the pH is low the patient has acidemia. If the Pco_2 value is elevated, it must be determined whether the acidemia is secondary to carbon dioxide build-up (i.e., respiratory acidosis) or accumulation of metabolic acids (i.e., metabolic acidosis). To make this determination, it should be noted that each 10-mm Hg change in maternal Pco_2 causes 0.08 pH units to move in the opposite direction. Any pH changes that exceed this guideline suggest metabolic processes. For in-

Table 12-8

Acid-Base Balance

Initial acid-base changes ⇒ buffers
     $Paco_2$ <35 constitutes respiratory alkalosis
     $Paco_2$ >45 constitutes respiratory acidosis
Rapid compensatory mechanisms
     CO_2 is affected through ventilation changes (lungs)
Slower compensatory mechanisms
     HCO_3^- is affected through filtering/reabsorption changes (kidneys)

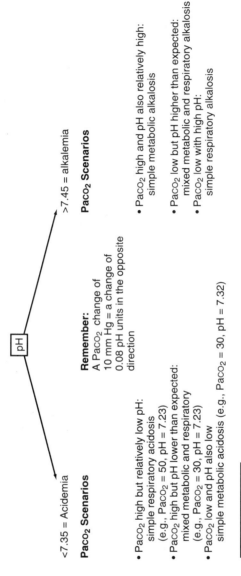

Figure 12-1

Approach to arterial blood gas interpretation.

pH

<7.35 = Acidemia

Paco₂ Scenarios

- Paco₂ high but relatively low pH:
  simple respiratory acidosis
  (e.g., Paco₂ = 50, pH = 7.23)
- Paco₂ high but pH lower than expected:
  mixed metabolic and respiratory
  (e.g., Paco₂ = 30, pH = 7.23)
- Paco₂ low and pH also low
  simple metabolic acidosis (e.g., Paco₂ = 30, pH = 7.32)

Remember:
A Paco₂ change of
10 mm Hg = a change of
0.08 pH units in the opposite
direction

>7.45 = alkalemia

Paco₂ Scenarios

- Paco₂ high and pH also relatively high:
  simple metabolic alkalosis
- Paco₂ low but pH higher than expected:
  mixed metabolic and respiratory alkalosis
- Paco₂ low with high pH:
  simple respiratory alkalosis

> ### Table 12-9
> **Anion Gap (AG)**
>
> Total positively charged ions = Total negatively charged ions
> $[Na^+] + [K^+] = [HCO_3^-] + [Cl^-] + [Unmeasured\ anions]$
> $$\uparrow$$
> Anion gap
>
> $AG^* = [Na^+] - [HCO_3^-] + [Cl^-]$
> Normal AG = 11 ± 3
>
> ---
> *Owing to potassium's relatively small contribution, it is frequently not included in calculations of AG.

stance, if the pH falls from the normal 7.40 value to 7.32 and the P_{CO_2} rises from its normal baseline of 40 to 50 mm Hg, the abnormal pH is deemed to be secondary to carbon dioxide accumulation due to respiratory acidosis.

Standard laboratory tests generally favor the detection of cations (sodium, potassium) over anions (chloride, bicarbonate), creating an artifactual deficiency of anions known as the "anion gap" (Table 12–9). In reality, the actual numbers of cations and anions are roughly equal; thus electrical neutrality in the body is maintained. The unmeasured anions that compose the anion gap are largely metabolic acids (e.g., lactate). As a result, metabolic acidosis generally causes the anion gap to widen as metabolic acids accumulate during certain pathologic conditions (i.e., diabetic ketoacidosis, hypoxia). Conversely, metabolic alkalosis occurs when acid (i.e., stomach acid, etc.) is depleted by nasogastric suction, prolonged vomiting, or diuretic therapy (Tables 12–10 through 12–12). Normal blood gas values as assessed during pregnancy are listed below:

Pa_{O_2}	104–108	(same as "nonpregnant value")
Pa_{CO_2}	27–32	(nonpregnant value 38–45)
HCO_3^-	18–31	(nonpregnant value 24–31)
pH	7.4–7.45	(alkalosis of pregnancy)

Respiratory Emergencies

Acute Pulmonary Edema

Acute pulmonary edema occurs when fluid transudates from the alveolar capillaries into the alveolar spaces. This is the result of

---

Table 12–10

Treatment of Metabolic Acidosis

Ensure adequate oxygenation, ventilation, perfusion pressure, oxygen delivery. Treatment of metabolic acidosis is aimed at correcting the underlying cause; however, if the pH is <7.2 it may be reasonable to administer sodium bicarbonate. Generally, half the total base deficit (TBD) is given.

TBD = Base excess × 0.2 × body weight (kg)

Table 12–11

Metabolic Alkalosis*

Urinary chloride

<10 mmol/L "NaCl responsive"   >20 mmol/L "NaCl resistant"
          ↓   ↓
Gastrointestinal (vomiting,   Excess mineralocorticoid activity
   nasogastric suction, etc.)
Diuretic therapy   Profound K^+ depletion

*The body generally tolerates metabolic acidosis better than metabolic alkalosis.

Table 12–12

Treatment of Metabolic Alkalosis

Correct underlying pathophysiology.
Halt ongoing acid loss.
A trial of NaCl or KCl may be attempted if urinary chloride is less than 10 mmol/L.
For some patients, a carbonic anhydrase inhibitor (e.g., acetazolamide) may be useful.
For severe alkalosis, consider four options:
   Dilute HCl infusion via central vein (0.05 mmol/L of HCl not exceeding 300 mL/hr).
   Oral arginine HCl (300 mL of 10% solution infused over 60 min).
   Ammonium chloride infusion (1000 mL of 2% solution infused over 8 hr). Avoid in the presence of liver dysfunction, to avoid ammonia toxicity.
   Hemodialysis.

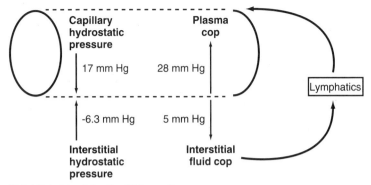

Total Out 17 + 6.3 + 5 = 28.3 mm Hg
Total In   28 mm Hg
Net Outward Force = 0.3 mm Hg
cop, colloid oncotic pressure

Figure 12–2

Normal capillary exchange in the lungs.

a net imbalance of the Starling forces that push fluid out of the pulmonary capillaries and the forces that keep fluid inside (Fig. 12–2). The end result is a foamy transudate in the alveoli, which creates a barrier to oxygenation. Treatment is directed at clearing the alveoli by unloading the pulmonary vasculature and increasing the inspired concentration of oxygen (Table 12–13). For severe pulmonary edema, endotracheal intubation, mechanical ventilation, and positive end-expiratory pressure (PEEP) may be necessary to improve the situation. The underlying disease process that is responsible for pulmonary edema must also be treated.

Venous Air Embolism

Typically an intraoperative complication, air embolism can happen whenever the lumen of a vein is exposed to the atmosphere, thus allowing air to be siphoned into the central circulation. It is heralded by hypoxemia, hypotension, and cardiovascular collapse. Diagnosis is supported by the presence of a "windmill murmur," Doppler auscultation of the right ventricle, and echocardiography.

The treatment includes immersing the operative site in saline and supporting the circulation with vasopressors, inotropes, and

---

Table 12-13

Treatment of Acute Pulmonary Edema

1. Elevate mother's head and chest to improve ventilation.
2. Oxygen: Administer via nonrebreather face mask at 10 L/min or with continuous positive airway pressure (CPAP). Intubation may be required for severe cases (see Tables 12–19, 12–20).
3. Nitroglycerin (optional depending on clinical circumstance): Apply 2 inches of paste to chest or administer sublingually (1/150) until IV access is secured. For patients with IV access, morphine sulfate (5 mg) may be used. Avoid morphine in the presence of altered consciousness, increased intracranial pressure, or chronic severe pulmonary disease.
4. Continuous pulse oximetry and cardiac monitoring.
5. Furosemide (40 mg IV); repeat as necessary. Do not use more than 120 mg within 1 hr. (This improves pulmonary lymphatic drainage and reduces preload by initiating diuresis.) Give slowly to minimize ototoxicity.
6. Monitor blood pressure and fetal heart rate tracing.
7. Digoxin as clinically indicated: Initial dose 0.5–1.0 mg IV, give in 0.2 mg increments followed by increments of 0.25 mg q4–6h as needed.
8. Cardioversion as clinically indicated.
9. Continuous electronic fetal monitoring.

---

fluids (Table 12–14). A catheter placed into the right atrium may be used to aspirate the air. The patient should be placed in the left lateral recumbent position (to trap the embolus in the right atrium) and ventilated with 100% oxygen.

Bronchial Asthma

Asthma is characterized by bronchial smooth muscle hyperactivity and hypertrophy wherein the bronchus becomes obstructed

---

Table 12-14

Supportive Measures for Venous Air Embolus

1. Flood surgical field with saline. Discontinue nitrous oxide. Position surgical site below level of the right atrium.
2. Administer 100% oxygen.
3. Aspirate through multiorifice central venous catheter.
4. Raise central venous pressure
   a. Volume load
   b. Pressors.
5. Place patient in left lateral decubitus position to trap embolus in right atrium.

Table 12–15

Asthma Pathophysiology

Early-Phase Response

- Peak: 30–60 min; duration: hours
- Release of histamine and other inflammatory mediators
  - Bronchial smooth muscle contraction
  - Increased vascular permeability
  - Epithelial injury
  - Vasodilatation

Late-Phase Response

- Peak: 5–6 h; duration: hours–days
- Influx of neutrophils, eosinophils, basophils
- Inflammation
- Desquamation of ciliated epithelium
- Viscous mucus plugging

in response to stimulation of the bronchial epithelium. Chemical mediators of this reaction have been described, the final common pathway being release of mediators (i.e., histamine) that provoke spasm and hypersecretion of the airways (Table 12–15). The result is impaired air movement and gas exchange. Treatment is directed at relaxing the bronchial smooth muscle and neutralizing chemical mediators (Table 12–16).

Adult Respiratory Distress Syndrome

The adult respiratory distress syndrome (ARDS) is a condition for which conventional mechanical ventilation cannot achieve normal ventilation or oxygenation. In this setting, the alveolar-arterial difference exceeds 200 mm Hg and the chest film shows diffuse, bilateral infiltrates. This condition requires judicious use of drugs and careful manipulation of maternal ventilatory parameters (Table 12–17).

Respiratory failure of any cause (Table 12–18) almost invariably requires endotracheal intubation and mechanical ventilation (Tables 12–19, 12–20). At some point ventilatory support no longer is needed. Determining the proper time for discontinuing ventilatory support may be difficult. Intermittent mandatory ventilation (IMV) has been helpful as a technique for "weaning" pregnant women. The general strategy is to reduce to FIO_2 to 0.3 to 0.4 and the PEEP to 5 cm H_2O while decreasing the

---

Table 12–16

Treatment of Acute Asthma

1. Oxygen: couple with continuous pulse oximetry, cardiac monitoring, and electronic fetal monitoring. Obtain arterial blood gas analysis as needed.
2. Beta-adrenergic agents:
   Subcutaneous: Terbutaline, 0.25 mg q15min × 3
   or
   Epinephrine, 0.3 mL of 1:1000 solution q20min × 3.
   Nebulizer: Metaproterenol, 0.3 mL of 5% solution q4h.
3. Aminophylline: 5 mg/kg loading dose followed by 0.5–0.7 mg/kg/hr, IV.
4. Corticosteroids:
   Inhaler: Beclomethasone, 2–5 puffs b.i.d.–q.i.d.
   Intravenous: methylprednisolone, 60–80 mg q6–8h.
5. Treat acidosis with dilute bicarbonate (pH <7.20).
6. Mechanical ventilation for refractory cases only (may provoke bronchospasm).
7. Bronchoscopy and lavage are rarely used. May be useful for patients with voluminous mucous secretions, epithelial sloughing, and airway plugging.
8. General anesthesia is used rarely and as last resort.

Table 12–17

Acute Respiratory Distress Syndrome

Criteria

Alveolar–arterial difference ≥200 mm Hg.
Bilateral pulmonary infiltrates on chest film.
Pulmonary wedge pressure ≤18 mm Hg.

Therapeutic Goals

Ensure adequate oxygen delivery.
Avoid barotrauma and oxygen toxicity.
Avoid compromising cardiovascular status.

Therapeutic Strategies

During mechanical ventilation use low tidal volumes (i.e., 6 mL/kg).
Limit respiratory frequency.
Maintain airway pressures ≤35 cm H_2O.
Accept elevated $Paco_2$ levels.
Use lowest Fio_2 possible (0.50 maximum).
Consider use of PEEP. Do not exceed pressures of 15 cm H_2O.

Table 12-18

Acute Respiratory Failure (ARF)

"Mind Your *P*s and *A*s"

*P*ulmonary edema
*P*neumothorax
*P*ulmonary embolus, also amniotic fluid embolus, venous air embolus
*P*neumonia
*P*ulmonary contusion (trauma)
*A*spiration pneumonitis
*A*sthma
*A*RDS
*A*naphylaxis/allergic reactions
*A*irway obstruction

Table 12-19

Indications for Endotracheal Intubation (Remember ATOP)

*A*cute respiratory failure (e.g., ARDS)
Pulmonary *T*oilet
Acute airway *O*bstruction (e.g., trauma, allergic reaction)
Airway *P*rotection (e.g., altered consciousness)

Table 12-20

Criteria for Mechanical Ventilation with Acute Respiratory Failure (ARF)

"You Must M-O-V-E with ARF!"

1. *M*echanical (remember 15-25-35)
   Vital capacity <15 mL/kg
   Maximal inspiratory force (MIF) < -25 cm H_2O
   Respiratory rate >35/min
2. *O*xygenation
   Pao_2 <70 mm Hg with Flo_2 0.40
   A-a gradient >350 mm Hg with 100% O_2
3. *V*entilation
   $Paco_2$ >55 mm Hg (except in chronic hypercapnia)
   Dead-space / tidal volume ratio (Vd/Vt) >0.6
4. *E*nd-inspiratory lung inflation inadequate for adequate gas exchange.

Table 12–21

General Strategies for Treating ARF

1. Increase supplemental oxygen.
2. Aggressive medical therapy directed at underlying pathophysiology may include:
   diuretics (furosemide)
   beta$_2$ agonists
   anticholinergic agents
   steroids
3. Aggressive chest physiotherapy
4. Change of position
5. Continuous positive airway pressure (CPAP). Make sure patients:
   are awake and alert (use cautiously if patient has full stomach)
   have airway protective reflexes intact
   are not retaining CO_2
   are not in need of positive-pressure ventilation
   do not exceed 10 cm H_2O

Table 12–22

Anaphylaxis

Presentation

Hypotension, tachycardia.
Wheezing.
Rash, flushing.

Management

Eliminate or impede contact with triggering agent.
Maintain airway; intubate as clinically necessary (Table 12–20).
100% oxygen.
Rapid volume expansion.
Epinephrine, 0.3 mL of 1:1000 dilution, SC *or*
　　　　　　　10 mL of 1:10,000 dilution via endotracheal tube
Inhaled beta$_2$ agonists.
Methylprednisolone, 125 mg IV.
Diphenhydramine, 50 mg IV or IM.
Consider continuous epinephrine infusion (0.02 μg/kg/min) if
　patient's condition does not stabilize.
Continuous electronic fetal monitoring.

number of ventilator-assisted breaths to one or two per minute before successful extubation. Table 12–21 illustrates general strategies for treating acute respiratory failure.

Anaphylaxis

An acute anaphylactic reaction (Table 12–22) is a vigorous, overwhelming immune-mediated reaction to a given antigen. It is viewed by some as a systemic version of asthma. In fact, asthma is frequently one of the early manifestations of anaphylaxis. An acute anaphylactic reaction is characterized by hypotension, tachycardia, and bronchospasm. It is a life-threatening emergency that demands immediate, aggressive intervention (Table 12–22).

Aspiration of Gastric Contents

Aspiration is a dangerous, potentially lethal problem. During gestation, esophageal sphincter tone is reduced, gastric emptying is slowed, the gastric angle is altered, and the risk of aspiration increased. The risk is compounded by the use of general anesthesia and by other conditions that alter the consciousness of the mother. As pulmonary damage from aspiration of stomach contents is proportional to the acidity of the aspirated materials,

---

Table 12–23

Managing Aspiration

Trendelenburg position with head turned to side.
Suction upper airways.
Place cuffed endotracheal tube.
Suction lower airways via endotracheal tube.
Administer 100% oxygen; use mechanical ventilation (with PEEP).
Arterial blood gas, continuous pulse oximetry.
Chest x-rays.
Place nasogastric tube to empty stomach contents.
Non-particulate antacid.
H_2 blocker (metoclopramide or cisapride).
Bronchoscopy as needed to remove particulate matter.
Beta$_2$ agonists to treat bronchospasm.
Intermittent pulmonary toilet, as needed.
Supportive measures as needed (i.e., pressors, etc.).
Continuous electronic fetal monitoring.

a common strategy for reducing the risk involves administration of nonparticulate antacids before induction of general anesthesia. Treatment of acute aspiration is outlined in Table 12–23.

■
Bibliography

Cohen JJ: Disorders of hydrogen ion metabolism. In Early LE, Gottschalk CE (eds): Strauss and Welt's Diseases of the Kidney, ed 3, vol II. Boston: Little, Brown, 1979.

Cohen JJ, Kassirer JP: Acid-Base. Boston, Little, Brown, 1982.

Nunn JF: Applied Respiratory Physiology, ed 3. Boston: Butterworths, 1987.

Pare JAP, Fraser RG: Synopsis of Diseases of the Chest. Philadelphia: W.B. Saunders, 1983.

West JB: Respiratory Physiology: The Essentials, ed 3. Baltimore: Williams & Wilkins, 1985.

West JB: Ventilation/Blood Flow and Gas Exchange, ed 4. London: Blackwell Scientific Publications, 1985.

JAMES BERNASKO AND

MANUEL ALVAREZ

Acute Renal Failure in the Obstetric Intensive Care Patient

Renal failure is an uncommon complication of pregnancy. The majority of cases of renal impairment that manifest clinically during pregnancy are the result of chronic renal disease antedating the pregnancy. While the incidence of acute renal failure (ARF) requiring dialysis is estimated to be less than 1 in 10,000 to 15,000 pregnancies, an accurate estimate of the incidence of milder degrees of renal failure is prohibitive. ARF is seen more often during the postpartum period for two reasons. First, certain peripartum events place pregnant patients at increased risk for insults to renal function. Second, when a patient with a preexisting medical illness suffers an exacerbation, the tendency of the obstetric care provider is to effect delivery with the hope of simplifying maternal and fetal management. It is important, however, to recognize that the delivery process itself may place the mother at even greater risk of death. In fact, when ARF occurs early in the period of fetal viability, the interests of both mother and fetus are often better served by delaying delivery until renal function and fetal prognosis improve. Table 13–1 reviews relevant physiologic and anatomic alterations imposed by pregnancy. A working knowledge and clear understanding of these changes are paramount to the timely recognition and treatment of acute renal disorders during pregnancy. Tables 13–2 and 13–3 outline the various causes of ARF.

◼ Antepartum Renal Failure

All patients who present for prenatal care should be appropriately screened for preexisting medical diseases with a thorough history, physical examination, and blood and urine analyses. Even in the absence of a history of renal disease, persistent proteinuria, pyuria, glycosuria or hematuria should prompt a more detailed search for abnormalities of renal function or struc-

---

Table 13–1

Relevant Alterations in Maternal Physiology and Anatomy During Pregnancy

Cardiovascular
  Increased total body water (≈6–8 L)
  Increased blood volume (≈45%)
  Increased cardiac output (≈50%)
  Decreased systemic vascular resistance (≈20%)
Uterine
  Increased uterine blood flow (≈900%)
  Increased fraction of cardiac output perfusing uterus—2% nonpregnant versus 17% pregnant
  Increased uterine size (extrinsic compression of inferior vena cava and ureters)
Renal
  Increased effective renal plasma flow (ERPF) (≈75% by 16 weeks' gestation; declines late in third trimester)
  Increased glomerular filtration rate (GFR) (≈50% by 5–7 weeks' gestation; no decline in late pregnancy)
  Increased creatinine clearance (normal for pregnancy is 150–200 mL/min)
  Increased sodium retention (≈1000 mEq/L; distributed to fetus, placenta, and maternal interstitial and intravascular fluids)
  Increased plasma aldosterone levels (increased from 100–200 ng/L to 200–700 ng/L by late pregnancy)
  Increased potassium retention (≈350 mEq/L)
  Increased renal loss of vitamin B_{12} and folate
  Increased renal glucose excretion (primarily because of increased GFR)
  Decreased plasma osmolality (decreases by 10 mOsm/kg by the fifth week of gestation to 270–280 mOsm/kg)
  Decreased filtration fraction (GFR/ERPF) until late third trimester, when it returns to nonpregnant values of 20%–21%
  Decreased serum BUN (≈25%; falls to 8–9 mg/dL by end of first trimester)
  Decreased serum creatinine (decreases to 0.7 mg/dL by first trimester and further to 0.5–0.6 mg/dL by late pregnancy)
  Decreased serum uric acid (decreases to 2.0–3.0 mg/dL until 24 weeks' gestation, then reaches nonpregnant norms by late pregnancy)
  No change in urine protein loss during pregnancy (normal 100–300 mg/24 hr)

Table 13–2

Causes of Acute Renal Failure

Prerenal (decreased renal perfusion)
  A. Decreased systemic blood pressure
    1. Intravascular volume depletion (e.g., hemorrhage, third space losses, diuretics)
    2. Decreased cardiac output (e.g., decreased preload [venous pooling, pump failure] cardiomyopathy, myocardial infarction, valvular disease)
    3. Shock syndromes (e.g., sepsis, anaphylaxis)
  B. Hepatorenal syndrome
  C. Autoregulatory failure (e.g., angiotensin-converting enzyme [ACE] inhibitors, nonsteroidal antiinflammatory drugs [NSAIDS]).
  D. Disseminated intravascular coagulopathy (e.g., injury from fibrin degradation products)
Renovascular
  A. Glomerular disease
    1. Primary (e.g., membranoproliferative) glomerulonephropathy
    2. Immune-mediated nephritis (e.g., systemic lupus erythematosus, Goodpasture's syndrome).
    3. End-organ disease (e.g., chronic diabetes mellitus, chronic hypertension)
    4. Polycystic disease
  B. Acute tubular necrosis
    1. Nephrotoxins: exogenous (e.g., aminoglycosides, radiocontrast agents, chemotherapy, heavy metals, animal poisons, organic chemicals); endogenous (e.g., uric acid, oxalate, myeloma protein)
    2. Prolonged ischemia
    3. Rhabdomyolysis
    4. Hemoglobinuria
    5. Reflux nephropathy
  C. Interstitial disease
    1. Allergic (e.g., drug-induced—diuretics, antibiotics, NSAIDS, methyldopa)
    2. Infective (e.g., chronic pyelonephritis)
    3. Metabolic (e.g., hypercalcemia)
  D. Massive bilateral cortical necrosis
Postrenal (obstructive)
  A. Tumor, stone, clot, necrotic debris in urinary tract
  B. Extrinsic compression of ureters (e.g., retroperitoneal tumor/hemorrhage, uterine fibroid, surgical ligation)

Table 13-3

Causes of Renal Failure Unique to Pregnancy

Severe preeclampsia or eclampsia
Abruptio placentae
Prolonged intrauterine fetal demise
Acute fatty liver of pregnancy
Amniotic fluid embolism
Septic abortion
Postpartum idiopathic ARF
Postpartum hemorrhage

ture. Ideally, any patient with a medical illness that could adversely affect kidney function should have renal function assessed prior to conception and at least once each trimester. Pre- and postconception counseling and subsequent care should be accomplished by consultation with both a nephrologist and a maternal-fetal medicine specialist. These patients are at especially high risk for spontaneous pregnancy loss, anemia, malnutrition, intrauterine growth restriction, preterm labor, hypertension, preeclampsia, and rapid deterioration of renal function. Not infrequently, pregnancy is a time when the patient with end-stage renal disease may first need dialysis or require more frequent treatments. Although creatinine clearance typically improves during the second trimester, diligent close monitoring of both mother and fetus should continue throughout the third trimester to ensure early detection of any potential complication. For patients who require multiple hemodialysis treatments during pregnancy, chronic ambulatory peritoneal dialysis (CAPD) offers several advantages over hemodialysis, including ease of catheter placement, avoidance of anticoagulation and acute fluctuations in drug levels, and a more constant fluid and electrolyte balance. In addition, hemodialysis is more likely to be associated with uterine contractions and fetal distress resulting from hypotension-induced placental insufficiency. Scrupulous attention should be paid to aseptic care of the peritoneal dialysis catheter to prevent peritonitis. The goal of dialysis is to maintain serum blood urea nitrogen (BUN) and creatinine below 70 mg/dL and 5 mg/dL, respectively. The optimal time for delivery depends on both maternal and fetal status. Although it is often possible to delay delivery until fetal viability, many of these pregnancies deliver before term. After 32 weeks' gestation, when neonatal survival and subsequent morbidity are favorable, embarking toward heroic measures to prolong pregnancy in the face of maternal or fetal compromise is both unsafe and unwise.

Postpartum Renal Failure

When renal failure occurs during the postpartum period there is often a clear precipitating event. The importance of anticipating the development of renal failure cannot be overemphasized. Any clinical circumstance that predisposes the gravid patient to significant renal insult warrants measures aimed at promptly detecting evidence of impending renal failure (e.g., strict intake and output assessment, serial serum BUN and creatinine evaluations). In the classic clinical presentation, a progressive serial increase in serum BUN and creatinine is observed, coupled with a marked reduction in urine production. It is important to remember that anuria does not always accompany renal failure and that the clinical symptoms of uremia are often late findings. Table 13–4 outlines a systematic approach to the diagnosis of ARF.

Urine electrolyte measurement remains one of the most useful tests in the differential diagnosis of ARF (see Table 13–4). In the absence of diuretic therapy, high urine osmolality and creatinine values or low sodium suggests prerenal, rather than intrinsic renal, failure. Urinalysis in patients with acute tubular necrosis (ATN) usually reveals moderate proteinuria, tubular cell casts, and coarsely granular pigmented casts. White cell casts are more suggestive of renal infection. Heavy proteinuria suggests acute glomerulonephritis or vasculitis. Anemia would suggest either recent hemorrhage or chronic renal disease. Eosinophilia often is associated with allergic interstitial nephritis. For the oliguric or anuric patient who fails to respond appropriately to initial fluid resuscitation (i.e., output ≥ 0.5 mL/kg/hr), invasive hemodynamic monitoring should be seriously considered to guide further volume replacement (see Chapters 1 and 27).

Dialysis

Hemodialysis is usually the preferred method of dialysis for pregnant and postpartum patients who require short-term renal replacement therapy. Treatment may be carried out over 4 to 6 hours (traditional intermittent hemodialysis) or over 12 to 24

Table 13-4

Diagnosis of Acute Renal Failure in Pregnancy

History of Precipitating Factor(s)

Begin intake-output assessment immediately.

Anuria (<100 mL/24 hr)
1. Complete urinary tract obstruction
2. Bilateral renal arterial or venous occlusion
3. Bilateral cortical necrosis
4. Overwhelming acute tubular necrosis
5. Severe acute glomerulonephritis

Oliguria (100–500 mL/24 hr)
1. Prerenal azotemia
2. Tubular necrosis
3. Interstitial nephritis
4. Glomerulonephritis
5. Partial or intermittent obstruction

Nonoliguria/polyuria (>500 mL/24 hr)
1. Tubular necrosis
2. Interstitial nephritis
3. Partial or intermittent obstruction

Physical Examination

Seek evidence of:

Fluid retention (e.g., hypertension, rales on lung auscultation, hyperdynamic circulation)

Fluid depletion (e.g., hypotension, decreased skin turgor)

Uremic syndrome (e.g., altered sensorium, pericarditis, bleeding diathesis)

Bladder palpation (consider obstruction in catheter drainage)

Laboratory Investigation

Urine sediment,* urine electrolytes,* urine creatinine,* urine osmolality*

Complete blood count

Coagulation profile (prothrombin and partial thromboplastin times)

Serum electrolytes, osmolality, BUN, creatinine, calcium, phosphorus, protein, liver transaminases

Specialized tests (e.g., antinuclear antibody, anti–double-stranded DNA antibodies, anti-Smith antibodies, renal sonogram, biopsy, arteriogram, ureteral cannulation)

*Test	Prerenal Azotemia	Acute Renal Failure	Obstruction
Urine osmolality	>500	<400	<400
Urine sodium	<20	>40	>40
Fractional excretion of sodium: (Urine sodium × Plasma creatinine) / (Plasma sodium × Urine creatinine)	<1%	≥2%	≥2%
Urine sediment	Normal, occasional granular casts	Granular casts, cellular debris	Normal sediment

hours (continuous hemodialysis/hemofiltration). Although the indications for both modalities are similar, continuous therapy is often better tolerated and more efficient. Continuous renal replacement therapy can be performed either by an arteriovenous-driven circulation (continuous arteriovenous hemofiltration/hemodialysis) or by a pump-driven circulation (continuous venovenous hemofiltration/hemodialysis). The advantages of the latter include avoidance of arterial cannulation, minimal treatment-induced hypotension, decreased anticoagulation requirements, less frequent iatrogenic fetal distress, avoidance of abrupt changes in drug, electrolyte, or temperature levels, and less risk of air or clot embolization. It is important to remember that frequent dialysis may be associated with considerable nutritional losses (6 to 9 gm of amino acids per treatment and 5 gm/hr of glucose when using a glucose-free dialysate). Prophylactic dialysis to maintain BUN and creatinine below 70 mg/dL and 5 mg/dL, respectively, together with provision for adequate essential amino acids and glucose, may improve survival.

Table 13–5

General Management Guidelines for Acute Renal Failure in the Pregnant Patient

Prompt identification of the cause of ARF
Institute timely therapy
Consult with a perinatologist and a nephrologist on diagnosis and management
Position the gravida with abdomen partially tilted to left (improve renal blood flow)
Avoid significant hypertension or hypotension
Avoid major fluid or electrolyte imbalance
Maintain adequate nutrition
Maintain close communication with family

Fetal surveillance
  >24 wk, continuous monitoring
  <24 wk, intermittent monitoring
  Biophysical profile assessment as indicated
  Consider maternal steroid administration for acceleration of fetal lung maturity
Maintain capability for emergency cesarean delivery for persistently abnormal fetal testing
Early evaluation for dialysis

Table 13–6

Management Protocol for Acute Renal Failure

1. Volume status
    a. Consider pulmonary artery catheterization for close assessment of volume status
    b. Fluid intake: 6–8 mL/kg + urine output
    c. Lasix, 40–80 mg IV, to assist in fluid balance (max. daily dose 600 mg)
    d. Dialysis for fluid overload (cardiac failure)
2. Hyperkalemia
    a. $K^+ \geq 8.0$ mEq/L or electrocardiographic changes (other than peaked T waves)
        1. Calcium gluconate, 10–20 mL of 10% solution
        2. 10 U regular insulin and 50 mL 50% glucose
        3. Sodium bicarbonate, 50–150 mEq/L (if patient is not volume overloaded)
        4. Dialysis
        5. Cardiac monitor
    b. $K^+ = 6.8$–7.9 mEq/L
        1. 10 U regular insulin and 50 mL 50% glucose
        2. Sodium bicarbonate, 50–150 mEq/L (if patient is not volume overloaded)
        3. Kayexalate, 20–30 gm every 2–4 hr PO, 50–100 gm per rectum
        4. Dialysis
        5. Cardiac monitor
    c. $K^+ = 5.6$–6.8 mEq/L
        1. Kayexalate as in step b,
            and/or
        2. Dialysis
3. Acidosis: Maintain bicarbonate >15 mEq/L and pH >7.2
    a. Euvolemic patient: Normal bicarbonate − patient's bicarbonate × 0.6 × wt (kg) = Dose of sodium bicarbonate to totally correct deficit (start with 50% of this calculated dose to avoid total correction)
    b. Volume-overloaded, hypernatremic, or severely catabolic patient: Dialysis with high-bicarbonate dialysate
4. Hyponatremia
    a. Serum sodium >125 mEq/L: Restrict free water
    b. Serum sodium 120–125 mEq/L: Dialysis
    c. Serum sodium <120 mEq/L: Dialysis with high-sodium dialysate; administration of hypertonic saline during dialysis
5. Hypocalcemia: Administer IV calcium only if Chvostek's sign or carpopedal spasm is present. Oral supplements to maintain serum calcium >7.5 mg% and to keep phosphorus <5.5 mg%.

Table continued on opposite page

Table 13–6

Management Protocol for Acute Renal Failure
Continued

6. Nutrition
   a. Management without dialysis: ≥100 gm glucose, 25–50 kcal/kg/d, 0.6 gm protein/kg ideal body weight, up to 1.5 gm/kg if BUN can be kept <100 mg/dL or if the patient is still pregnant.
   b. Management with dialysis
      1. Oral intake: 1–1.5 gm of protein/kg; 25–50 kcal/kg to prevent catabolism, potassium 50 mEq, sodium 2 gm in the form of food or enteral-elemental diet preparations; supplemental multivitamins
      2. Total parenteral nutrition (TPN): 25–50 kcal/d, 70% as glucose with 1–1.5 gm protein/kg/d; 40% of protein as essential amino acids; maximum lipid is 500 mL of a 10% intralipid solution; supplemental multivitamins; electrolytes added as indicated by lab values
7. Adjust drug doses for renal failure:

Glomerular filtration rate	Suggested reduction in daily dose
10–50 mL/min	Aminoglycosides 65–50% Digoxin 75–25% Insulin 25% Cefazolin 50%
<10 mL/min	Aminoglycosides 75% Digoxin 90–75% Insulin 50% Cefazolin 75%

8. Indications for dialysis:
   a. Uremia: BUN >100 mg/dL or uremic symptoms
   b. Volume overload (congestive heart failure)
   c. Hyperkalemia unresponsive to other measures
   d. Severe metabolic acidosis
   e. Pericarditis or pericardial effusion
   f. Need for TPN, blood products, or other fluid in excess of what can be tolerated with conservative therapy
   g. Seizures, severe mental status changes
   h. Hypermagnesemia >7 mEq/L unresponsive to other measures

Adapted from Hou S: Acute and chronic renal failure in pregnancy. In Clark SL, Cotton DB, Hankins GDV, et al.: Critical Care Obstretrics, ed 2. New York: Blackwell Scientific Publications, 1991.)

Prognosis

The prognosis for resolution of acute renal dysfunction during pregnancy depends on baseline renal function, the nature of the renal injury, and prompt identification and adequate treatment of the underlying cause. While acute tubular necrosis usually resolves completely within 1 to 3 weeks, bilateral cortical necrosis may be irreversible in as many as 20% of cases. Nonoliguric renal failure has a milder course and better prognosis than oliguric renal failure. When renal dysfunction antedates the pregnancy, long-term prognosis depends more on the rate of decline of renal function before the pregnancy than on the specific underlying illness.

Summary

The diagnosis and management of ARF during pregnancy requires a multidisciplinary team approach (see Tables 13–5 and 13–6). Liberal use of consultation with internal medicine, nephrology, and maternal-fetal medicine specialists is encouraged. Prompt identification of the cause of ARF, coupled with the timely institution of appropriate therapy, is the cornerstone of the successful management of this disease during pregnancy.

Bibliography

Clark SL, Cotton DB, Hankins GDV, et al. (eds): Critical Care Obstetrics, ed 2. New York: Blackwell Scientific Publications, 1991.
Hall JB, Schmidt GA, Wood LDH (eds): Principles of Critical Care. New York: McGraw-Hill, 1991.
Rippe JM, et al. (eds): Intensive Care Medicine, ed 2. Boston: Little, Brown, 1991.

GARY A. DILDY AND

STEVEN L. CLARK

14

Amniotic Fluid Embolism

Amniotic fluid embolism (AFE) is an unpreventable and unpre-dictable complication of obstetrics classically characterized as a syndrome of acute peripartum hypoxia, hemodynamic collapse, and coagulopathy.

This syndrome was first described in the medical literature in 1926 by Meyer and was characterized more fully in the 1941 classic monograph by Steiner and Lushbaugh. The incidence of AFE has been reported to be between 1 in 8000 and 1 in 80,000 pregnancies. Reporting data from the United States Vital Statistics between the years 1968 and 1973, Resnik and coworkers de-scribed an incidence of 1 in 47,300 to 1 in 63,500. AFE causes approximately 11% to 13% of the maternal deaths in the United States and is the most common cause of peripartum death. The maternal mortality rate remains as high as 80%.

AFE usually occurs around the time of delivery but has been reported to occur also after legal abortion or transabdominal amniocentesis. The route of delivery (vaginal versus cesarean section) does not appear to affect the risk of occurrence.

The exact cause of AFE is not known, and much remains to be learned about this dangerous syndrome. Because AFE is so rare and any single institution may encounter only a few cases during the course of time, Clark initiated a National Registry for AFE in 1988. In 1995, the analysis of the National Registry was reported in *The American Journal of Obstetrics and Gynecology.*

■ Pathophysiology

AFE has been described as a biphasic process. Initially profound hemodynamic and oxygenation alterations occur, followed by the development of a consumptive coagulopathy in 40% of cases. It was once thought that AFE was the result of passage of a large volume of amniotic fluid through the venous circulation into the right side of the heart and pulmonary vasculature, producing pulmonary hypertension, hypoxemia, and death.

More recently, however, investigators have suggested that AFE is the result of an immune-mediated process similar to anaphylactic and septic shock. The precise mechanism still remains undetermined.

In the analysis of the AFE National Registry, it was found that 70% of cases occurred during labor (but before delivery) and 30% of cases after (the majority within 5 minutes of) delivery. Several cases occurred during cesarean section without prior labor. Seventy-eight percent of cases occurred after ruptured membranes; thus, in the minority membranes were intact.

The diagnosis of AFE is usually made by clinical presentation (vide infra). Previous reports have attempted to confirm diagnosis by aspirating blood from central venous or Swan-Ganz catheter ports; however, it has been shown that squamous cells may be aspirated through central lines in subjects thought *not* to have the syndrome of AFE.

The analysis of the National Registry reported the most common signs and symptoms of AFE to be hypotension, fetal distress, pulmonary edema, and respiratory distress syndrome. Cardiopulmonary arrest occurred in a significant number of cases, the initial dysrhythmia being electromechanical dissociation, bradycardia, ventricular tachycardia/ventricular fibrillation,

Table 14–1
Signs and Symptoms of Amniotic Fluid Embolism

Cardiovascular	Respiratory	Hematologic	Utero-placental Fetal	Other
Hypotension* Cardiopulmonary arrest† Transient hypertension	Pulmonary edema† ARDS† Cyanosis† Dyspnea Broncho-spasm Cough Chest pain	Coagulop-athy†	Fetal distress* Atony	Seizure Headache

*Always present.

†>50% of cases.

Adapted from Clark SL, et al: Amniotic fluid embolism: Analysis of the national registry. Am J Obstet Gynecol 1995;172:1158–1169.

Table 14–2

Diagnostic Criteria for Amniotic Fluid Embolism

1. Acute hypotension or cardiac arrest
2. Acute hypoxia (defined as dyspnea, cyanosis, or respiratory arrest)
3. Coagulopathy (defined as laboratory evidence of intravascular consumption, fibrinolysis, or severe clinical hemorrhage in the absence of other explanations)
4. Acute signs and symptoms have onset during labor, cesarean section, dilatation and evacuation, or within 30 min post partum
5. Absence of any other significant confounding condition or potential explanation for the signs and symptoms observed

Data from Clark SL, et al: Amniotic fluid embolism: Analysis of the National Registry. Am J Obstet Gynecol 1995; 172:1158–1169.

and asystole. Other reported signs and symptoms included cyanosis, coagulopathy, dyspnea, seizures, uterine atony, bronchial spasm, transient hypertension, cough, headache, and chest pain. Table 14–1 lists the most common signs and symptoms of amniotic fluid embolus. Tetanic uterine contractions have been observed and are thought to be secondary to the initial hemodynamic response, a result, rather than a cause, of AFE. It has also been observed that a larger proportion of male fetuses is associated with this disorder; this is similar to the observation of a higher proportion of male fetuses with the syndrome of RhD sensitization. The diagnosis of AFE is usually made on clinical grounds; diagnostic criteria suggested by Clark and coworkers in 1995 are listed in Table 14–2.

■ Differential Diagnosis

When the peripartum patient develops acute severe hypoxia, hemodynamic collapse with hypotension, and clinical or laboratory coagulopathy, the diagnosis of AFE should be considered. It should be emphasized, however, that the clinical manifestations of this syndrome are variable and all classic criteria may not be present. Nevertheless, in the absence of classic criteria, other possible diagnoses should not be overlooked. The differential diagnosis of AFE is listed in Table 14–3.

Table 14–3
Differential Diagnosis of Amniotic Fluid Embolism

Septic shock	Pulmonary
Acute myocardial	thromboembolism
infarction	Placental abruption
Aspiration pneumonia	Anesthetic accident

Evaluation

A woman suspected of developing AFE should undergo immediate laboratory and radiographic evaluation (Table 14–4). Arterial blood gases should generally be obtained, noting the inspired oxygen concentration, to observe for development of hypoxia, hypercarbia, and acidosis. A complete blood count and coagulation studies may reveal the presence of microangiopathic red blood cell changes, prolonged coagulation times (prothrombin and partial thromboplastin) times, hypofibrinogenemia, thrombocytopenia, elevated fibrin degradation products, and if tested, decreased factor levels.

Chest x-ray findings are usually nonspecific, but in 70% of cases pulmonary edema is evident. Reported electrocardiographic findings include tachycardia—and in some cases ST-segment and T-wave changes or a right ventricular strain pattern.

Observations from patients undergoing pulmonary artery catheterization reveal a high incidence of *left-sided* heart failure (Table 14–5). This is contrary to what would be expected with pulmonary vascular obstruction and may be explained by myocardial hypoxia or a direct toxic myocardial effect of amniotic fluid.

Table 14–4
Evaluation of Suspected AFE

Arterial blood gas	Blood type and
CBC and platelets	cross-match
Prothrombin and partial	Chest radiography
thromboplastin times	12-lead
Fibrinogen and fibrin split products	electrocardiogram

Table 14–5

Hemodynamic Indices (Mean ± SD) in Non-Pregnant Women, Normal Women in the Third Trimester, and Women with Amniotic Fluid Embolism (AFE)

	MPAP mm Hg	PCWP mm Hg	PVR dynes-sec-cm^{-5}	LVSWI gm-m-M^{-2}
Non-pregnant (n = 10)	11.9 ± 2.0‡	6.3 ± 2.1†	119 ± 47†	41 ± 8†
Normal third trimester (n = 10)	12.5 ± 2.0‡	7.5 ± 1.8†	78 ± 22†	48 ± 6†
AFE (n = 15)	26.2 ± 15.7¶	18.9 ± 9.2¶	176 ± 72¶	26 ± 19¶

MPAP, mean pulmonary artery pressure; PCWP, pulmonary capillary wedge pressure; PVR, pulmonary vascular resistance; LVSWI, left ventricular stroke work index.

Data from
†Clark SL, et al: (Am J Obstet Gynecol 1989;161:1439–1442.)
‡Clark SL, et al: (unpublished data)
¶Clark SL, et al: Central hemodynamic alterations in amniotic fluid embolism. (Am J Obstet Gynecol 1988;158:1124–1126) and unpublished data from the National AFE Registry.

■ Management

The management of AFE is nonspecific and supportive (Fig. 14–1). Oxygen should be administered to maintain a normal oxygen saturation, and a pulse oximeter is useful in continuous oxygen saturation monitoring of the critically ill patient. Oxygen should be administered by face mask or by positive pressure via an endotracheal tube for an unconscious patient or a conscious one with severe hypoxemia.

Of course, cardiopulmonary resuscitation (CPR) measures should be instituted immediately for cardiorespiratory arrest. Issues related to CPR during pregnancy are discussed in Chapter 17. When a patient suffers cardiac arrest and does not respond to resuscitative measures in the first several minutes, perimortem cesarean section should be performed as soon as possible (see Chapter 17).

Hemodynamic support is necessary to treat hypotension and shock. Blood volume expansion with crystalloids or blood component therapy is instituted, as indicated. Pressor agents such as

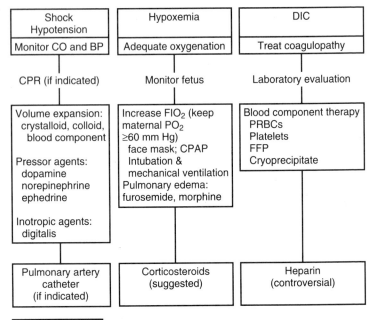

Shock Hypotension	Hypoxemia	DIC
Monitor CO and BP	Adequate oxygenation	Treat coagulopathy
CPR (if indicated)	Monitor fetus	Laboratory evaluation
Volume expansion: crystalloid, colloid, blood component Pressor agents: dopamine norepinephrine ephedrine Inotropic agents: digitalis	Increase FIO_2 (keep maternal PO_2 $\geq$60 mm Hg) face mask; CPAP Intubation & mechanical ventilation Pulmonary edema: furosemide, morphine	Blood component therapy PRBCs Platelets FFP Cryoprecipitate
Pulmonary artery catheter (if indicated)	Corticosteroids (suggested)	Heparin (controversial)

Figure 14–1

Management of amniotic fluid embolism. CO, cardiac output; BP, blood pressure; CPR, cardiopulmonary resuscitation; FIO_2, inspired oxygen concentration; ET, endotracheal; DIC, disseminated intravascular coagulation; PRBCs, packed red blood cells; FFP, fresh-frozen plasma; CPAP, continuous positive airway pressure.

dopamine, norepinephrine, and ephedrine may be useful to maintain blood pressure, but no specific agent is known to be superior to the others in this clinical situation (Table 14–6). Because of the common occurrence of left ventricular failure, inotropic support with digoxin should be considered in nonhypoxic patients. Pulmonary artery catheterization may provide important information for the clinical management of patients who are hemodynamically unstable.

Pulmonary edema is very common and must be treated with careful attention to intake and output of fluids. Corticosteroids may be helpful in the setting of AFE, as the syndrome may be immune mediated; however, the clinical efficacy of corticosteroids is unproven at this time. Hydrocortisone may be administered (500 mg intravenously every 6 hours) until the patient

Table 14-6

Pharmacologic Agents Used to Treat Amniotic Fluid Embolism

Agent	Mechanism of Action	Dosage	Comments
Dopamine	Dopaminergic (0.5–5.0 μg/kg/min) vasodilation of renal and mesenteric vasculature β₁-adrenergic (5.0–10.0 μg/kg/min) increased myocardial contractility, SV, CO α-adrenergic (15–20 μg/kg/min) increased general vasoconstriction	2–5 μg/kg/min and titrate to BP and CO	Protect from light. Do not use if injection is discolored
Norepinephrine	α-adrenergic—peripheral vasoconstriction β-adrenergic—inotropic stimulator of the heart and dilator of coronary arteries	Initial dose 8–12 μg/min and titrate to blood pressure	Contraindicated in hypovolemic hypotension
Ephedrine	α and β sympathomimetic effects increase blood pressure	25–50 mg SQ or IM 5–10 min if necessary	Peripheral actions partly secondary to release of norepinephrine
Digoxin	Improved contractility of myocardium	0.5 mg IV push and 0.25 mg q4h × 2, then 0.25–0.37 mg/day	Narrow toxic-to-therapeutic ratio, especially with potassium depletion
Hydrocortisone sodium succinate	Naturally occurring glucocorticoid, modifies immune system response to diverse stimuli	500 mg IV q6h until condition stabilizes	Sodium retention and hypernatremia may occur if administered beyond 48–72 hr

*Refer to package insert for further information regarding preparation, contraindications, dosage, etc.

responds or expires. The use of furosemide to improve diuresis is supported.

When coagulopathy occurs, it is treated with blood component therapy, as indicated by laboratory parameters (see Chapter 4). An ample supply of packed red blood cells, platelets, fresh frozen plasma, or cryoprecipitate should be available through the blood bank. Rodgers and Heymach recommend the use of cryoprecipitate for repletion of plasma fibronectin. Heparin should not be used in the face of disseminated intravascular coagulation (DIC) secondary to AFE.

As noted above, as for any critically ill patient at risk for severe hypoxemia, an oxygen saturation monitor may be helpful. Electronic fetal heart rate monitoring should be employed if the fetus is undelivered and of viable age. During the initial phase of hemodynamic collapse and hypoxemia, profound fetal bradycardia may be noted. The response of the fetal heart rate to maternal medical therapy may be evaluated with electronic fetal heart rate monitoring. If the baby is viable, the decision must be made whether to proceed with operative delivery.

■ Prognosis

Maternal mortality rates were once as high as 80%, but more recently the figure of 61% was reported in the National Registry. Many of the women who survive AFE suffer permanent neurologic disabilities secondary to the effects of profound hypoxia. Death usually occurs at the time of cardiopulmonary arrest; however, in some cases the diagnosis of brain death may lead to discontinuation of life support after initial resuscitation and successful stabilization. As would be expected, women who survived without experiencing cardiac arrest have a higher rate of normal neurologic outcomes than did those who survived cardiac arrest (15% versus 8%). Long-standing sequelae of AFE include neurologic complications such as partial vision loss and hemiplegia. Acute renal failure may occur secondary to hypotension or DIC (see Chapter 13).

Neonatal survival has been reported most recently at 79%, with 50% of those surviving being neurologically intact. The shorter the arrest-to-delivery interval, the better is the rate of intact survival. This emphasizes the importance of proceeding promptly with delivery if after cardiac arrest initial resuscitative measurements are not successful within a few minutes.

■ Summary

AFE is a rare, but usually fatal, syndrome unique to obstetric patients. It is unpredictable and unpreventable. Early recognition and supportive management should optimize the maternal and fetal outcomes; however, maternal and fetal morbidity and mortality remain extremely high, despite appropriate aggressive interventions. Treatment is focused on correction of hypotension, hypoxemia, and coagulopathy. If maternal cardiac arrest occurs before delivery and if resuscitation measures are not immediately successful, the fetus should be delivered, if it is viable, as soon as possible, to optimize chances of fetal survival and neurologic normalcy.

■ Bibliography

Azegami A, Mori N: Amniotic fluid embolism and leukotrienes. Am J Obstet Gynecol 1986; 155:1119–1124.

Chung AF, Merkatz IR: Survival following amniotic fluid embolism with early heparinization. Obstet Gynecol 1973; 42:809–814.

Clark SL: Arachidonic acid metabolites and the pathophysiology of amniotic fluid embolism. Semin Reprod Endocrinol 1985; 3:253–257.

Clark SL: New concepts of amniotic fluid embolism: A review. Obstet Gynecol Surv 1990; 45:360–368.

Clark SL: Amniotic fluid embolism. Crit Care Clin 1991; 7:877–882.

Clark SL: Successful pregnancy outcomes after amniotic fluid embolism. Am J Obstet Gynecol 1992; 167:511–512.

Clark SL, Cotton DB, Gonik B, et al: Central hemodynamic alterations in amniotic fluid embolism. Am J Obstet Gynecol 1988; 158:1124–1126.

Clark SL, Hankins GDV, Dudley DA, et al: Amniotic fluid embolism: Analysis of the National Registry. Am J Obstet Gynecol 1995; 172:1158–1169.

Clark SL, Montz FJ, Phelan JP: Hemodynamic alterations associated with amniotic fluid embolism: A reappraisal. Am J Obstet Gynecol 1985; 151:617–621.

Clark SL, Pavlova Z, Greenspoon J, et al: Squamous cells in the maternal pulmonary circulation. Am J Obstet Gynecol 1986; 154:104–106.

Dildy GA, Clark SL: Cardiac arrest during pregnancy. Obstet Gynecol Clin North Am 1995; 22:303–314.

Guidotti RJ, Grimes DA, Gates W: Fatal amniotic fluid embolism during legally induced abortion. Am J Obstet Gynecol 1981; 141:257–261.

Hankins GDV, Snyder RR, Clark SL, et al: Acute hemodynamic and respiratory effects of amniotic fluid embolism in the pregnant goat model. Am J Obstet Gynecol 1993; 168:1113–1130.

Johnson TRB, Abbasi IA, Urso PJ: Fetal heart rate patterns associated with amniotic fluid embolism. Am J Perinatol 1987; 4:187–189.

Resnik R, Swartz WH, Plumer MH, et al: Amniotic fluid embolism with survival. Obstet Gynecol 1976; 47:295–298.

Rodgers GP, Heymach GJ: Amniotic fluid embolism. JAMA 1986; 256:14.

Steiner PE, Lushbaugh CC: Maternal pulmonary embolism by amniotic fluid. JAMA 1941; 117:1245–1344.

Vanmaele L, Noppen M, Vincken W, et al: Transient left heart failure in amniotic fluid embolism. Intensive Care Med 1990; 16:269–271.

SHIRLEY K. SAWAI

Acute Fatty Liver of Pregnancy

Acute fatty liver of pregnancy (AFLP) was once considered fatal. Before 1980, reported maternal and fetal mortalities were as high as 75% and 85%, respectively. Greater awareness of the disease and improved diagnostic capabilities have proved that the disorder is more common and less fatal than was previously thought. The maternal mortality rate today is 14% and the fetal mortality rate 8% to 10%. Maternal deaths are attributed to sepsis, aspiration, renal failure, circulatory collapse, or gastrointestinal bleeding. The incidence of AFLP is 1 in 13,000 deliveries, and it is most common in the late third trimester (mean gestational age, 35 to 36 weeks). Cases have been been reported as early as 26 weeks and as late as immediately post partum.

Obstetric Risk Factors for AFLP:

- First pregnancy
- Preeclampsia (20%–47%)
- Male fetus (75%)
- Twin gestation (14%)
- Fetal long chain 3-hydroxyacyl-CoA dehydrogenase

Survivors of AFLP usually recover without sequelae, and recurrence is extremely rare.

■ Pathophysiology

The cause of AFLP is unknown. Disease characteristics similar to those of tetracycline-induced hepatic failure, microvesicular fatty infiltrative disorders of Reye's syndrome, and valproic acid toxicity suggest a common cause. Carnitine deficiency, mitochondrial injury, free fatty acid content of the liver, and defective removal of plasma lipoproteins have all been implicated. Recent information suggests an association of fetal long chain 3-hydroxyacyl-CoA dehydrogenase deficiency with maternal AFLP. The end result is fat accumulation and ammonia production by the hepatocytes, and eventually coagulopathy and hypoglycemia secondary to progressive hepatic failure.

Grossly, the liver appears small, soft, and yellow. Within 2 weeks of clinical onset, liver biopsy reveals pale, ballooned centrilobular hepatocytes with microvesicles containing free fatty acids (seen on oil red O stain) arranged around a normal-looking nucleus. The periportal areas are spared, and there is no evidence of necrosis or inflammation like that seen with preeclampsia. The kidney, pancreas, brain, and bone marrow may also demonstrate similar infiltrations of fat and vacuolization. Figure 15–1 demonstrates these findings in a photomicrograph.

Early symptoms of AFLP may be nonspecific, such as anorexia, nausea, vomiting, malaise, fatigue, headache, and ab-

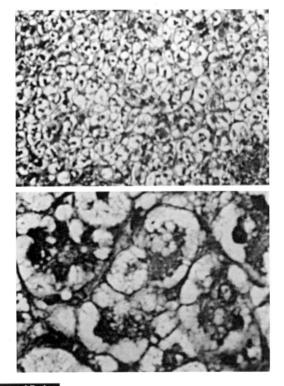

Figure 15-1

Acute fatty liver of pregnancy, microvesicular fat (hematoxylin and eosin)—*top* × 200; *bottom* × 400). (Schorr-Lesnick B, Lebovics C, Dworkin B, et al: Liver disease unique to pregnancy. Am J Gastroenterol 1991; 86:659–670.)

Table 15–1

Clinical Presentation of Acute Fatty Liver of Pregnancy

Sign/Symptom	Prevalence (%)
Abdominal pain	50–60%
Anorexia	————
Ascites	————
CNS aberrations (altered sensorium, asterixis, confusion, disorientation, psychosis, restlessness, seizures)	60–80%
DIC	55%
Edema	————
Fatigue	————
Gastroinestinal bleeding	20–60%
Headache	————
Hypertension	————
Jaundice	70%
Malaise	————
Nausea and vomiting	50–60%
Oliguria	40–60%
Petechiae	————
Premature labor	————
Pyrexia (late)	50%
Tachycardia	50%
Vaginal bleeding	————

dominal pain. As the disease progresses, jaundice becomes evident, and in severe cases oliguria, gastrointestinal bleeding, and central nervous system (CNS) aberrations consistent with hepatic encephalopathy and coma may ensue. Hypertension and edema are frequently seen since AFLP is often associated with preeclampsia. Abdominal examination reveals right upper quadrant or midepigastric tenderness. Hepatomegaly and splenomegaly are uncommon (Tables 15–1 and 15–2).

Diagnostic Tests

The severity of the disease and the specific organ systems affected determine the degree of laboratory abnormalities. More advanced stages of the disease are reflected by disseminated intravascular coagulation (DIC), renal insufficiency, elevated ammonia levels, and hypoglycemia. Table 15–3 reviews the effects

Table 15–2

Complications of Acute Fatty Liver of Pregnancy

Pancreatitis
Infection (iatrogenic)
Coagulopathy (DIC)
  Anemia
  Gastrointestinal bleeding
  (20–60%)
  Hemorrhage
  Vaginal bleeding
Kidney failure
  Oliguria (40–60%)
  Hyperuricemia

Liver Failure
  Acidosis
  Ascites
  Hepatic encephalopathy/coma
  Hypoglycemia
  Hypovolemia
Edema (pulmonary)
  Hypoxia

Memory aid: PICKLE

of normal pregnancy on liver function tests, and Table 15–4 summarizes the expected laboratory abnormalities in a patient with AFLP.

Diagnostic imaging for AFLP includes computed tomography (CT), in which fatty infiltration of the liver is revealed as diffuse, low-density areas, and magnetic resonance imaging (MRI), in which the same areas are recorded with increased signal intensity. Although ultrasonography is not helpful in making the diagnosis of AFLP, its usefulness is in eliminating other more

Table 15–3

Effect of Normal Pregnancy on Liver Function Tests

Values *not affected* by normal pregnancy
  Aminotransferases (AST/SGOT, ALT/SGPT)
  Gamma-glutamyl transpeptidase
  5′ Nucleotidase
  Lactic dehydrogenase
  Prothrombin time

Values *decreased* in normal pregnancy
  Albumin (↓ 30% by term)

Values *elevated* in normal pregnancy
  Alkaline phosphatase (↑ twofold)
  Bilirubin (1.0 mg/dL)
  Globulins
  Cholesterol (↑ 20–60%)
  Fibrinogen (↑ 50%)
  Transferrin

Table 15-4

Expected Laboratory Abnormalities in AFLP

Biochemical
- ↑ Alkaline phosphatase
- ↑ Ammonia
- ↑ Amylase
- ↑ Bilirubin (usually <10 mg/dL)
- ↑ BUN (as high as 50–100 mg/dL)
- ↑ Creatinine
- ↑ Amniotransferases (usually <500 U/mL)
- ↑ Uric acid

Hematologic
- Abnormal peripheral smear (normoblasts, target cells, basophilic stippling, toxic granulations, giant platelets)
- ↓ Hematocrit/hemoglobin (anemia)
- ↓ Antithrombin III (<10% activity)
- ↓ Clotting factors
- ↑ Fibrin split products
- ↓ Fibrinogen
- ↓ Platelets
- ↑ Prothrombin & partial thromboplastin times
- ↑ WBC count (20,000–30,000/μL)

Urinalysis
- ↓ Creatinine clearance
- ↑ Proteinuria
- ↓ Urine sodium
- ↑ Urobilinogen

common hepatobiliary causes of jaundice such as biliary obstruction.

The definitive diagnosis of AFLP is made by liver biopsy. Biopsy, however, is contraindicated with evidence of coagulopathy and should be reserved for making the diagnosis when the course of disease is atypical.

■ Differential Diagnosis

Table 15–5 presents a comparison of the common liver diseases of pregnancy. The clinical presentation and laboratory results in AFLP may be difficult to distinguish from those of preeclampsia. In fact, preeclampsia may be superimposed on AFLP in 30% of cases. Both entities may present with hypertension, edema, proteinuria, coagulopathy, elevated transaminase values, and

Table 15-5

Liver Disease During Pregnancy: A Clinical Comparison of Relevant Disorders

	Acute Viral Hepatitis	Thrombotic Thrombocytopenia Purpura	HELLP Syndrome/ Preeclampsia/Eclampsia	Fatty Liver of Pregnancy
Onset (trimester)	Variable	Usually post partum; late II, early III	II/III (after 20th week)	III; usually after 35th week
Clinical findings	Malaise, nausea/vomiting, jaundice	Nausea/vomiting (30%), abdominal pain (30%), hypertension, Fever (~ 102°F), altered mental status, neurologic symptoms (almost 100%)	Hypertension, edema, proteinuria, nausea, abdominal pain, jaundice, ± convulsions, oliguria, coagulopathy	Nausea, vomiting, abdominal pain, jaundice, confusion, coma, ± fever, ± hemorrhage, ± preeclampsia
Laboratory				
Transaminase	↑↑ > 1000	± ↑	Slight to 100 × ↑	Slight to 10 × ↑
Alkaline phosphatase	↑		2–3 × ↑	Up to 10 × ↑
Bilirubin (mg/dL)	↑ 5–40×	↑ (Unconj.)	≤ 10.0 (unconj.)	Up to 30 × ↑
Prothrombin time	± ↑	Normal	± ↓	2 × ↑
Other	⊕ Hepatitis serology; → antithrombin III	± ↑ WBC, schistocytes, normoblasts, thrombocytopenia <50,000; creatinine normal to 5 × ↑; ± proteinuria; ± ↑ uric acid; normal antithrombin III; subendothelial and intraluminal hyaline consisting of platelets and fibrin (skin or gingival biopsy)	↓ Antithrombin III activity, microangiopathic hemolysis, proteinuria, thrombocytopenia, ↑ uric acid, ↑ BUN, creatinine	↑ Ammonia; ↓ antithrombin III activity; ↑ WBC (20,000–30,000); hypoglycemia; thrombocytopenia, coagulopathy; ↑ uric acid; proteinuria; ↑ BUN, creatinine
Liver biopsy	Marked inflammation and necrosis	Unknown	Periportal fibrin deposits, hemorrhagic hepatocellular necrosis and inflammation	Centrilobular microvesicular fat, cholestasis
Treatment	Supportive therapy	Fresh-frozen plasma, plasma exchange therapy, antiplatelet agents (dipyridamole, aspirin), prednisone	$MgSO_4$, antihypertensive agents, may require delivery	Immediate delivery, supportive care
Perinatal mortality	Minimal ↑	← ↑	Moderate ↑	Marked ↑
Maternal mortality	Minimal ↑	Unknown	Moderate ↑	Marked ↑
Recurrence in subsequent pregnancy	No	Unknown	Yes	No

⊕, positive

Table 15-5

Liver Disease During Pregnancy: A Clinical Comparison of Relevant Disorders (Continued)

	Hyperemesis Gravidarum	Hemolytic Uremic Syndrome	Intrahepatic Cholestasis	Hepatic Hemorrhage
Onset (trimester)	I	Variable	III	III
Clinical findings	Nausea/vomiting, ± jaundice	Nausea/vomiting (almost 100%), hypertension (more common than with TTP), acute renal failure	Pruritus, ± jaundice	Nausea/vomiting, acute abdominal pain, jaundice, usually associated w/ preeclampsia/HELLP
Laboratory				
Transaminase	3 × ↑ (≤ 200)	± ↑	5 × ↑ (< 250)	≤500 or ↑ ↑ transaminases
Alkaline phosphatase	2 × ↑	—	7-10 × ↑ (≤ 1000)	—
Bilirubin (mg/dL)	≤3.5	↑ (unconj.)	<5.0	—
Prothrombin time	Normal	—	2 × ↑	—
Other	+ Ketones, electrolyte abnormalities, occasional ↑ thyroid function tests	± ↑ WBC, schistocytes, normoblasts, thrombocytopenia, ↑ creatinine, ± proteinuria, ↑ uric acid	Bile acids 10–100 × ↑	Anemia, thrombocytopenia, proteinuria
Liver biopsy	Normal	Unknown	Centrolobular cholestasis	Normal
Treatment	Supportive	Fresh-frozen plasma, plasma exchange, hemodialysis, antiplatelet agents (dipyridamole, aspirin), prednisone	Cholestyramine, phenobarbital, vitamin K, aluminum-containing antacids, corticosteroids	Conservative therapy for nonprogressive hematoma, may require surgery
Perinatal mortality	No ↑	↑	Minimal ↑	↑
Maternal mortality	No ↑	↑	No ↑	↑
Recurrence in subsequent pregnancy	Yes	Unknown	Yes	No

renal insufficiency. Preeclampsia usually has a more insidious onset, whereas AFLP presents more acutely, with sudden nausea and vomiting in 75% of cases, right upper quadrant pain in 50% to 60% of cases, and jaundice in more than 70%. In contrast, only 40% of patients with preeclampsia present with nausea and vomiting or right upper quadrant pain. In addition, only 20% of patients with preeclampsia experience clinically apparent jaundice. It is important to differentiate AFLP and preeclampsia/HELLP (*h*emolytic anemia, *e*levated *l*iver function tests, and *l*ow *p*latelets) syndrome from liver diseases of other causes, since delivery is curative with these conditions.

Fulminant viral hepatitis and AFLP may present with similar clinical manifestations; however, hepatitis can occur in any trimester, is usually associated with much higher serum transaminase values, and can be diagnosed definitively with serologic studies.

Cholestasis of pregnancy is also more common during the third trimester; however, pruritus is the more characteristic symptom and serum transaminase and serum bilirubin measurements are less dramatically elevated. There is often a family history or similar syndrome with the use of oral contraceptives. Seventy to eighty percent of jaundice in pregnancy is due to hepatitis or cholestasis of pregnancy.

AFLP is also difficult to distinguish from thrombotic thrombocytopenic purpura (TTP), since four of the five characteristics of TTP (fever, thrombocytopenia, CNS symptoms, renal impairment, microangiopathic hemolytic anemia) may also be observed with AFLP. Coombs' test–negative microangiopathic hemolytic anemia is not present in AFLP. Proteinuria and hypertension may occur with TTP; however, clotting abnormalities are absent, antithrombin III activity is normal, and renal abnormalities are less striking (BUN $\leq$ 40 mg/dL and creatinine $\leq$ 3 mg/dL).

Renal impairment is the principal feature seen with hemolytic uremic syndrome (HUS). Secondary hypertension can create a clinical picture similar to that of preeclampsia or AFLP.

Gastrointestinal symptoms are encountered in the majority of patients with HUS; in contrast, only 30% of TTP patients present with nausea, vomiting, or abdominal pain. Similar symptoms may occur in 50% to 75% of patients with AFLP. Coagulopathy and CNS symptoms are not typical of HUS.

■ Management

The primary therapy for AFLP is delivery of the fetus with attentive, supportive intensive care (Table 15–6). The mode of delivery is determined by the following considerations:

Table 15–6

ABCs of Management of AFLP

A dmit to intensive care unit

B reathing:	If comatose, provide a secure airway and maintain effective ventilation. Evaluate arterial blood gas. Provide supplemental oxygen as needed.
C NS:	Decrease endogenous ammonia by: • Protein restriction (dietary) • Neomycin 6–12 gm/d PO to decrease presence of ammonia-producing bacteria • Magnesium citrate 30–50 mL PO or enema to evacuate nitrogenous wastes from colon
D IC:	Correct coagulopathy with vitamin K, fresh-frozen plasma, packed RBCs, or platelets (see Chapters 2 and 4)
E lectrolytes:	Correct abnormalities (see Chapter 27)
F luids:	Dextrose 20% to 25% by NG or IV to provide 2000–2400 cal/24 hr & correct hypoglycemia (maintain serum glucose >60 mg%). (dextrose 20%, 125 mL/hr, gives 1980 cal/24 hr)
G I:	Prevent GI hemorrhage with antacids, citric acid solution, 30 mL q6hr; H_2 blockers (ranitidine, 50 mg IV q 6–8 hr, or cimetidine 30 mg IV q 6–8 hr); sucralfate 1 gm PO q6hr (& correction of coagulopathy)
H epatic:	Avoid medications that require hepatic metabolism (e.g., general anesthesia, narcotics)
I nfection:	Aggressive surveillance for and treatment of nosocomial infections: • Pneumonia from aspiration or ventilator contamination • Urosepsis from indwelling bladder catheter • Bacteremia from prolonged IV catheter • Consider prophylactic antibiotics
J oint effort care team:	Consult internal medicine, nephrology, and gastroenterology
K idneys:	Maintain urine output (≥0.5 mL/kg/hr) Avoid hypovolemia Consider hemodialysis
L aboratory tests (see Table 15–4)	Frequency of assessment is dictated by clinical condition of patient. DELIVER THE FETUS!

1. Maternal and fetal status.
2. Fetal size and presentation.
3. Favorability of the patient's cervix for induction of labor.
4. Maternal coagulation status.
5. Presence or absence of cerebral edema.
6. Anticipated duration of labor.

If clinically feasible, vaginal delivery should be effected to mini-mize the risk of complications known to be associated with surgical delivery. Should cesarean delivery become necessary and if the hypocoagulable state of the patient precludes conduc-tion anesthesia, general anesthetic agents that are not hepato-toxic should be used. Continued patient deterioration despite successful delivery and supportive care is extremely uncommon. Exchange transfusion, hemodialysis, plasmapheresis, extracor-poreal perfusion, and liver transplantation should be considered as alternative adjunctive treatments in these circumstances.

■
Bibliography

Duff P: Acute fatty liver of pregnancy. *In* Clark SL, Cohen DB, Hankins GDV, et al (eds): Critical Care Obstetrics, ed 2. Boston: Blackwell Scientific Publications, 1991.

Schorr-Lesnick B, Lebovics E, Dworkin B, et al: Liver diseases unique to pregnancy. Am J Gastroenterol 1991; 86:659–670.

Sims HF, Brackett JC, Powell CK, et al: The molecular basis of pediatric long chain 3-hydroxyacyl-CoA dehydrogenase deficiency associated with maternal acute fatty liver of pregnancy. Proc Natl Acad Sci USA 1995; 92:841–845.

Watson WJ, Seeds JW: Acute fatty liver of pregnancy. Obstet Gynecol Survey 1990; 45:585–593.

HARRY S. TAMM

16

Neurologic Emergencies During Pregnancy

A variety of neurologic emergencies occur during pregnancy, but many are secondary to uncommon diseases that obstetricians are unlikely to encounter in practice. In this chapter I focus on three common disorders: seizures, stroke, and intracerebral hemorrhage.

■ Seizure Disorders

Seizures affect 1% to 2% of the population and can usually be well controlled with appropriate medication. Nevertheless, they represent a significant cause of obstetric morbidity. The threat they pose to both mother and fetus is a dilemma for which there are only incomplete solutions.

Most women with epilepsy have to cope with the consequences of their disease for a lifetime. Pregnancy, however, causes added anxiety because it puts a second—dependent—life in jeopardy. A humane therapeutic approach requires that the physician address the mother's fears in a direct and considerate fashion. The importance of such candor and concern should not be underestimated.

Women can be told that although the course of established seizures in pregnancy cannot be predicted with certainty, their seizure frequency during the preceding 9 months is the best indicator. If they have been seizure free during this period, the risk is significantly diminished.

Knowledge of changes in antiepileptic drug pharmacokinetics during pregnancy is crucial. During this time, plasma clearances of most drugs increase, probably owing to a combination of decreased gastrointestinal absorption and increased hepatic metabolism. If levels are not carefully monitored, uncontrolled seizures may occur, even in women who were previously asymptomatic.

Seizures pose a potentially greater threat to the fetus than to the mother. The most intuitively obvious concerns are those related to changes in placental hemodynamics and oxygenation that occur during generalized tonic-clonic seizures, in addition to the threat of direct physical trauma. Less obvious but equally serious is the risk posed by a variety of antiepileptic drugs.

Fetal malformations more commonly occur during first trimester in utero exposure to antiepileptic medication, but the risk of malformations is increased for children of epileptic mothers, independent of drug exposure. This fact affects treatment decisions, which must therefore be tailored more to the individual than to any defined "recipe."

The most commonly reported malformations are finger and nail hypoplasia, orofacial clefts, and dysmorphic facies. Whereas similar changes were once referred to as the "fetal hydantoin syndrome," it is now understood that these features are not specific to phenytoin, and can occur with exposure to many different agents. Two drugs, however, are distinctively teratogenic. Trimethadione, a little used antiepileptic, causes a well-described dysmorphic syndrome, and sodium valproate causes neural tube defects in 1% to 2% of children whose mothers receive it during the first trimester of pregnancy.

In practice, it is probably best for mothers with incompletely controlled convulsive seizures to continue taking anticonvulsants throughout pregnancy. If they have been seizure free for 2 years before pregnancy and have normal electroencephalograms (EEGs), a case can be made for attempting discontinuation, but relative risks must be clearly outlined. When medications are to be continued, valproate should be avoided during the first trimester if possible, and because higher malformation rates and morbidity are associated with the use of multiple antiepileptic agents, drug regimens should be simplified. Specifically, patients should be maintained with the smallest doses of the fewest medications that control seizures. Monotherapy is extremely desirable. Additionally, since antiepileptics interfere with folate availability and decreased folate stores are associated with higher malformation rates, supplemental folic acid (0.5–1.0 mg/day) should be administered. Adjustments in medication dosage depend on changes in measured drug levels and clinical course. Table 16–1 lists common antiepileptic drugs and their indications.

■
Status Epilepticus

Generalized status epilepticus occurs most often in patients with known seizures who either fail to take their medications prop-

Table 16–1

Commonly Used Antiepileptic Medications

Drug	Indications	Usual Dosage	Pharmacokinetics in Pregnancy	Therapeutic Level (μg/mL)
Carbamazepine (Tegretol)	Generalized tonic-clonic seizures, partial simple and complex seizures, secondary generalized seizures	400–1200 mg in two or three divided doses	Total levels decrease late in pregnancy, but free levels do not	4–10
Phenytoin (Dilantin)	Generalized tonic-clonic seizures, partial simple and complex seizures, secondary generalized seizures, status epilepticus	300–600 mg/d as single dose	Increased clearance can result in increased dose requirements	10–20 (free phenytoin level 1–2)
Phenobarbital	Generalized tonic-clonic seizures	60–240 mg/d as single dose	Plasma clearance can increase	10–35
Divalproex sodium (Depakote)	Absence seizures	500–2500 mg/d in two or three divided doses	Not known	50–100
Gabapentin (Neurontin)	Partial simple seizures, partial complex seizures, secondary generalized seizures	900–1800 mg/d in three divided doses	Varies with creatinine clearance	Not followed routinely

erly or who suffer a superimposed insult that triggers an exacer-bation. Alteration of antiepileptic drug metabolism during preg-nancy is another possible explanation.

Status epilepticus is truly a life-threatening emergency, and treatment must be instituted and carried through with an eye to the clock, since the likelihood of long-term adverse central nervous system consequences increases with the interval until control is achieved.

The principal threat of generalized status epilepticus is lactic acidosis and cardiovascular instability, but prolonged seizures can also result in irreversible—and sometimes devastating—brain injury as a result of both hypoxia and cellular changes induced by prolonged electrical excitability. Early diagnosis is critical. The initial goal of therapy is to establish a stable airway and adequate intravenous access. Diagnostic studies, including drug levels in previously treated patients, additional blood work for metabolic abnormalities, computed tomography (CT) or magnetic resonance imaging (MRI) brain scan, lumbar puncture, and EEG are performed when appropriate to exclude a revers-ible superimposed disorder whose treatment might include mea-sures other than antiepileptic medication. Examples of such disorders are hypoglycemia, meningitis, and intracerebral hem-orrhage. The importance of rapid administration of medication cannot be overstated. A suggested timetable for the treatment of status epilepticus is summarized in Table 16–2.

■ Stroke

The treatment of stroke remains an enigma for neurologists. In the past, most attention focused on the issue of anticoagulation. Today, anticoagulation is the treatment of choice for a limited number of stroke mechanisms. In the majority of cases, however, it does not improve outcome. The thrust of current research concerns thrombolytic and "neuroprotective" agents. Thrombo-lytic agents may have a short therapeutic window. Neuroprotec-tive agents appear to have greater promise, since logic would suggest that treatment can be successful even when initiated some time after the ictus. These drugs are intended to prevent the cascade of biochemical events that lead to neuronal death. Nevertheless, as a practical matter, diagnosis and timely treat-ment are the most important tenets in the context of pregnancy.

Doctors in other specialties tend to take the "a stroke is a stroke" approach to this disease, but, clearly, proper treatment

From Epilepsy Foundation of America: Treatment of status epilepticus. JAMA 1993; 270:854–859.

Table 16–2

Suggested Timetable for the Treatment of Status Epilepticus

Time, Minutes	Action
0–5	Diagnose status epilepticus by observing continued seizure activity or one additional seizure.
	Give oxygen by nasal cannula or mask; position patient's head for optimal airway patency; consider intubation if respiratory assistance is needed.
	Obtain and record vital signs at onset and periodically thereafter; control any abnormalities as necessary; initiate EEG monitoring.
	Establish IV line; draw venous blood samples for glucose level, serum chemistries, hematology studies, toxicology screens, and determination of antiepileptic drug levels.
6–9	If hypoglycemia is established or a blood glucose determination is not available, administer glucose. In adults, give 100 mg of thiamine first, followed by 50 mL of 50% glucose by direct push into the IV. In children, the dose of glucose is 2 mg/kg of 25% glucose.
10–20	Administer either 0.1 mg/kg of lorazepam at 2 mg/min or 0.2 mg/kg of diazepam at 5 mg/min by IV. If diazepam is given, it can be repeated if seizures do not stop after 5 minutes. If diazepam is used to stop the status, phenytoin should be administered next to prevent recurrent status.
21–60	If status persists, administer 15–20 mg/kg of phenytoin no faster than 50 mg/min in adults and 1 mg/kg/min in children by IV; monitor ECG and blood pressure during infusion. Phenytoin is incompatible with glucose-containing solutions. The IV should be purged with normal saline before the phenytoin infusion.
>60	If status does not stop after 20 mg/kg of phenytoin, give additional doses of 5 mg/kg to a maximum of dose of 30 mg/kg. If status persists, give 20 mg/kg of phenobarbital by IV at 100 mg/min. When phenobarbital is given after benzodiazepine, the risk of apnea or hypopnea is great and assisted ventilation is usually required. If status persists, give anesthetic dose of drugs such as phenobarbital or pentobarbital; ventilatory assistance and vasopressors are virtually always necessary.

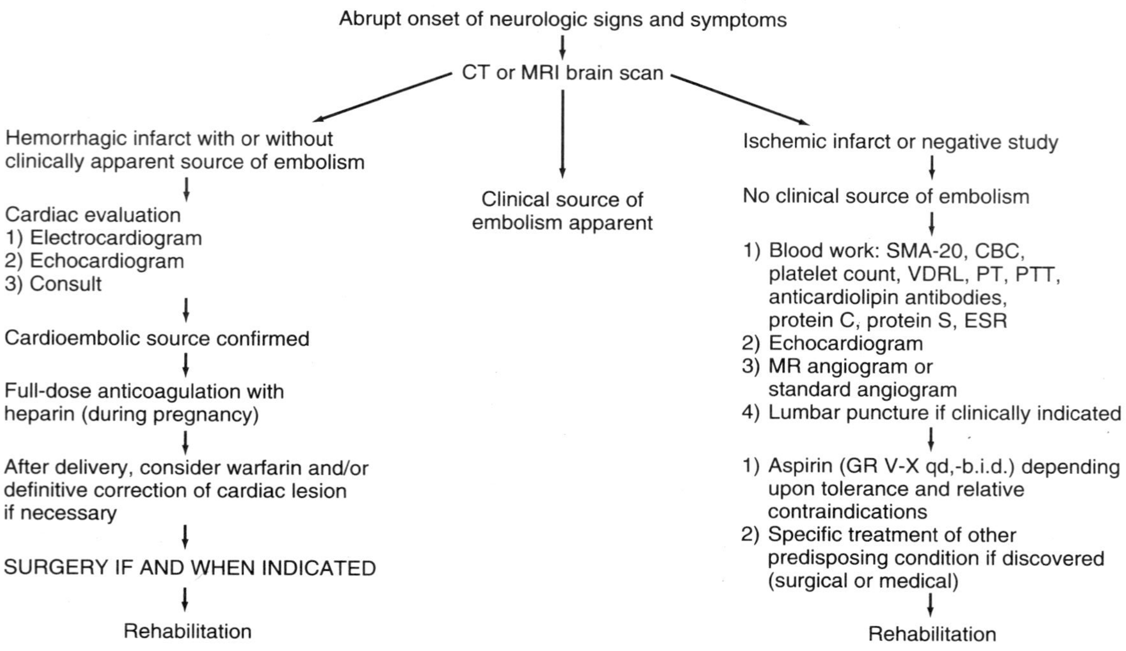

Abrupt onset of neurologic signs and symptoms

CT or MRI brain scan

Hemorrhagic infarct with or without clinically apparent source of embolism

Cardiac evaluation
1) Electrocardiogram
2) Echocardiogram
3) Consult

Cardioembolic source confirmed

Full-dose anticoagulation with heparin (during pregnancy)

After delivery, consider warfarin and/or definitive correction of cardiac lesion if necessary

SURGERY IF AND WHEN INDICATED

Rehabilitation

Clinical source of embolism apparent

Ischemic infarct or negative study

No clinical source of embolism

1) Blood work: SMA-20, CBC, platelet count, VDRL, PT, PTT, anticardiolipin antibodies, protein C, protein S, ESR
2) Echocardiogram
3) MR angiogram or standard angiogram
4) Lumbar puncture if clinically indicated

1) Aspirin (GR V-X qd,-b.i.d.) depending upon tolerance and relative contraindications
2) Specific treatment of other predisposing condition if discovered (surgical or medical)

Rehabilitation

Figure 16-1   Algorithm for treatment of stroke.

requires an understanding of the pathophysiologic mechanism, and varies accordingly. The classic approach to stroke has been to divide it into three categories: thrombotic, embolic, and hemorrhagic. Since hemorrhagic infarct is almost always embolic and is a different lesion from that of intracerebral hemorrhage, only the first two mechanisms are discussed here. Figure 16–1 provides a general algorithm for treatment of stroke.

■ Thrombotic Stroke

Thrombotic stroke cannot be distinguished with certainty utilizing clinical parameters, though its greater likelihood can be assumed in the absence of associated valvular heart disease (not including mitral prolapse). Its most common cause is atherosclerosis, which is uncommon in the obstetric population. Certain common diseases and environmental factors may increase the risk, however. These include hypertension, diabetes, hypercholesterolemia, drug exposure (e.g., cocaine), infection, collagen vascular disease, smoking, and alcohol abuse. In addition, there is a group of relatively rare coagulation disturbances collectively known as the "antiphospholipid antibody syndrome" (lupus anticoagulant, anticardiolipin antibody) that can be operative in this age group and whose presence should therefore be considered. Table 16–3 summarizes the common causes of thrombotic stroke during pregnancy.

Whereas diagnosis is usually simple, requiring only a good history and physical examination plus brain CT or MRI (findings are often negative during the first 24 hours), treatment depends

---

Table 16–3

Common Causes of Thrombotic Stroke in Pregnancy

> Hypertension
> Diabetes
> Hypercholesterolemia
> Drug exposure (e.g., cocaine)
> Infection
> Collagen vascular disease
> Smoking
> Alcohol abuse
> Antiphospholipid antibody syndrome

to an extent on identification of risk factors previously described. Certain general principles still apply.

Simple stroke without intracranial hypertension does not represent a threat to the fetus, and primary attention needs to be given to the mother. Secondary vascular instability would constitute the exception to this rule. When the diagnosis is confirmed, close attention should be paid to a number of simple matters. Since cerebral autoregulation is altered after a stroke, measures should be taken to ensure that the ischemic area is maximally perfused. Until 24 hours of neurologic stability has been documented by examination, the patient should be kept as flat as possible in bed. Though there is uncertainty about this issue, it is probably best to monitor blood sugar values and to attempt to keep them below 120 mg/dL. In addition, blood pressure is an important treatable parameter. In the context of eclampsia, there is good reason for concern about allowing it to reach dangerously high levels. Absent this disorder, higher pressures are preferable, as they improve cerebral perfusion. Indeed, systolic pressures of 180 to 200 mm Hg are tolerated well in this circumstance, assuming the caveat for eclampsia, with its risk for intracerebral hemorrhage, is observed.

The use of heparin in acute thrombotic stroke is unwarranted. It has no proven value in this setting for any of the mechanisms described and does not lessen the ultimate neurologic deficit. Its use carries increased risk of hemorrhagic conversion of bland infarction, and it should be avoided. Though warfarin is likely effective in preventing recurrence in women with antiphospholipid antibody syndrome, it is potentially teratogenic, and the decision to treat must be individualized.

■
Embolic Stroke

Embolic stroke (infarction) most often occurs in the setting of known valvular heart disease, cardiomyopathy, or cardiac rhythm disturbance. Atrial fibrillation is a frequently predisposing rhythm, even in the absence of valvular dysfunction. Intravenous drug users are especially at risk for bacterial endocarditis, but in an age of immunosuppression, less virulent organisms need to be considered under appropriate circumstances.

While it is likely that a careful physical examination will expose a murmur or abnormal rhythm, silent lesions also occur in young people, and cardiac consultation with echocardiography may be required to exclude entities such as atrial myxoma and septal defect predisposing to paradoxical embolus.

The approach to embolic stroke is essentially the same as that for thrombosis, once the diagnosis has been established. When there is a cardiac source of clot, however, anticoagulation becomes more important. It should be reemphasized that heparinization does nothing to improve the outcome of a stroke that has already occurred. Its utility is in the prevention of recurrence. Since the risk of hemorrhagic conversion is as high as 20%, caution should be the watchword of decision making. Indeed, conversion can result in development of intracranial hypertension and can be life threatening. If the infarct is small (lacunar or occupying the territory of a small branch vessel) and blood pressure is controlled, then heparin is safe, and it should be started. If the infarct is large, use of full dose anticoagulation with heparin should be delayed for 7 to 10 days. Since hemorrhage usually occurs as a result of reflow into the infarcted area, this delay allows repair of injured vascular endothelium. Aspirin is less effective than heparin or warfarin for prevention but those who cannot take these drugs can still use it and expect to benefit.

■
Intracerebral Hemorrhage

Intracerebral hemorrhage differs from hemorrhagic stroke in that it represents release of blood into a normal brain rather than one that has previously suffered an infarct. Like stroke, it has many causes and certain distinctive clinical features. In pregnant women it is often seen in the context of eclampsia, and that diagnosis should be considered when the timing and clinical findings are suggestive, but other causes will be discussed. Table 16–4 summarizes the common causes of intracerebral hemorrhage during pregnancy.

Table 16–4

Common Causes of Intracerebral Hemorrhage in Pregnancy

Ruptured berry aneurysm (usually occurring in late trimester; age >30) and subarachnoid in location

Ruptured arteriovenous malformation (usually occurring in early trimester <20 wk; age <25), intracerebral in location

Hypertension: preeclampsia-induced hemorrhage usually appears in the deep hemispheric gray matter (thalamus, putamen, globus pallidus), pons, and cerebellum

Intracerebral hemorrhage presents abruptly, but its onset is more frequently heralded by headache than is stroke. Focal findings such as hemiparesis or aphasia may predominate early, but signs of intracranial hypertension are the key to the diagnosis. Signs of particular importance include papilledema, altered level of consciousness, changes in respiratory pattern (e.g., Cheyne-Stokes), bilaterality (quadriparesis, diffuse hyperreflexia, upgoing toes), and pathologic motor activity (flexor or extensor posturing). Diagnostic impressions can be confirmed with non-contrast brain CT, which is the most useful tool in this regard because it is simple, is tolerated well, and is without risk as long as the fetus is protected from radiation exposure.

The most common causes of intracerebral hemorrhage include ruptured berry aneurysm, ruptured arteriovenous malformation (AVM), and hypertension (pregnancy-induced or of other causes). Berry aneurysm frequently presents with subarachnoid, rather than intracerebral, hemorrhage. Manifestations then include headache, nausea, vomiting, and stiff neck. CT makes the distinction. Since early rebleeding is associated with a mortality rate of 40 to 60%, rapid treatment of the offending lesion is paramount. Angiography confirms the presence of the aneurysm, which should be surgically repaired as quickly as possible. The presence of an intracerebral hematoma and intracranial hypertension may well delay surgery because of unacceptable morbidity and mortality for the mother. At the same time, it is important to consider the threat to the fetus. If the fetus is independently viable, delivery may be a reasonable option. Earlier on in the pregnancy, however, the risks to the fetus are the anesthetic and hemodynamic effects, but generally, modern techniques protect the child and neurosurgery should not be delayed if the mother's life is in jeopardy.

Ruptured AVM threatens the mother when the hemorrhage is large and intracranial hypertension occurs. When the hemorrhage is smaller, however, and the only deficit is focal, a more conservative approach can be followed. Though brain CT or MRI may well demonstrate the vascular abnormality, cerebral angiography is still needed for accurate definition of the lesion. In this setting, risk of rebleeding is considerably less than that of aneurysm, and it is perfectly reasonable, if the patient is stable, to offer supportive care and delay surgical correction until a time deemed optimally safe for both mother and child.

The approach to supportive care for these two entities is somewhat different. After surgical correction of an aneurysm that has resulted in subarachnoid hemorrhage, systolic pressures of up to 200 mm Hg are acceptable because they play a role in the prevention of possibly fatal vasospasm. Simultaneous administration of the calcium channel blocker nimodipine is a standard of therapy. In the case of a ruptured AVM, when the primary lesion is intracerebral blood, an attempt should be made to normalize blood pressures. Hypotension, on the other hand, may lead to ischemic brain injury and should be avoided. Systolic pressures in the 120- to 140-mm Hg range are generally acceptable.

Hypertensive intracerebral hemorrhage can usually be distinguished from its relatives by its appearance on CT. The diagnosis is often difficult to distinguish on clinical grounds, and since all of these entities are associated with secondary blood pressure elevations, the observation of hypertension is not, by itself, useful. These bleeds, whether the result of pregnancy-induced hypertension or not, tend to occur in specific locations, including the deep hemispheric gray matter (thalamus, putamen, globus pallidus), pons, and cerebellum. The only site for which surgical intervention has been consistently effective is the cerebellum, and, there, rapid decompression before the onset of irreversible secondary brain stem compression is an emergent need. Before surgery, and with hemorrhage in the other locations, treatment is medical and the most important issue is control of intracranial hypertension.

With hypertensive intracerebral hemorrhage, blood pressure control is an obvious concern and the approach is the same as that for ruptured AVM. Overcontrol, however, can lead to inadequate cerebral perfusion and more extensive deficits. Undercontrol, while undesirable, does not as a rule lead to an increase in hemorrhage size or to rebleeding. These hemorrhages are the result of the rupture of small, deep penetrating cerebral vessels, and the bleed itself tends to tamponade the vessels so that these are one-time events of very brief duration.

A treatment algorithm for intracerebral hemorrhage is provided in Figure 16–2. Please note that less common mechanisms—such as bleeding dyscrasias, sickle cell disease, and embolic choriocarcinoma—are not addressed and would require a more individualized approach.

■
Miscellaneous Neurologic Conditions

Several other neurologic diseases that might lead to emergent situations in the obstetrics population deserve brief mention in

Abrupt onset headache, focal symptoms, deteriorating level of consciousness

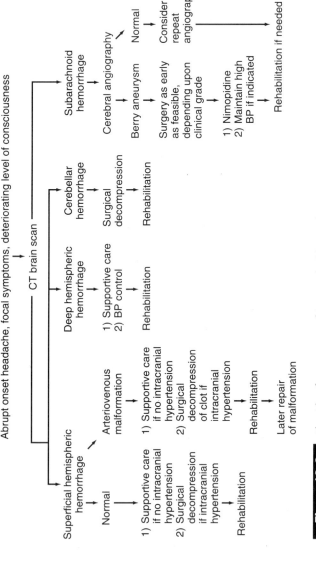

Figure 16-2   Algorithm for treatment of intracerebral hemorrhage.

this chapter. These are multiple sclerosis, Guillain-Barré syndrome, and myasthenia gravis.

Multiple sclerosis is a common neurologic diagnosis that tends to affect women more frequently than men. Its course during pregnancy is variable, and, like the disease itself, unpredictable. Still, most women can deliver successfully, and it would be unfortunate to advise a woman who wants children to avoid pregnancy because of this disease. Because no treatment is fully proven, most neurologists take a symptomatic approach, and caution must be exercised with the use of potentially teratogenic medications. Acute exacerbations are often treated with steroids. In the last two years, two new preventive agents, interferon beta 1A and 1B, have been approved, and it is likely that we will begin to see discussions of their impact on pregnancy. Though their effects on the human fetus are not known, they have a dose-related abortifacient effect on rhesus monkeys, and patients need to be aware of this fact.

Myasthenia gravis is less common than multiple sclerosis but is sometimes encountered in obstetric practice. Its course is not predictably altered by pregnancy, and standard medications, with the exception of the immunosuppressive agent azathioprine, do not adversely affect the fetus. On the other hand, magnesium sulfate, a neuromuscular blocker, can precipitate a myasthenic crisis. Offspring should be monitored closely for the development of neonatal myasthenia. Fortunately, this is a transient disorder that disappears as acetylcholine receptor antibody levels decrease.

The incidence of *Guillain-Barré syndrome,* an acute polyradiculoneuropathy that rapidly leads to quadriparesis—and occasionally to respiratory failure—is not increased during pregnancy, nor should pregnancy affect the standard approach to treatment. This includes control of autonomic instability (principally blood pressure), ventilatory support when needed, and either plasmapheresis or intravenous immunoglobulin therapy. These modalities should not pose any serious threat to the fetus.

■ Maternal and Fetal Operative Concerns

Obstetricians are rightly concerned about conditions that could adversely affect a fetus during neurosurgical repair of lesions that cause intracranial hypertension. These most frequently include aneurysm, AVM, and intracerebral hemorrhage itself. In the operating suite, treatment consists of inducing controlled hypotension and hypothermia. Experience would indicate that

Table 16–5

Summary of Maternal and Fetal Operative Concerns

Controlled hypothermia generally is tolerated well by the fetus.
Controlled hypotensive anesthesia may adversely affect the fetus.
  Consider delivery of near-term fetus before neurosurgery.
  Otherwise, employ intraoperative fetal monitoring and manipulate
  blood pressure to improve fetal oxygen delivery as perceived
  appropriate.
Reserve cesarean delivery for obstetric indications only.

hypothermia is tolerated well by the fetus and need not be considered a serious threat. Medically induced controlled hypotension, however, can adversely affect the fetus. If the fetus could be delivered with the expectation of excellent survival and low morbidity from prematurity (see Chapter 26), delivery before maternal neurosurgical repair would be advisable. In other circumstances, however, as long as close fetal monitoring is maintained during the operative procedure and rapid response is initiated in the form of blood pressure control to facilitate improved fetal oxygen delivery, the fetus generally does well.

In the same setting, the question of cesarean section versus vaginal delivery is also a legitimate one. Investigators have suggested that because the physiologic blood pressure increases associated with the stresses of labor and delivery are counterbalanced by parallel increases in cerebrospinal fluid pressure, the overall transluminal vascular pressure is unchanged. Therefore, vaginal delivery, utilizing epidural anesthesia and outlet forceps to shorten the second stage of labor, appears to offer no additional neurologic risk over elective cesarean section. Cesarean delivery, therefore, should be reserved for obstetric indications only. Table 16–5 summarizes these operative concerns.

■
Bibliography

Donaldson JO: Neurology of Pregnancy, ed 2. London, W.B. Saunders Co. Ltd, London, 1989.

Epilepsy Foundation of America: Treatment of status epilepticus. JAMA 1993; 270:854–859.

Johnson RT, Griffin JW: Current Therapy in Neurologic Disease, ed 4. Chicago, Mosby–Year Book, 1993.

Wyllie E: The Treatment of Epilepsy, Principles and Practice. Philadelphia, Lea & Febiger, 1993.

THOMAS M. BAJO

Cardiopulmonary Resuscitation of the Pregnant Patient

A number of textbook chapters and review articles discuss cardiopulmonary resuscitation (CPR) of pregnant patients. This chapter is similar to those, but I emphasize the resuscitation of the hospitalized gravid patient whose fetus is of gestational age adequate to survive outside the mother.

Cardiopulmonary arrest is uncommon during pregnancy. The precise incidence is unknown, but it has been reported to occur once in every 30,000 pregnancies. Events so rare have resulted in no published randomized controlled clinical trials of CPR during pregnancy. Much of the information comes from animal model studies and from years of accumulated anecdotal human cases. Advanced cardiac life support (ACLS) guidelines have been developed principally for sudden death from ischemic heart disease, a relative rarity during pregnancy. Most sudden deaths in pregnancy are related to embolism, anesthesia, or cerebrovascular accidents. Medical progress has increased the number of women who successfully complete pregnancy, despite underlying medical illness. Although underlying medical illness may increase the risk of sudden death, intrapartum death most often occurs in previously healthy women. The unpredictability and rarity of sudden death during pregnancy make any preparation difficult. It is my opinion that the single most important factor in improving the survival chances of mother and baby is an *organized, time-conscious team approach*.

■ Code Arrest Team

Cardiopulmonary arrest in the labor and delivery area of the hospital tends to be a chaotic event. It is imperative that there be an organized team approach with tasks performed in a time-conscious manner. The code team will have, at minimum, these members:

    Code team leader
    Airway person
    Chest compression person
    Vascular access person
    Drug administration person
    Drug preparation person
    Event recorder
    Physician to perform cesarean delivery
    Neonatologist/pediatrician

Each individual on the team should understand his or her particular assignment. The equipment needed is that which is necessary to sustain ACLS, to perform cesarean delivery, and to resuscitate the newborn infant. It is the responsibility of the code team leader to direct team members according to the situation and to be cognizant of time since the mother's death.

■
Pathophysiology of Cardiopulmonary Arrest in Pregnancy

Cardiopulmonary arrest results in maternal and fetal injury secondary to the precipitating illness and to the dramatic decrease in nutrient supplies. The nutrient deficit most dramatically associated with tissue injury appears to be oxygen. Although, theoretically, there are many mediators of this injury, it is the dramatic reduction in oxygen delivery to the tissues that precipitates the injury.

From a most simplistic point of view, the cardiopulmonary adaptations to pregnancy allow a balanced delivery of oxygen (Do_2) to the mother's tissues and to the uterus. Analogous to the mother's circulation, the fetal cardiovascular adaptations during life in-utero allow balanced delivery of oxygen (Do_2) to the fetal tissues and delivery of blood to the umbilical and placental circulation. The uteroplacental unit is responsible for the exchange of gas from mother to fetus (Fig. 17–1). Adequate maternal and fetal tissue oxygen consumption (Vo_2) necessary to maintain tissue viability depends on maintenance of adequate gas exchange from mother to fetus and maintenance of adequate oxygen delivery (Do_2) to the tissues. Clinical experience and animal experimentation indicate that, during normal pregnancy,

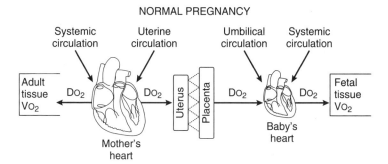

Maternal and fetal oxygen delivery during normal pregnancy.

maternal systemic and uterine oxygen delivery exceed the minimal level necessary to sustain maternal and fetal life. This allows for various maternal conditions to occur that may decrease maternal tissue and uterine oxygen delivery without affecting maternal or fetal tissue oxygen consumption.

During cardiopulmonary arrest (Fig. 17–2) oxygen delivery

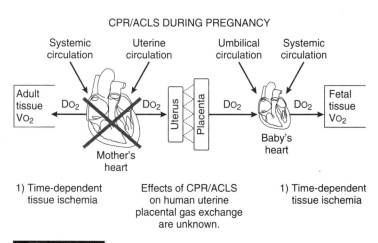

Maternal and fetal oxygen delivery during cardiopulmonary arrest.

to maternal tissues and the uterus is dramatically reduced or eliminated completely. There are few maternal or fetal adaptations to such severe reductions in oxygen delivery that allow maintenance of tissue viability. Tissue death begins in minutes.

■ Goals of Cardiopulmonary Resuscitation During Pregnancy

The principal goal of CPR is to restore spontaneous breathing and circulation quickly. This can be viewed as a two-step process, although the actual events often occur simultaneously. Once a stable rhythm is achieved, emphasis is placed on maintaining adequate oxygen delivery (Cardiac output × Arterial oxygen content), so that both maternal and fetal oxygen consumption can be maintained (Table 17–1).

It should be understood that the precipitating event leading to cardiopulmonary arrest during pregnancy is difficult to determine at the time of arrest. Additionally, as stated previously, ACLS guidelines have been designed principally for resuscitation after sudden death caused by ischemic heart disease. It is helpful to consider the arrested pregnant patient as having a severe form of shock, often with moderate or severe hypoxemic lung disease. Using the broad categories of shock as cardiogenic, hypovolemic, obstructive, and distributive provides a quick method of mentally determining the genesis of the arrest. It also

---

Table 17–1

Goals of CPR-ACLS

Establish stable rhythm
Drugs
Cardioversion
Electrical pacing

Maintain oxygen delivery (cardiac output × Cao_2)

Think	Treatment
Cardiogenic	Fluids
Hypovolemic	Drugs
Obstructive	Chest compression
Distributive	Airway/oxygen
	Other

Table 17–2

Pregnancy CPR (Ideal)

A. ACLS maneuvers should benefit mother and baby.
B. Fetal monitoring should be available.
C. Continue ACLS and deliver baby to improve maternal and fetal survival based on responses to A and B.

---

provides an opportunity to modify the ACLS guidelines based on what you think is the precipitating event.

The actual success rate of CPR during pregnancy is not known. In nonpregnant patients chest compression is estimated to result in cardiac output equal to approximately 30% of normal. It has been demonstrated in normal late pregnancy that the supine position results in decreased stroke index. This is probably secondary to inferior vena cava compression by the gravid uterus. It can be understood, then, that chest compression in the supine pregnant patient can result in dramatic decreases in oxygen delivery to maternal tissues. Additionally, similar to caval compression, gravid uterine aortic compression results in decreased uterine—and therefore decreased fetal—oxygen delivery. It is recommended that, during CPR, manual displacement of the uterus to the left be attempted. Others suggest placing the patient in 15- to 30-degrees left lateral tilt position. The latter movement makes chest compression more difficult and probably less effective.

No available studies evaluate the systemic or uterine blood flow during optimal cardiopulmonary resuscitation in pregnant humans. Ideal CPR of the pregnant patient is tempered by the reality of the situation (Tables 17–2, 17–3).

Table 17–3

Pregnancy CPR (Reality)

Code arrest is a rare event.
Precipitating event is often difficult to identify.
Difficult to predict mother's response to ACLS.
Fetal monitoring is difficult.
Need to *make time-dependent decisions* for fetal-maternal viability.
No systematic studies of CPR/ACLS on pregnant animals or humans.

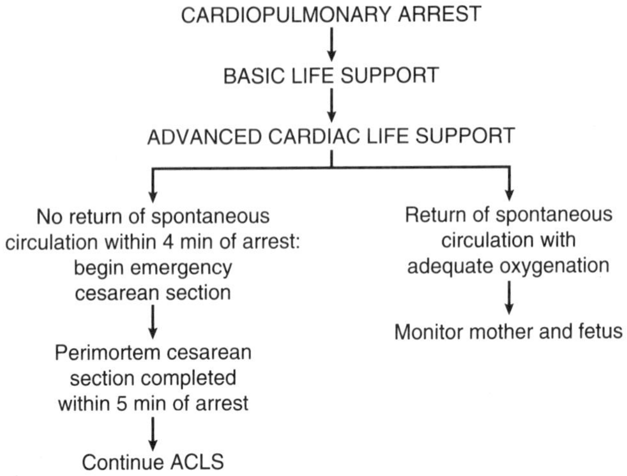

CARDIOPULMONARY ARREST
↓
BASIC LIFE SUPPORT
↓
ADVANCED CARDIAC LIFE SUPPORT

No return of spontaneous
circulation within 4 min of arrest:
begin emergency
cesarean section
↓
Perimortem cesarean
section completed
within 5 min of arrest
↓
Continue ACLS

Return of spontaneous
circulation with
adequate oxygenation
↓
Monitor mother and fetus

Figure 17–3

Summary of the basic conceptual management of maternal cardiopulmonary arrest.

Table 17–4

Interval from Death of Mother Until Perimortem Cesarean Delivery of Surviving Infants: 1900 to 1985

Interval (min)	Patients (No.)	Percent
0–5	42 normal infants	70
6–10	7 normal infants	13
	1 mild neurologic sequela	
11–15	6 normal infants	12
	1 severe neurologic sequela	1.7
16–20	1 severe neurologic sequela	
21+	2 severe neurologic sequelae	
	1 normal infant	3.3

Adapted from Katz VL, Dotters DJ, Droegemueller W: Perimortem cesarean delivery. Obstet Gynecol 1986; 68(4):511.

As stated at the beginning of this section, the goal of CPR is to restore spontaneous ventilation and circulation. If this is achieved quickly, both mother and fetus can be monitored further. The duration of CPR that can be continued without severe injury to the mother and fetus is not known. Statements such as, "Good CPR provides adequate maternal and fetal oxygen delivery" are not supported in the medical literature. If spontaneous circulation with adequate arterial oxygenation is not achieved within minutes of cardiopulmonary arrest, serious consideration needs to be given to performance of perimortem cesarean section (Figure 17–3).

■
Perimortem Cesarean Section

Perimortem cesarean section is performed to save the life of the mother and baby. Review of the published literature (Table 17–4) shows that the baby has the greatest chance of being healthy if it is delivered within 5 minutes after the mother's cardiopulmonary arrest. Additionally, both animal experimental and human clinical experience have shown that a mother's cardiovascular function can improve dramatically after emergency delivery.

Currently, the recommendation is to complete delivery of the baby by emergency cesarean section no more than 5 minutes after spontaneous circulation ceases.

Memory Aid: "The Four-Five Rule"

Begin the perimortem cesarean section 4 minutes after the mother's cardiac arrest to have the baby delivered no later than 5 minutes after cessation of spontaneous circulation.

Tables 17–5 through 17–12 review basic life support techniques and ACLS, as resources for readers.

Text continued on page 249

Table 17-5

Adult One-Rescuer CPR

1. Determine responsiveness and activate the EMS system (911)

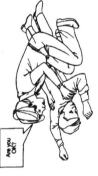

Tap or gently shake the victim and shout, "Are you OK?"

If trauma to the head and neck is visible or suspected, the victim should be moved *only if absolutely necessary.*

2. Airway

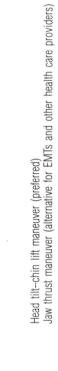

Head tilt–chin lift maneuver (preferred)

Jaw thrust maneuver (alternative for EMTs and other health care providers)

Table continued on opposite page

3. Breathing (assess 3–5 sec)

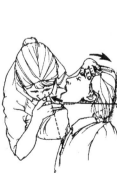

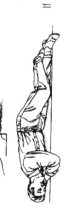

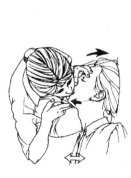

Look: For rise and fall of the chest
Listen: For air escaping during exhalation
Feel: For the flow of air

If the victim is breathing, place in the recovery position.

If the victim's airway is obstructed, follow the "foreign body–airway obstruction management" sequence.
If the victim is not breathing, *deliver two slow breaths, each lasting 1½–2 sec.*

Table continued on following page

Table 17-5

Adult One-Rescuer CPR *Continued*

4. Circulation (assess 5–10 sec)

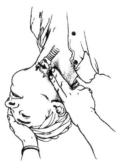

Check for a carotid pulse.

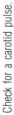

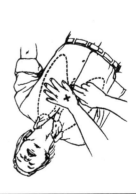

If carotid pulse is *present* but the victim is not breathing, *deliver one breath every 5–6 sec (10–12/min).*

If a carotid pulse is *absent*, begin chest compressions.
- Position hands on lower half of sternum.
- Depress sternum approximately 1½–2 in (for average adult).
- Perform 15 external chest compressions for every two ventilations at a rate of 80–100/min ("one and, two and, three and, four and,...").

Table continued on opposite page

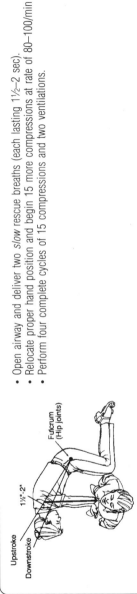

Upstroke
Downstroke
1½–2"
Fulcrum
(Hip joints)

- Open airway and deliver two *slow* rescue breaths (each lasting 1½–2 sec).
- Relocate proper hand position and begin 15 more compressions at rate of 80–100/min
- Perform four complete cycles of 15 compressions and two ventilations.

5. Reassessment

After four cycles of compressions and ventilations (15:2 ratio), reassess patient, checking the carotid pulse for 3–5 sec.

If pulse is not felt, resume CPR and reassess pulse and breathing every few minutes.

If pulse *is* present, check for breathing.

- If breathing *is* present, continue monitoring victim's pulse and breathing.
- If breathing *is not* present, continue rescue breathing at a rate of 10–12 breaths per minute and monitor pulse.

If the victim resumes breathing and regains a pulse *and trauma is not apparent or suspected*, roll victim onto his/her side so that head, shoulders, and torso move simultaneously without twisting.

6. Recovery position

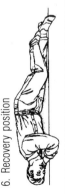

Source: American Heart Association.

Table 17-6

Asystole

CPR
Assess ventilation
Assess pulses with compressions
↓
Confirm rhythm in another lead
↓
Intubate (confirm tube placement)
Assess breath sounds
Observe chest rise
↓
Establish IV access, large-bore IV
Normal saline or lactated Ringer's
Antecubital or external jugular
↓
Consider possible causes
H(× 4)AD
*H*ypoxia
*H*ypokalemia
*H*yperkalemia
*H*ypothermia
*A*cidosis (preexisting)
*D*rug overdose
↓
Consider immediate transcutaneous pacing
↓
Epinephrine, 1 mg (1:10,000) IV q 3–5 min (or 2–2.5 mg ET) or alternative*
For ET dosing, use epinephrine, 1:1000 solution
Mix 2 mg epinephrine (2 mL) and dilute in syringe with 8 mL normal saline
↓
Atropine 1 mg IV q 3–5 min to maximum of 3 mg (or 2–2.5 mg ET)
For ET dosing, using multidose vial (0.4 mg/mL), mix 5 mL atropine with 5
mL of normal saline for 2.0-mg dose
↓
Consider termination of efforts
*Dosing Alternatives
Recommended: 1 mg q 3–5 min
Intermediate: 2–5 mg IV push, q 3–5 min
Escalating: 1 mg, 3 mg, 5 mg (IV 3 min apart)
High: 0.1 mg/kg IV push q 3–5 min

Source: The American Heart Association.

Table 17-7

Sustained Ventricular Tachycardia with a Pulse

Stable	Unstable	Pulseless
Suppress with lidocaine	"Sick" = Synchronized • Chest pain • Dyspnea • Ischemia • Infarction	"Dead" = Defibrillation Pulseless VT Pulseless, apneic
	"Dying" = Defibrillation • Hypotension • Unconscious • Pulmonary edema	Treat using VF algorithm.
ABCs, O_2, IV	ABCs, O_2, IV	Defib with 200, 200–300, 360 J
Lidocaine, 1–1½ mg/kg, may be repeated with 0.5–0.75 mg/kg q 5–10 min to max 3 mg/kg	Consider meds	
Procainamide, 20–30 mg/min, to max dose of 17 mg/kg	Administer sedation whenever possible	
Bretylium, 5–10 mg/kg infusion over 8–10 minutes	Unsynchronized countershock 100–200–300–360 J	
Synchronized countershock 100–200–300–360 J	Lidocaine, 1–1½ mg/kg	
	Unsynchronized countershock 360 J	
	After 5–10 min, lidocaine, 0.5–0.75 mg/kg... Check pulse and rhythm between each shock	

Stable column (continued):

ABCs, O_2, IV

Lidocaine, 1–1½ mg/kg, may be repeated with 0.5–0.75 mg/kg q 5–10 min to max 3 mg/kg

Procainamide, 20–30 mg/min, to max dose of 17 mg/kg

Bretylium, 5–10 mg/kg infusion over 8–10 minutes

Synchronized countershock 100–200–300–360 J

Unstable column:

Administer sedation whenever possible

Synchronized countershock 100–200–300–360 J

Lidocaine bolus (1–1½ mg/kg if initial bolus was NOT given prior to countershock, 0.5–0.75 mg/kg if initial bolus WAS given prior to countershock)

Check pulse and rhythm between each shock

IF VF occurs during the course of synchronization:
*Check pulse
*Check rhythm
*Turn off the synchronizer switch
*Defibrillate

Source: The American Heart Association.

Table 17–8

Ventricular Fibrillation Pulseless Ventricular Tachycardia

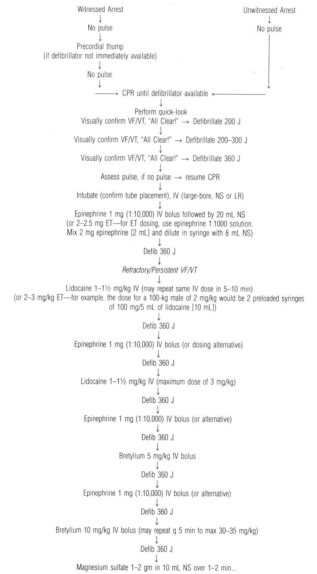

Source: The American Heart Association.

Table 17–9

Pulseless Electrical Activity (PEA)

CPR
Assess ventilation
Assess pulses with compressions
↓
Intubate (confirm tube placement)
Assess breath sounds, observe chest rise
↓
Establish IV access, large-bore IV
Normal saline or lactated Ringer's
Antecubital or external jugular
500 mL fluid challenge
↓
Assess blood **flow** using Doppler
↓
Consider underlying causes
↓

MATCH(× 5)ED

*M*yocardial Infarction (massive acute)
*A*cidosis (severe)
*T*ension pneumothorax
Peri*C*ardial tamponade
*H*ypoxia (severe)
*H*ypothermia
*H*ypovolemia
*H*yperkalemia
*H*ypermagnesemia
Pulmonary *E*mbolism (massive)
*D*rug overdose
↓
Epinephrine 1 mg (1:10,000) IV q 3–5 min* (or dosing alternative)
(or 2–2.5 mg ET—for ET dosing, use epinephrine 1:1000 solution
Mix 2 mg epinephrine [2 mL] and dilute in syringe with 8 mL NS)
↓
If bradycardic, atropine 1 mg IV every 3–5 min to max dose of 3 mg (or
2–2.5 mg ET—for ET dosing, using multidose vial [0.4 mg/mL], mix 5
mL of atropine with 5 mL of normal saline for 2.0-mg dose)

*Dosing Alternatives
Recommended: 1 mg every 3–5 min
Intermediate: 2–5 mg IV push, every 3–5 min
Escalating: 1–3–5 mg (IV 3 min apart)
High: 0.1 mg/kg IV push 3–5 min

Source: The American Heart Association.

Table 17-10

Symptomatic Bradycardia

Symptoms:

Chest pain
Shortness of breath
↓ Level of consciousness
Signs/symptoms of shock
Pulmonary congestion
Congestive heart failure
Acute myocardial infarction

Symptomatic *Narrow-QRS* Bradycardia	Symptomatic *Wide-QRS* AV Block
• Sinus bradycardia • Junctional rhythm • Second-degree AV block, type I • Third-degree (narrow QRS) ABCs, O$_2$, IV ↓ Atropine 0.5–1.0 mg IV q 3–5 min to maximum dose of 2–3 mg ↓ Transcutaneous pacemaker ↓ Dopamine infusion 5–20 μg/kg/min ↓ Epinephrine infusion 2–10 μg/min ↓ Isoproterenol infusion 2–10 μg/min	• Second-degree AV block, type II • Third-degree (wide-QRS) ABCs, O$_2$, IV ↓ Atropine may be considered ↓ Transcutaneous pacemaker (prepare for transvenous pacemaker) ↓ Dopamine infusion 5–20 μg/kg/min ↓ Epinephrine infusion 2–10 μg/min

Source: The American Heart Association.

Table 17–11

Narrow QRS Tachycardia (PSVT)

Stable	Unstable
ABCs, O$_2$, IV ↓ Vagal maneuvers ↓ Adenosine 6 mg *rapid* IV bolus Consider ↓ dose in patients on dipyridamole (Persantine) Consider ↑ dose in patients on theophylline ↓ If needed, after 1–2 min: Adenosine 12 mg *rapid* IV bolus (may repeat in 1–2 min if needed) ↓ Verapamil 2.5–5.0 mg *slow* IV bolus ↓ If needed, after 15–30 minutes: Verapamil 5–10 mg *slow* IV bolus ↓ Consider digoxin, β-blockers, diltiazem	ABCs, O$_2$, IV ↓ Consider medications ↓ Consider sedation ↓ Synchronized countershock 50, 100, 200, 300, 360 J

Atrial Fibrillation/Atrial Flutter with a *Rapid* Ventricular Response

Stable	Unstable
ABCs, O$_2$, IV ↓ *Consider:* Diltiazem β-blockers Verapamil Digoxin Procainamide Quinidine Anticoagulants	ABCs, O$_2$, IV ↓ Consider medications ↓ Administer sedation whenever possible ↓ *Atrial Flutter* Synchronized countershock 50, 100, 200, 300, 360 J *Atrial Fibrillation* Synchronized countershock 100, 200, 300, 360 J

Source: The American Heart Association.

Table 17-12

Wide-Complex Tachycardia of Uncertain Origin

Stable	Unstable
ABCs, O_2, IV	ABCs, O_2, IV
↓	↓
Lidocaine 1–1½ mg/kg IV bolus	Consider meds
↓	↓
In 5–10 min:	Administer sedation whenever
Lidocaine 0.5–0.75 mg/kg IV bolus	possible
q 5–10 min to max 3 mg/kg	↓
↓	*Synchronized* countershock
Adenosine 6 mg *rapid* IV bolus	100, 200, 300, 360 J
Consider ↓ dose in patients on	
dipyridamole (Persantine)	
Consider ↑ dose in patients on	
theophylline	
↓	
If needed, in 1–2 min adenosine 12	
mg *rapid* IV bolus	
↓	
If needed, in 1–2 min adenosine 12	
mg *rapid* IV bolus	
↓	
Procainamide 20–30 mg/min	
(max 17 mg/kg)	
Bretylium 5–10 mg/kg *infusion* in	
50 mL of IV solution over 8–10	
min ...	

Source: The American Heart Association.

■ Bibliography

Creasy RK, Resnik R: Placental respiratory gas exchange and fetal oxygenation. *In* Creasy RK, Resnik R (eds): Maternal-Fetal Medicine: Principles and Practice. Philadelphia: W.B. Saunders, 1994.

Elkayam U, Gleicher N: Cardiac Problems in Pregnancy: Diagnosis and Management of Maternal and Fetal Disease, ed 2. New York: Alan R. Liss, 1990, p 809.

Katz VL, Dotter DJ, Droegemueller W: Perimortem cesarean delivery. Obstet Gynecol 1986;68(4):571.

Meschia G: Safety margin of fetal oxygenation. J Reprod Med 1985; 30(4):308.

Strong TH, Lowe RA: Perimortem cesarean section. Am J Emerg Med 1989;7:489–494.

18

DANIEL F. O'KEEFFE

Trauma in Pregnancy

Pregnant trauma victims present a variety of complex medical problems. The major causes of maternal injury are vehicular accidents, falls, and penetrating injuries. Fetal loss due to trauma in the first trimester is rare because the fetus is usually well-protected by the bony pelvis, the uterus, and amniotic fluid. In the second and third trimesters, the uterus emerges from the pelvis, becoming an intraabdominal organ and a relatively immobile target that is vulnerable to abdominal trauma.

Pregnancy is associated with a number of normal physiologic and anatomic alterations that can affect the severity of injury and the presenting signs and symptoms. Thus, it is prudent for the practitioner to be aware of the differences between nongravid and gravid trauma victims.

■ Cardiovascular System Changes

Anatomic and Functional

1. Heart shifts upward, anteriorly and to the left.
2. Louder heart sounds are produced.
3. The first apical and second pulmonic sounds are accentuated.
4. Left axis deviation occurs on electrocardiographic (ECG) tracings.
5. Benign S-T–segment depression and T-wave flattening on ECG tracings.

Hemodynamic

1. Pulse increases 15% to 20%.
2. Cardiac output increases 30% to 40%.
3. Systemic vascular resistance decreases 20% to 30%.
4. Colloid oncotic pressure decreases 15%.
5. No change in mean arterial pressure occurs.
6. No change in pulmonary capillary wedge pressure occurs.
7. No change in left ventricular stroke work index occurs.

Owing to the hemodynamic changes of pregnancy, 25% to 30% of a gravida's blood volume may be lost before signs or symptoms of hypotension develop. Moreover, the patient may maintain her own cardiovascular status at the expense of decreased perfusion to the uterus. As a result, the fetus may demonstrate adverse responses to maternal hypovolemia before the mother does.

■ Respiratory System Changes

Anatomic

1. Diaphragm elevates approximately 4 cm.
2. Thoracic circumference increases 5 to 7 cm.
3. Large airways dilate.
4. Capillaries engorge; respiratory tract mucosa becomes friable.
5. Vascularity increases; trauma is more likely to provoke bleeding.
6. Submucosal tissue hypertrophies. Nose breathing can be impaired.
7. Radiographic lung markings increase and may simulate mild pulmonary edema.

Pulmonary Function Tests and Volumes

1. Tidal volume (TV) increases 45%.
2. Inspiratory capacity (IC) increases 10%.
3. Expiratory reserve volume (ERV) decreases 20%.
4. Residual volume (RV) and functional residual capacity (FRC) decrease 20%.
5. Vital capacity (VC) and inspiratory reserve volume (IRV) are unchanged.

Volumes Memory Aid

"*IC* the *TV* is increased"
"*IRV* the *VC* is unchanged"
"All other volumes are decreased"

Dynamic Ventilatory Changes

1. Lung compliance increases.
2. Minute ventilation increases 50%.
3. Respiratory rate increases 10%.
4. Basal metabolic rate increases 15%; hypoxia develops more rapidly.
5. Supine positions decrease FRC and partial pressure of oxygen (Po_2).

Arterial Blood Gas Analysis in Pregnancy

1. Po_2 increases slightly, if at all (104–108 mm Hg)
2. Partial pressure of carbon dioxide (Pco_2) decreases (27–32 mm Hg)
3. pH increases slightly (7.40 to 7.45).*
4. Base excess decreases.*
5. Buffer base decreases (HCO_3^- 18–31 mm Hg).*

■ Gastrointestinal Tract Changes

1. Acidity and volume of gastric secretions increase.
2. Gastric motility is reduced and emptying time is delayed. Gastroesophageal sphincter tone decreases. The risk of aspiration during pregnancy is increased.
3. With advancing gestation, the intestines are displaced into the upper abdomen.
4. Stretching of the abdominal wall by the enlarging uterus diminishes sensitivity to peritoneal irritation.
5. The abdomen becomes compartmentalized during pregnancy, making peritoneal lavage the diagnostic procedure of choice.
6. Small and large bowel motility decrease.
7. Serum alkaline phosphatase and cholesterol levels increase considerably.
8. Liver function values increase slightly.

■ Urinary Tract Changes

1. Renal pelvis and ureters are mildly dilated during pregnancy. This effect is more pronounced in the right kidney and ureter.

---

*"Respiratory alkalosis" of pregnancy is maintained.

2. The bladder becomes an intraabdominal organ by the 15th week of gestation.
3. Effective renal plasma flow increases 80%.
4. Glomerular filtration rate increases 50%.

■
Genital Tract Changes

1. Uterine blood flow at term is approximately 500 to 700 mL/min.
2. The uterus is not autoregulated and is incapable of increasing blood flow in response to decreasing maternal blood pressure.

Many of the normal laboratory values during pregnancy are different from nongravid values (Table 18–1).

Table 18–1	
Hematologic Changes During Pregnancy	
Variable	**Variation**
RBC volume	↑ 30%
Plasma volume	↑ 50%
Total volume	↑ 45%
Hemoglobin	↓ 1–2 gm/dL
Hematocrit	↓ 4–5%
WBC	↑ 3000
Platelets	↓ 40,000/mm³
Sodium	↓ 5–10 mEq/L
Potassium	↓ Slightly
Calcium	↑ Slightly
Chloride	↓ Slightly
Bicarbonate	↓ 3–5 mEq/L
Albumin (concentration)	↓ 20%
Amylase	↑ 50–100%
BUN	↓ 50%
Creatinine	↓ 30%
Creatinine clearance	↑ 50%
RBC sedimentation rate	↑ 4×
Total protein concentration	↓ 10%

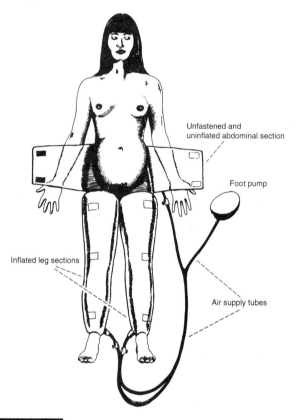

Figure 18–1

Military antishock trousers.

Management Principles for Pregnant Trauma Patients

The early management of the pregnant trauma victim is crucial. The initial stabilization differs very little whether the victim is pregnant or not:

1. Determine ventilatory and cardiovascular status and institute appropriate treatment.
2. Position patient in a left lateral tilt or use lateral displacement of the uterus to optimize uteroplacental blood flow.

3. Hypovolemia should be treated aggressively with use of lactated Ringer's or normal saline solution. A fluid replacement ratio of 3:1 of crystalloid to blood loss is prudent.
4. The MAST suit (military antishock trousers) is a pneumatic device that is sometimes used to treat abdominal bleeding or hypovolemia (Fig. 18–1). The trousers have three separate chambers that can be inflated or deflated independently, two for the legs and one for the abdomen. After the first trimester of pregnancy, the abdominal compartment is not utilized, owing to the potential for undue increases in intrauterine pressure, which may acutely diminish uteroplacental blood flow.

   Use of the device (Table 18–2) in properly selected patients can increase perfusion of vital organs and reduce the need for crystalloid and blood products and may reduce the incidence of acute tubular necrosis and adult respiratory distress syndrome; however, use of the trousers may be associated with maternal hypoventilation, lactic acidosis, and hyperkalemia. Skin breakdown at unprotected pressure points has also been reported. The suit may also worsen cardiogenic shock. Thus, the lowest MAST pressure that produces an acceptable maternal blood pressure

---

Table 18–2

Use of the MAST Suit

Application and inflation
1. Remove all clothing below the waist and place a Foley catheter.
2. Pad all potential pressure points.
3. After the first trimester do not inflate abdominal compartment.
4. Monitor vital signs and urine output.
5. Monitor for lactic acidosis at pressures >40 mm Hg.

Duration of use
1. 12–24 hr after bleeding has stopped.
2. Try to limit use to 48 hr.

Procedure for deflation
1. Monitor vital signs and urine output.
2. Deflate gradually—up to 60 minutes may be required.
3. Infuse fluids as needed to support blood pressure during deflation.
4. Monitor for metabolic washout (see text).
5. Deflate very slowly in the setting of increased intracranial pressure.

Table 18–3

Estimated Radiation Exposure (millirads)

Abdominal x-ray*	289 (per film)
Bilateral venography*	610
Chest fluoroscopy*	71
Chest x-ray*	8–9 (per film)
Intravenous pyelography*	407 (per film)
Lumbar spine x-ray	275 (per film)
Pelvic x-ray*	41 (per film)
Perfusion lung scan (^{99m}Tc MAA)	6–18
Pulmonary angiography	
Brachial route	<50
Femoral route	405
Radioisotope venography	205
Ventilation lung scan (^{133}Xe)	3–20

*Ovarian radiation.

Adapted from Penfil RL, et al: Genetically significant dose in the United States population from diagnostic medical roentgenology. Radiology 1968; 90:209, and Ginsberg JS, et al: Risk to the fetus of radiologic procedures used in the diagnosis of maternal venous thromboembolic disease. Thromb Haemost 1989; 61:189.

should be used. All pressure points should be well-padded. When pressures above 40 mm Hg are required, maternal arterial pH should be monitored and bicarbonate administered as needed. Upon deflation of the suit, metabolic "washout" with transient decreases in maternal pH may occur.

5. Any necessary diagnostic tests, including full radiologic assessment, should be used to optimize maternal outcome; however, when practical, abdominal shielding should be used (Table 18–3).

6. In the viable-aged fetus, continuous fetal heart rate monitoring should be used.

■
The Role of the Obstetrician as Consultant for Mother and Fetus

1. The obstetric care provider should be a source of information about the changes in maternal physiology and anatomy during pregnancy.

2. The obstetric care provider should interpret the laboratory

results in light of pregnancy and should evaluate the status of the fetus using real-time ultrasound, fetal heart rate monitoring, Kleihauer-Betke, and other appropriate tests.
3. Careful record keeping should be done to ensure that entries are accurate, detailed, and timely.

It is important to remember that a direct blow to the abdomen is not necessary to cause fetal-maternal hemorrhage or abruption. Sudden decelerative injuries may also provoke placental separation. For example, the shearing forces and uterine distortion produced by the sudden compression of a waist-anchored seatbelt are sufficient to produce abruption. Cardiotocographic monitoring after the 20th week of pregnancy can be helpful in predicting abruptio placentae. In my practice, 4 hours of cardiotocographic monitoring for frequent uterine contractions (more than eight per hour) or changes in the fetal heart rate (late decelerations or loss of beat-to-beat variability) is sufficient to predict which patients will have abruptio placentae

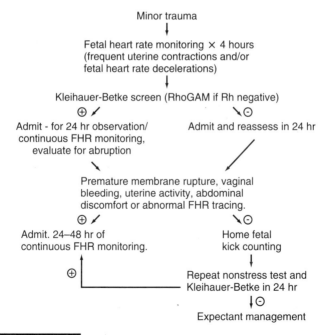

Figure 18-2

Management of noncatastrophic minor trauma in pregnancy.

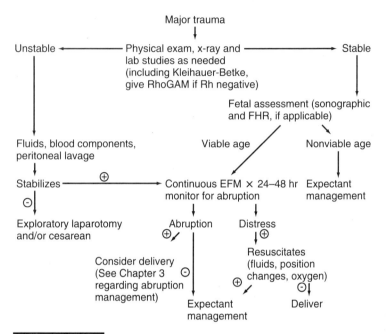

Figure 18–3

Management of noncatastrophic major trauma in pregnancy. FHR, fetal heart rate; EFM, electronic fetal monitoring.

as a consequence of blunt abdominal trauma. If noncatastrophic trauma does not produce an adverse outcome within 48 hours of the traumatic event, it is unlikely to do so thereafter (Fig. 18–2).

Perimortem Cesarean Delivery

New data suggest that perimortem cesarean delivery for a mother in cardiopulmonary arrest during the late second or third trimester should be done within 4 minutes of maternal death to increase both the mother's and the fetus's chances for survival. Resuscitation is difficult with a gravid abdomen, and evidence suggests that when cesarean delivery is performed survival rates for mother and fetus may be better owing to favorable alterations in maternal hemodynamics upon evacuation of the uterus (Fig. 18–3). The reader is referred to Chapter 17 for discussion of cardiopulmonary resuscitation during gestation.

■
Bibliography

Bonica JJ: Maternal anatomic and physiologic alterations during pregnancy and parturition. In Bonica JJ, McDonald JS (eds): Principles and Practice of Obstetric Analgesia and Anesthesia, ed 2. Baltimore, Williams & Wilkins, 1995.

Kuhlmann RS, Cruikshank DP: Maternal trauma during pregnancy. Clin Obstet Gynecol 1994;37:274–291.

Pearse CS, Magrina JF, Finley BE: Use of MAST suit in obstetrics and gynecology. Obstet Gynecol Survey 1984;39:416–422.

JOHN P. ELLIOTT

Transport of the Critically Ill Obstetric Patient

Transport of sick or injured patients to specialized treatment facilities has awaited advances in vehicle development, as distance and speed of travel determine the benefit of this measure. Invention of the automobile, airplane, and helicopter were each instrumental in improving outcome—for military casualties and eventually for civilian emergencies. Baxt and Moody demonstrated the benefit to trauma patients of stabilization and fast transport. Comparing patients transported by ground ambulance with those transported by helicopter they demonstrated a 52% reduction in mortality in the group transported by helicopter. Neonatal transport evolved as the concept of regionalization was applied to perinatal care. Maternal transport eventually proved to be even more efficacious in reducing overall morbidity, mortality, and cost of care.

The broad goal for the concept of regionalization is to make complex technologic perinatal care available to every patient within a designated region though not specifically available in each hospital. The level of care provided at any individual hospital is determined by the availability of technology, skilled nursing and medical personnel, and other related support services. When transport becomes necessary, the issue is not quality of care but the level of available technology and support.

■ Indications for Maternal Transport

Maternal transport to a tertiary facility should be considered when:

1. The facility immediately available to the patient is not sufficient to manage the patient's actual or predicted obstetric, medical, or surgical complications
   or

2. There is reasonable expectation of the birth of one or more infants who may require neonatal care more intensive than that available at the patient's current location
or
3. The patient's obstetric, medical, or surgical condition requires continuous attendance by trained personnel not available at the patient's medical facility.

Low analyzed 463 maternal transports in the United States over a 6-month period, noting prematurity as the primary reason for transport in 330 (71%) cases, hemorrhage in 79 (17%), pregnancy-induced hypertension in 41 (9%), and eclampsia in 8 (2%). In a study done by the author, acute maternal medical complications were the indication for transport in 360 of 1541 maternal patients (23.4%) transported in Arizona over an 18-month period. Fifty-two percent had hypertensive crises, 36% had hemorrhage, 6% were trauma victims, and 3% had respiratory compromise. *Thus, about 25% of transported maternal patients have critical care diagnoses.* In many of these instances, the fetus is at greater risk than the mother. This would include abdominal trauma to the mother, severe preeclampsia, feto-maternal hemorrhage, eclampsia, diabetic ketoacidosis, and maternal respiratory failure.

◼ Obstetric Intensive Care During Transport

In general, critical care complications in obstetric patients should first be stabilized at the referring hospital before transport. Hypertensive emergencies such as severe preeclampsia should be treated with magnesium sulfate to stabilize the neuromuscular irritability that can lead to eclamptic seizures. In addition, diastolic hypertension should be lowered to 90 to 100 mm Hg by administration of intravenous hydralazine or labetalol. Third trimester bleeding due to either placenta previa or abruptio placentae can cause hypovolemic shock and disseminated intravascular coagulopathy (DIC). The estimated blood loss should be replaced with a crystalloid solution such as normal saline or lactated Ringer's solution in a 3:1 ratio (3 mL of crystalloid for each milliliter of blood loss). Maternal intravascular volume is increased by about 40%; therefore, signs and symptoms of shock may not be apparent until blood loss reaches 2000 to 2500 mL. Magnesium sulfate may be used for tocolysis of uterine contractions. DIC is treated with blood component therapy.

During transport and depending on the high-risk circumstance, in-flight therapy with fluids, blood or blood products, oxygen, magnesium sulfate, hydralazine, or labetalol and left-side recumbent positioning may be utilized to help ensure maternal and fetal safety. Table 19–1 illustrates typical standing orders for maternal transport.

■ Maternal Trauma

Transport of the pregnant trauma victim requires special knowledge and skills of the transport team. The uterus may be injured even though no signs of direct physical trauma are obvious. Abrupt deceleration with resulting contrecoup-type forces can be harmful to both the fetus and the placenta. In most cases of maternal trauma, every effort should be made to stabilize serious maternal injuries before transport. All pregnant patients after 20 weeks' gestation should be transported in left lateral tilt position to prevent hypotension from aorto-caval compression. Supine hypotension may significantly compromise maternal cardiac output and placental perfusion. Should the patient require a backboard for neck or back stabilization, the entire backboard can be effectively tilted to the left by placing rolled sheets or towels under the right side. The fetal heart rate should be auscultated in all cases of maternal traumatic injuries. The absence of fetal heart tones might be associated with abruption or fetal death. The uterus should be examined carefully for evidence of tenderness or rigidity and vaginal bleeding appropriately identified.

The Emergency Medical System (EMS) in the United States is efficient at triage and directing trauma victims to designated trauma centers. When considering transport from an accident scene of a gravida after 20 weeks' gestation, the EMS system often fails to recognize that the fetus also needs to be treated at an appropriate level facility. Level I trauma patients in the second or third trimester of pregnancy (after 20 weeks), ideally should be transported to a hospital that combines level I trauma capabilities with level III obstetric and neonatal facilities.

■ The Obstetric Transport Crew

Transport of critically ill obstetric patients often requires more skilled personnel than the usual Advanced Life Support/Emer-
Text continued on page 269

Table 19–1

Maternal Transport Standing Orders

Premature Labor or Premature Rupture of Membranes (PROM), Multiple Pregnancy, Abnormal Presentations

Before transport:

1. Take BP, temperature, pulse, respirations, and fetal heart tones.
2. Assess contractions (frequency, duration, quality), status of membranes; time of PROM, color and if confirmed by nitrazine or ferning. If membranes intact, may perform vaginal exam as indicated by patient's labor pattern/affect. *If PROM, do not* do pelvic exam. Sterile speculum exam only, if in active labor and delivery is deemed imminent.
3. Administer meds as ordered by medical director.
4. Start IV (if absent) with 18- or 16-gauge needle; 1000 mL LR at 50–150 mL/hr (fluid restricting when necessary for magnesium sulfate administration).
5. Left/right lateral uterine displacement.
6. Record above data, obtain consent for transport, and obtain copies of patient's chart.
7. Assess maternal/fetal condition and call perinatologist, if necessary, for consultation and further orders.
8. Help facility prepare for birth, if imminent, and notify dispatch if neonatal transport team is needed.

During transport:

1. Vital signs with fetal heart tones q 15 min.
2. Administer tocolytics and other meds p.r.n.
3. Record above information.
4. Explain procedures to patient and family; reassure patient.

Terbutaline: 0.25 mg SC when contraction frequency is <q10 min, provided there are no contraindications such as maternal heart disease, maternal diabetes mellitus, shortness of breath, tachycardia of ≥120, or heavy maternal bleeding. *May repeat* 30–60 min.

Meperidine: 25–50 mg intravenous push (IVP) for labor pain. May repeat every hour. Observe BP closely. For other causes of pain, speak with medical director before giving meperidine.

Magnesium sulfate: intravenous piggyback (IVPB) 40 gm/1000 mL LR or 20 gm/500 mL LR, bolus 6 gm over 10 to 15 min. Follow with 3 gm/hr to suppress contractions; adjust as needed (6 gm bolus diluted ≤10% solution). May use 100-mL bag of LR or NS for $MgSO_4$ bolus.

Antidote to $MgSO_4$ overdose: Calcium gluconate, 500 mg to 1 gm IV push slowly. May repeat once if necessary. Observe BP closely.

Assess continually for adequate urine output, deep tendon reflexes (DTR), and respiratory rate/effort.

Table continued on following page

Table 19-1

Maternal Transport Standing Orders *Continued*

Preeclampsia or Eclampsia

Before Transport:
1. Take vital signs plus fetal heart tones and deep tendon reflexes.
2. Assess contractions (frequency, duration, quality), status of membranes (see Premature Labor or PROM, Multiple Pregnancy, Abnormal Presentation).
3. Right/left lateral uterine displacement.
4. Start IV. Mainline 1000 mL LR, infuse @ ≤100 mL/hr as indicated by hydration, cardiopulmonary status, etc. Hold total fluids at 75 mL/hr, if possible.
5. Mix $MgSO_4$ 40 gm/1000 mL, preferably LR (or 20 gm/500 mL) (6-gm bolus diluted to ≤10% IV solution). May use 100-mL bag of NS or LR for $MgSO_4$ bolus.
6. Administer meds as indicated by condition:
   $MgSO_4$, 4–6 gm IV bolus over 10–15 min, considering patient's weight, urine output, and deep tendon reflexes. $MgSO_4$ continuous infusion of 2–3 gm/hr.
7. Foley catheter p.r.n.; most often Foley is not needed if patient can void.
8. Record above information; obtain copy of chart; obtain consent to transport.
9. Assess maternal/fetal condition for transport and call perinatologist for consultation or further orders.

During transport:
1. Take vital signs with fetal heart tones q 15 min.
2. Administer meds p.r.n.
3. Explain procedures to patient and family.
4. Foley catheter p.r.n.

Emergency Medications

Hydralazine (first choice for hypertension): Give when diastolic BP ≥110 mm hg. Give 2–5 mg IV push q 15–20 min until BP begins to decrease. Stop when diastolic BP 90–100 mm Hg or a total of 30 mg is given. Consult medical director.

Labetalol: Give when diastolic BP ≥110 mm Hg. 10 mg (4 mL) over 2 min IV push. If desired effect not reached after 10 min, give 20 mg (8 mL) IV push. Call medical director.

Oxygen: 12 L by nonrebreathing mask p.r.n. maternal or fetal necessity.

Morphine: 2–5 mg slow IV for acute pulmonary edema with shortness of breath, dyspnea, chest pain, congestive heart failure.

Furosemide: 40 mg slow IV over 2–3 min for acute pulmonary edema with respiratory distress after hypertensive treatment has been initiated.

Table 19-1

Maternal Transport Standing Orders *Continued*

Eclamptic Emergency

Establish airway. Provide supplemental oxygen. Assist with bag/mask or endotracheal intubation for hypoventilation.

If seizure persists rebolus with $MgSO_4$, 2 gm more (total bolused $MgSO_4$ should not exceed 8 gm). If seizure still persists, give sodium amobarbital IV push 250 mg over 3–5 min. (Discuss with medical director.)

Hemorrhage (General)

Before transport:

1. Take vital signs and fetal heart tones.
2. Assess contractions, status of membranes, extent of bleeding, number of episodes, and amount of blood loss (weighing pads when possible).
3. Oxygen, 12 L by nonrebreathing mask.
4. Start IV with 16-gauge needle. Infuse 1 L LR using blood tubing to infuse at 125 mL/hr or as necessary to maintain adequate blood pressure and urine output >30 mL/hr (preferably 60 mL/hr).
5. With active bleeding or suspected abruption, strongly consider second IV line. Use 16-gauge catheter.
6. Check recent hemoglobin and hematocrit, type and cross-match (or screen).
7. May travel with blood infusing. Use NS to clear tubing.
8. Administer meds as ordered. (IV ritodrine and terbutaline contraindicated.) (See Premature Labor or PROM, Multiple Pregnancy, Abnormal Presentations for Tocolytics).
9. Foley catheter p.r.n.
10. Assess maternal-fetal condition for transport and call perinatologist p.r.n.
11. Record above information; obtain copy of chart and permit for transport.
12. No vaginal exam unless placenta previa has been clearly ruled out; then, if necessary, gentle vaginal exam or sterile speculum exam to document cervical status before departure.

During transport:

1. Take vital signs and fetal heart tones q 15 min or more often, as deemed necessary.
2. Check blood loss, keep pad count.
3. Record above.
4. Reassess patient and call perinatologist for consultation or further orders.

Acute Hemorrhage with Hypoperfusion

1. Oxygen, 12 L by nonrebreathing mask.
2. Start additional IV lines and increase IV fluids as needed.
3. MAST application as indicated (see Chapter 18).
4. Left/right lateral uterine displacement.
5. Elevate feet.
6. If hypotensive, consider ephedrine, 5–25 mg slow IV. Observe BP closely. (Call medical director.)

Table continued on following page

Table 19–1

Maternal Transport Standing Orders *Continued*

Acute Postpartum Hemorrhage

1. Pitocin, 40 U/L NS 125–150 mL/hr
2. Methylergonovine, 0.2 mg IM. Contraindicated in the presence of maternal hypertension.
3. 15-Methyl PGF$_{2\alpha}$, 0.25 mg IM. Contraindicated in the presence of maternal asthma. (Call medical director.)

Excessive Nausea and Vomiting

Promethazine, 25 mg IV.

Emergency Delivery

1. Perform emergency delivery if during transport it becomes imminent.
2. May perform small midline episiotomy if deemed necessary to prevent tearing.
3. Cut and clamp umbilical cord ½ in from stump.
4. Administer oxytocin, 10–20 units by dilute intravenous infusion after placenta is delivered.
5. Obtain cord blood when time permits.
6. Resuscitate newborn: (see Chapter 26) provide warmth, oxygen by bag and mask with intubation p.r.n. If estimated time of arrival is >20 min and situation permits, obtain Chem Strip for glucose.
7. For glucose <40, give dextrose 10% IV or gavage, if necessary. Give 2–4 mL/kg over 3–5 min.

Table 19–2

Maternal Flight Nurse Skills and Qualifications

Skills

Vaginal speculum examinations; cervical examination
Delivery: Carry appropriate equipment to perform both hospital and emergency field deliveries.
Advanced cardiac life support: All maternal flight nurses are certified in advanced cardiac life support procedures and protocols.
Intubation: All maternal flight nurses are trained through operating room experience to perform oral and nasal intubation in the field.

Qualifications/requirements

Basic and advanced cardiac life support providers.
Neonatal resuscitation provider.
National certification in obstetrics.
Three years of previous tertiary obstetric experience.
Successful completion of 8-wk maternal flight nurse course and examination.

Table 19–3

Equipment for Maternal Transport
Contents of Maternal Flight Nurse Delivery Bag

Bulb syringe
Suction trap
Self-inflating resuscitation bag
Infant and newborn mask
Infant hat
Pediatric stethoscope
Infant blanket pack
Portawarm mattress
Sterile gloves (6½, 7, 8)

Obstetric delivery kit:
  1 Chux
  Sterile gloves, size 7
  Cord clamps (2)
  Scissors (curved/straight) (2)
  Curved Kelly clamp
  Short ring forceps
  Plastic placenta bag
  Cloth towels (2)
  4 × 4's (2)
  Bulb syringe

Contents of Maternal Flight Nurse Pharmacy Bag

MgSO$_4$ 10 gm (2)	Ephedrine 50 mg (3)	Methylergonovine 0.2 mg (2)
Furosemide 20 gm (2)	Dextrose 50% 50 mL	Labetalol 100 mg (2)
Oxytocin 10 U (3)	Hydralazine 20 mg (2)	Terbutaline 1 mg (3)
MgSO$_4$ 10 gm (3)	D10W vial 5 mL (2)	Ammonium salts (2)
Normal saline 10 mL (3)	Hep-Lock	Promethazine HCl 25 mg (2)
		Albuterol, unit dose 2.5 mg (2)

Thermometer	Band-Aids	Alcohol swabs
TB syringe (2)	Needles	Labels
3-mL syringe (2)	10-gauge (3)	Hep-Lock cap
	22-gauge (3)	
	Filter (3)	

Dimenhydrinate (2)	Cord clamp (2)	Drug labels (4)
Narcotic sheets	Aspirin (2)	
	Acetaminophen (2)	Inventory

Bretylium 500 mg (2)	Epinephrine 1:1000 (3)	Atropine 1 mg (2)
Verapamil 5 mg (3)		Lidocaine 1 gm/50 mL (1)
		Sodium amobarbital 250 mg (1)
Epinephrine 1:10,000 (2)	Sodium bicarbonate 50-mL jet (1)	
Calcium gluconate 10% (1)	2% lidocaine 100-mg jet (2)	
Diphenhydramine (2)	Procainamide 1 gm (1)	Meperidine 100 mg (1)
		Diazepam 10 mg (4)
		Morphine 10 mg (1)
		Naloxone 0.4 mg (2)

Table continued on following page

Table 19–3

Equipment for Maternal Transport *Continued*

Contents of Top Portion Maternal Flight Nurse Medical Bag

3-mL syringe (2)	Alcohol wipes
TB syringe (2)	Virowipes
Insulin syringe	
Stopcock	
19-gauge needles	

Syringes	100 mL normal saline (2)
10 mL	
20 mL	
30 mL	
60 mL	

3-mL	
TB syringes (2)	Bite stick

Drug bag

Contents of Base Portion Maternal Flight Nurse Medical Bag

250 mL d$_5$W / 500 mL NS	1000 mL LR / 500 mL LR	Sterile speculum	

CARDIAC ELECTRODES	ORANGE	GREEN	YELLOW	STERILE GLOVES 7 & 8
	Laryngoscope handle	In self-seal bags	IV start kit	
	Blades		Nonsterile gloves	
	McIntosh (3, 4)	1. Chemstrips	Mainline tubing	
	Miller (0, 1, 3)	Alcohol wipes	IV catheters	
	Spare "C"	Lancets	16 gauge (3)	
	batteries (2)	Cotton balls	18 gauge (3)	
	Laryngoscope	2. KY jelly	24 gauge (2)	
	bulb	Betadine jelly	23-gauge	
	Xylocaine gel	Nitrazine	butterfly	
	Benzoin (2)	paper	T connector	
	1-in Adhesive	Tape-measure	Tourniquet	
	tape	3. Blood tubes:		
	10-mL syringe	Purple (2)		
		Red (2)		
		Vacutainer		
		Alcohol		
		Band-Aids		
		Tourniquet		
		Needles		
		Small self-		
		seal bag (2)		
		Urine dipstick		
		Plastic bags (2)		
		Flashlight		
		Peri pads (2)		

Table 19–3

Equipment for Maternal Transport *Continued*

Contents of Outside Pockets Maternal Flight Nurse Medical Bag

Top Handle Pocket
Micro Drip Extension set Stopcock 60-mL syringe Needles

Left	Top Center	Right Side

Micro Drip
Extension set
Blood tubing with
  pump
Salem sump
	Stethoscope
	Doppler and gel
	BP cuff
		Stylette
		  Adult
		  Pediatric
		End-tidal CO_2
		  detector

Zipper Bag

PEEP valve
Magill forceps
Oral airways
  Medium adult
  Small adult
  Infant
ET tubes
  2.0
  2.5
  3.0
  3.5
  7.0
  7.5
  8.0
  7.0 Endotrol
Beck Airway Airflow
  Monitor

Bottom Center
Emesis bag Adult BVM O_2 bag Leg BP cuff Charts (3) Self-inflating Ambu-bag Red isolation bag (1)

gency Medical technician ambulance crews provide. Modern maternal transport demands the advanced clinical skills of specialized transport nurses. These care providers may be cross-trained adult trauma nurses or dedicated obstetrics nurses. The personnel must have an excellent working knowledge of maternal physiology and the process of labor. Experience with obstetric drugs and fetal monitoring is also essential. The skills for facilitating advanced cardiac life support, interpreting electrocardiograms, and performing successful endotracheal intubation, if necessary, are important for a perinatal flight nurse to possess (Table 19–2). Table 19–3 illustrates the equipment recommended for use during perinatal transport plus a detailed plan for equipment organization and flight kit planning.

The comprehensive care of the critically ill obstetric patient during transport requires care providers who have detailed knowledge of the maternal physiologic adaptations as well as a comprehensive understanding of the disease processes unique to obstetrics. Coupling the concept of perinatal regionalization with a skilled perinatal transport service helps to improve survival and reduce morbidity for both mother and baby.

■
Bibliography

Baxt WG, Moody P: The impact of a rotocraft aeromedical emergency care service on trauma mortality. JAMA 1983; 249:3047–3051.

Elliott JP: Magnesium sulfate as a tocolytic agent. Am J Obstet Gynecol 1983; 147:277–284.

Elliott JP, Foley MR, Young L, et al.: Transport of obstetrical critical care patients to tertiary centers. J Reprod Med 1996; 41:171–174.

Elliott JP, O'Keeffe DF, Freeman RK: Helicopter transportation of patients with obstetric emergencies in an urban area. Am J Obstet Gynecol 1982; 143:157–162.

Elliott JP, Sipp TL, Balazs KT: Maternal transport of patients with advanced cervical dilatation—to fly or not to fly? Obstet Gynecol 1992; 79:380–382.

Elliott JP, Trujillo R: Fetal monitoring during emergency obstetric transport. Am J Obstet Gynecol 1987; 157:245–247.

Kanto WP, Bryant J, Thigpen J, et al: Impact of a maternal transport program on a newborn service. South Med J 1983; 76:834–837.

Katz VL, Hansen AR: Complications in the emergency transport of pregnant women. South Med J 1990; 83:7–10.

Knox GE, Schnitker KA: In-utero transport. Clin Obstet Gynecol 1984; 27:11–16.

Low RB, Martin D, Brown C: Emergency air transport of pregnant patients: The national experience. J Emerg Med 1988; 6:41–48.

Tsokos N, Newnham JP, Langford SA: Intravenous tocolytic therapy for long distance aeromedical transport of women in preterm labour in Western Australia. Asia-Oceania J Obstet Gynaecol 1988; 14:21–25.

LISA A. DADO

Anesthesia for the Obstetric Patient with Complications

20

A thorough understanding of the nature of the parturient's pain is the first step in providing optimal obstetric anesthesia care. Once the biology and pathophysiology of this special acute pain have been discussed, the benefits of analgesia for this pain will appropriately follow. Pharmacology of local anesthetics and related drugs is reviewed, with special emphasis on complications associated with their administration. A variety of techniques, including epidural, subarachnoid, and other regional techniques, are discussed and their benefits and complications reviewed. General anesthesia for cesarean section delivery is outlined. A variety of special patient considerations are addressed including: the preeclamptic patient, preterm mothers receiving tocolytics, human immunodeficiency virus (HIV)-positive mothers, coagulopathies, cardiac disease, and pulmonary disease.

■ Nature of the Patient's Pain

The current concept of pain focuses on the peripheral nervous system's relaying a stimulus to the central nervous system (CNS) for interpretion ("the somatosensory system"; Fig. 20–1). The peripheral system consists of afferent neurons embedded in body tissues and awaiting nociceptive (painful) stimuli. These afferent neurons, termed Ad (A-delta) and C fibers, extend into the spinal segments and form synapses at the dorsal spinal ganglion. Here, substance P is released, initiating the painful affect. From each spinal segment stimulated these messages ascend through one of two pathways—the lateral spinothalamic tract or the medial lemniscus tract—to the thalamus for further modulation. Once at the thalamus, inherent emotional and psychological regulation occurs. The data support the emphasis on the importance of perceptual factors that influence a patient's

Somatosensory System

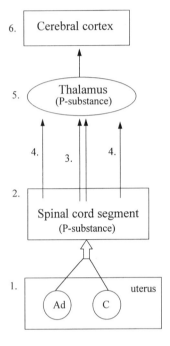

Figure 20-1

Schematic of the somatosensory system. 1. A-delta (Ad) and C fibers in body tissue, afferent nociceptor fibers. 2. Spinal ganglion. Substance P is released at receptor. Its function is to cause a "pain" affect. 3. Medial lemniscus tract (anterior ascending tract). 4. Lateral spinothalamic tract (anterior ascending tract). 5. Thalamus, the relay center for incoming sensory input from Ad and C fibers and psychological and emotional factors. 6. Cerebral cortex, integrating center from sensory input.

total experience of pain (Table 20–1). The psychodynamics of experience, motivation, anxiety, anticipation of pain, attention, personality, and ethnic and cultural factors all influence substance-P release, affecting the pain experience. From the thalamus, this information is synthesized in the sensory cortex for relay to the many effector sites that contribute to the pain response. Once pain has been perceived, the initiation of the pain response has neuroendocrine, behavioral, and psychological implications.

In humans, production of epinephrine increases 300% to 600% and of norepinephrine 200% to 400% during severe pain experienced in active labor. There is a 200% to 300% increase in cortisol levels, as well as increases in corticosteroid and adreno-corticotropic hormone levels reaching their peaks at or after delivery. During labor cardiac output increases 40% to 50%, and during painful contractions another 20% to 30%. The systolic and diastolic blood pressures also increase by 20 to 30 mm Hg. These increases in cardiac output and systolic blood pressure lead to a significant increase in left ventricular stroke work that

Table 20–1	
Pain Perception	
Psychological	Anxiety, fear, emotional arousal
Behavioral	Verbalization, motor activity
Neuroendocrine	Hyperventilation, maternal respiratory alkalosis
	Endocrine (stress) response
	$\uparrow$ Adrenocorticotropic hormone, $\uparrow$ cortisol
	$\uparrow$ Epinephrine & norepinephrine
	$\uparrow$ Lipolytic metabolism, metabolic acidosis
	Cardiovascular response
	$\uparrow$ Systemic vascular resistance
	$\uparrow$ Cardiac output
	$\uparrow$ Blood pressure
	$\uparrow$ Oxygen consumption
	$\uparrow$ Left ventricular stroke work
	Gastrointestinal function
	$\downarrow$ Gastric motility
	$\uparrow$ Risk for gastroesophageal reflux and aspiration
	$\uparrow$ Nausea and vomiting
	Urinary function
	$\downarrow$ Emptying, urinary retention, oliguria
Fetal effects	$\downarrow$ Uterine blood flow
	$\uparrow$ Fetal heart rate alterations

may be harmful to patients with preeclampsia, hypertension, cardiac valvular disease, pulmonary hypertension, or severe anemia.

Increased sympathetic activity increases metabolism and oxygen consumption and decreases gastrointestinal and urinary bladder motility. Respiratory rate is increased, with resultant respiratory alkalosis. The kidney compensates by excreting bicarbonate. $Paco_2$ levels below 25 to 27 mm Hg may result in increased uteroplacental resistance and reduced oxygen delivery to the fetus.

During peak contractions, there is a reduction of intervillous blood flow leading to a significant decrease in placental gas exchange. This exaggerates the already dramatic reduction in uterine blood flow secondary to the increases in norepinephrine and cortisol.

■
Effects of Analgesia

With blocking of nociceptive input, release of catecholamines, adrenocorticotropic hormone, and cortisol is reduced in the parturient (Table 20–2). Effective analgesia significantly reduces pain-related hemodynamic changes. Maternal cardiac output fluctuations are modulated and oxygen consumption is reduced. Gastric and bladder motility are not adversely affected by neuroblockade. Cautious epidural analgesia has been reported to provide a vasomotor-blocking effect that increases intervillous blood flow and oxygen delivery to the fetus.

The first stage of labor runs from the beginning of cervical dilatation and effacement until its completion. The second stage of labor extends from complete cervical dilatation until delivery of the infant. The third stage is delivery of the placenta.

During the first stage of labor pain is transmitted from spinal segments (pain fibers) T_{10} through L_1 and from S2 through S4 in the second and third stages (Fig. 20–2). It is important for the care provider to know from which spinal levels pain is transmitted at each stage of labor so as to direct analgesia appropriately. It is also important to consider that pain may also be due to some problem associated with the gestation, such as abruptio placentae, infection, adnexal torsion, or appendicitis, and that these may be *masked* if total neuroblockade is achieved from T4 to S5 at the onset of labor. Only segments related specifically to the pain of labor should be blocked (Table 20–3). Relatively decreased fetal perfusion has been reported to occur—both in the presence and absence of overt maternal hypotension—

Table 20–2

Analgesic Effects

Psychological	↓ Anxiety
	↓ Fear, ↑ emotional stability
Behavioral	↓ Motor activity
Neuroendocrine	↓ Respiratory alkalosis (maternal)
	↓ Catechol release
	↓ Cortisol
	↓ Adrenocorticotropic hormone
	↓ Metabolic acidosis (maternal)
	↓ Cardiac output
	↓ Oxygen consumption
	↓ Left ventricular stroke work
	Normal gastrointestinal function
	Normal urinary function
Fetal effects	↑ Uterine blood flow
	More stability in fetal heart rate tracing

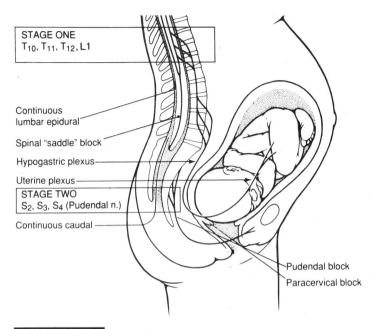

STAGE ONE
T_{10}, T_{11}, T_{12}, L_1

Continuous
lumbar epidural

Spinal "saddle" block

Hypogastric plexus

Uterine plexus

STAGE TWO
S_2, S_3, S_4 (Pudendal n.)

Continuous caudal

Pudendal block
Paracervical block

Figure 20–2

Note the completely separate pain fibers responsible for pain in the first and second stages of labor: T10–L1 vs. S2–S4. (From Bonica JJ, McDonald JS: Principles and Practice of Obstetric Analgesia and Anesthesia, ed 2. Baltimore: Williams & Wilkins, 1994.)

secondary to a sympathectomy-mediated reduction in uterine blood flow.

Pharmacology of Local Anesthetics and Related Drugs

The desired action of all local anesthetics is reversible blockade of nerve conduction and, therefore, of the cascade of events that produce the perception of pain. These drugs prevent the development of an action potential in a nerve by blocking sodium channels responsible for propagating a response in the nerve fiber (Fig. 20–3). Local anesthetics exist in both charged and uncharged forms. In the uncharged state, the drug crosses the lipid nerve membrane and enters the cell. Once in the cell, it reequilibrates into the charged form that is readily dissolved

Table 20–3

Innervation of Pelvic Viscera

Uterus	Motor fibers from parasympathetic pelvic nerves from S2–S4 and sympathetic sensory
Tubes/ovaries	Motor fibers from parasympathetic pelvic nerves from S2–S4 and sympathetic sensory fibers via the ovarian plexus from T12, L1
Broad ligament	Motor fibers from parasympathetic pelvic nerves from S2–S4 and sympathetic sensory fibers via the hypogastric plexus from T12, L1
Cervix	Motor fibers from parasympathetic pelvic nerves from S2–S4 and sympathetic sensory fibers via the hypogastric plexus from T12, L1
Vagina	Motor fibers from parasympathetic pelvic nerves from S2–S4 and sympathetic sensory fibers via the hypogastric plexus from T12, L1
Vestibule/hymen	Erectile vasodilator fibers from parasympathetic pelvic nerves from S2–S4
Labia	Posterior labial nerves S2, S3, and perineal branch of the posterior femoral cutaneous nerves S1–S3
Clitoris	Erectile vasodilator fibers from parasympathetic pelvic nerves from S2–S4
Perineum	Motor and sensory innervation from the pudendal nerve arising from S2–S4
Bladder	Sympathetic fibers from T11–L2 via the superior/inferior hypogastric plexuses control the sphincter and parasympathetic fibers from S2–S4 control filling and emptying of the bladder
Anus	Motor and sensory innervation from the pudendal nerve arising from S2–S4

From Bonica JJ, McDonald JS: Principles and Practice of Obstetric Analgesia and Anesthesia, ed 2. Baltimore: Williams & Wilkins, 1994.

in water. This charged form now reaches the sodium channels and blocks them from inside.

Ionization, the capacity for an uncharged species to assume a charged form, is the essential property of all local anesthetics. They are a combination of a weak base and a strong acid:

$$B + H^+ \rightleftharpoons BH^+$$

As a general principle, lowering the pH increases the ionized portion of drug and raising the pH increases the uncharged

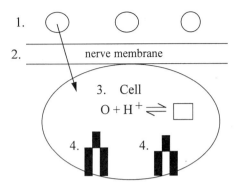

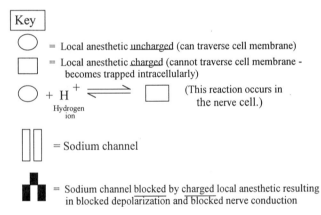

Figure 20–3

Local anesthetic action. 1, Uncharged local anesthetic passes through the (2) nerve membrane into the cell (3) where the local anesthetic gains a hydrogen ion (H$^+$) to become charged. 4, Sodium channel in the nerve cell blocked by the charged local anesthetic prevents the nerve from propagating a nerve impulse.

form. Since the local anesthetics are usually supplied in an acid medium, the addition of sodium bicarbonate increases the relative uncharged portion, allowing the drug to cross the nerve membrane more readily, resulting in quicker onset of block.

Usual Doses: Bupivacaine, 0.1 cc NaHCO$_3$/10 cc
Lidocaine, 1.0 cc NaHCO$_3$/10 cc

Table 20-4

Properties of Lidocaine and Bupivacaine Compared

Property	Lidocaine	Bupivacaine
Toxicity	↑ ↑	↑ ↑ ↑ ↑ ↑
pKa	7.9 (at pH 7.4, more drug in basic form)	8.16
Lipid solubility (directly related to speed of onset)	↑ ↑ ↑ ↑ ↑	↑ ↑
Protein binding	64%	95%
Elimination (half-life)	96 min	162 min
Maximum dose	5 mg/kg (7 mg/kg with epinephrine)	2 mg/kg
Toxicity (early effect)	Seizures	Cardiac arrest

Precipitation of the local anesthetic will occur if too much
NaHCO$_3$ is added. Comparative properties of lidocaine and bupivacaine are outlined in Table 20–4.

Protein binding is another property that is important to
understand. All local anesthetics bind to albumin and α_1-acid
glycoprotein (AAG). It is the free (unbound) portion of the drug
that is responsible for toxicity. In pregnancy, albumin levels are
depressed, so AAG binding becomes most important. AAG is
released in response to surgery, trauma, infection, and inflammation. Once AAG sites are saturated with local anesthetics, the
free drug levels progressively increase. Protein binding also
decreases with pH; therefore, in an acidotic environment a large
proportion of free drug is available that has the potential for
cardiac toxicity or neurotoxicity.

Absorption of local anesthetics refers to the movement of the
drug from the site of injection into the bloodstream. The more
vascular the area and the larger the total dose of anesthetic, the
higher the resulting serum level of the drug. The addition of a
vasoconstrictor (epinephrine) to the local anesthetic can decrease
the absorption—and, therefore, the toxicity—of the drug used.

Epidural Analgesia and Anesthesia

Lumbar epidural block is the most common form of analgesia
used to provide relief from the nociceptive pathways during the

stages of labor. The epidural space is the interval bounded superiorly by the foramen magnum, inferiorly by the lower end of the dural sac, anteriorly by the posterior longitudinal ligament, and posteriorly by the ligamentum flavum. The approach to the epidural space is dorsally through the skin, subcutaneous fat, supraspinous ligament, interspinous ligament, ligamentum flavum, and into the epidural space (Fig. 20–4).

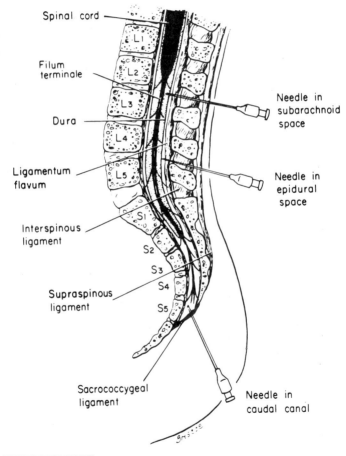

Figure 20-4

Lumbosacral anatomy showing needle depth for epidural and subarachnoid injections. (From Shnider SM: Anesthesia for Obstetrics, ed 3. Baltimore: Williams & Wilkins, 1993.)

The size of the epidural space varies along its course, the diameter being largest at the L2 interspace (range of the largest diameter, 4 to 9 mm). A simple maneuver that helps to open up the bony entrance to the epidural space is flexion of the lumbar spine (Fig. 20–5). The contents of the epidural space include fat, vertebral venous plexus, lymphatics, arteries, and dural spinal nerve projections. With the increase in intraabdominal pressure in pregnancy, the venous plexus becomes distended. This phenomenon, and the accompanying increase in epidural fat that occurs during pregnancy, functions to substantially reduce epidural volume. Therefore, pregnant patients usually require a smaller volume of local anesthetic than nonpregnant controls to produce a comparable level of blockade.

Once the epidural catheter is in place, local anesthetic is administered according to the appropriate pain pathway and corresponding stage of labor. In the first stage of labor, T10 block is sufficient. In the late first stage and the second stage the nerves to be blocked include the sacral area, so the parturient should be dosed in the semi-Fowler's position to allow downward spread of the local anesthetic. Finally, for predelivery and the third stage of labor the parturient may be seated upright (with a vena cava tilt) to secure sacral root spread of the drug (Fig. 20–6). This blockade may be achieved by intermittent bolus injections or by continuous infusion of drug with changes in patient positioning to alter the level of blockade.

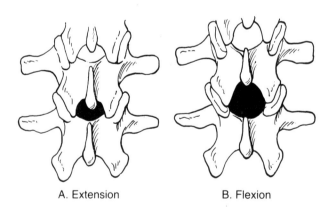

A. Extension   B. Flexion

Figure 20–5

Lumbar vertebrae. When spine is flexed *(B)*, the interlaminar space enlarges, increasing the ability to enter the epidural/subarachnoid space. (From Bonica JJ, McDonald JS: Principles and Practice of Obstetric Analgesia and Anesthesia, ed 2. Baltimore, Williams & Wilkins, 1994.)

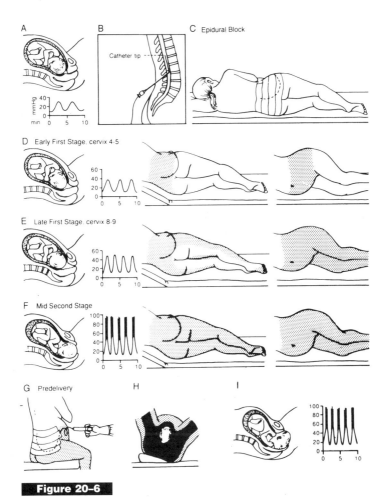

Figure 20–6

Lumbar epidural analgesia *(A–C)*. Epidural catheter may be placed early in the first stage of labor *(D)*. When the patient experiences labor pain, local anesthetic may be injected to achieve a T10–L1 neuroblockade *(E–F)*. In late first stage and mid-second stage of labor, the patient should be elevated 15 to 20 degrees to allow caudad spread of local anesthetic to achieve a T_{10}–S_5 block *(G–I)*. To ensure sacral root dispersion of local anesthetic, once flexion internal rotation of baby's head occurs more local anesthetic can be injected with the patient in the seated upright position with a left tilt to the pelvis. (From Bonica JJ, McDonald JS: Principles and Practice of Obstetric Analgesia and Anesthesia, ed 2. Baltimore: Williams & Wilkins, 1994.)

Table 20-5

Contraindications to Lumbar Epidural Analgesia/ Anesthesia

Absolute Contraindications

- Parturients who refuse the block or have great fear of spine puncture. In our experience, many patients who initially are concerned about epidural block consent to be managed with this technique after being properly informed. However, if they still refuse, it is an absolute contraindication to the technique.
- Administrator unskilled in carrying out the procedure, managing the parturient, and promptly treating complications.
- Infection at the puncture site or in the epidural space.
- Severe hypovolemia from hemorrhage, dehydration, or malnutrition.
- Coagulopathies.
- Lack of resuscitation equipment in the immediate area ready for *prompt* use.

Relative Contraindications

Failure of the obstetrician to appreciate how the procedure influences the management of labor.

A very rapid or precipitate labor, or any case that requires immediate anesthesia.

From Bonica JJ, McDonald JS: Principles and Practice of Obstetric Analgesia and Anesthesia, ed 2. Baltimore: Williams & Wilkins, 1994.

With the uppermost level of analgesia at T10, the five lowermost vasomotor segments supplying the pelvis, lower trunk, and limbs are interrupted, causing decreases in total peripheral resistance, venous return, and cardiac output. In normal parturients this insult induces a reflex cardiovascular response directed toward maintaining systemic blood pressure. Preload of an adequate intravenous crystalloid infusion, keeping the parturient on her side, and minimizing the dose of the local anesthetic all reduce the adverse decrease in blood flow to the pelvis and its structures.

High epidural anesthesia that extends from T4 to S5 is associated with significant interruption of vasomotor segments, resulting in significant hypotension. Again, fluid preload and lateral tilt of the parturient can augment the reflex corrective responses of the cardiovascular system in this situation. Extending the epidural blockade above spinal level T10 is unnecessary and counterproductive for the normally laboring patient. If epidural analgesia needs to be changed to anesthesia for cesarean section, these risks are necessary and measures to prevent them should be instituted. In addition, in most circumstances ephedrine is the best vasopressor to augment blood pressure without reducing blood supply to the uterus. Contraindications to lumbar epidural analgesia and anesthesia are reviewed in Table 20–5; the advantages and disadvantages of regional analgesia and anesthesia in Table 20–6.

Table 20–6

Advantages and Disadvantages of Regional Analgesia/Anesthesia

Advantages

In contrast to opioids, regional analgesia produces complete relief of pain in most parturients.

The hazards of pulmonary aspiration of gastric contents inherent in general anesthesia are diminished and can even be eliminated.

Provided it is administered properly and no complications occur, regional analgesia/anesthesia causes no serious maternal or neonatal complications.

Administered at the proper time, it does not impede the progress of labor during the first stage.

Continuous techniques can be extended for delivery and may even be modified for cesarean section.

Regional analgesia permits the mother to remain awake during labor and delivery so that she can experience the pleasure of actively participating in the birth of her child.

Regional anesthesia for cesarean section also permits the mother to be awake and to bond immediately with the newborn.

Provided the mother is doing well, the anesthesiologist can leave her and resuscitate the newborn if this is necessary.

Disadvantages

Regional techniques require greater administrator skill than does administration of systemic drugs or inhalation agents.

Technical failures occur even in experienced hands.

Certain techniques produce side effects (e.g., maternal hypotension) that, if not treated promptly and properly can progress to complications in the mother and fetus.

Techniques that produce perineal muscle paralysis interfere with the mechanism of internal rotation and increase the need for instrumental delivery.

These procedures can be carried out only in the hospital.

From Bonica JJ, McDonald JS: Principles and Practice of Obstetric Analgesia and Anesthesia, ed 2. Baltimore: Williams & Wilkins, 1994.

Table 20–7	
Intrathecal Opioids:	
Recommended Treatment for Side Effects	
Side Effect	Treatment
Itching	Benadryl, 25 mg IV
	Propofol, 10 mg IV
	Naloxone, 40 μg IV
Nausea and vomiting	Reglan, 10 mg IV
	Propofol, 10 mg IV
	Naloxone, 40 μg IV
	Zofran, 4 mg IV
Hypotension	IV fluids
	Ephedrine, 5–25 mg slow IV
Urinary retention	Catheterization
	Naloxone, 400 μg IV

A combined spinal and epidural analgesia technique provides rapid onset of spinal opioid analgesia plus the flexibility of epidural blockade. Sufentanil, 10 μg, or fentanyl, 25 μg, injected spinally when the epidural catheter is inserted, can reliably give several hours of analgesia to patients in the early first stage of labor (less than 5 cm dilation). The continuous infusion of a weak local anesthetic (0.125% or 0.0625% bupivacaine) with small doses of a narcotic (sufentanil, 1 to 2 μg/mL, or fentanyl, 5 to 10 μg/mL) can provide good perineal analgesia for later stages of labor. If needed, higher concentrations of bupivacaine or lidocaine can be bolused for more complete nerve blockade. Less motor blockade, less hypotension, smaller volume of local anesthetic (with less risk of toxicity), and faster onset of analgesia are all benefits of this combined technique. The side effects of intrathecal opioids and corresponding treatment are listed in Table 20–7.

■
Other Regional Analgesic and Anesthetic Techniques

There are two important techniques to discuss that may be used by the obstetric care provider to provide analgesia when obstetric anesthesia coverage is not available. Although these techniques are relatively easy to execute, a thorough knowledge of the anatomy, physiology, and effects of local anesthetics on mother and fetus is paramount.

■ Bilateral Pudendal Nerve Block

This block is an effective blockade for the second and third stages of labor, blocking the sacral nerves S3 through S5 (Fig. 20–7). The transvaginal approach points the needle behind the sacrospinous ligament, aiming toward the ischial spine. Up to

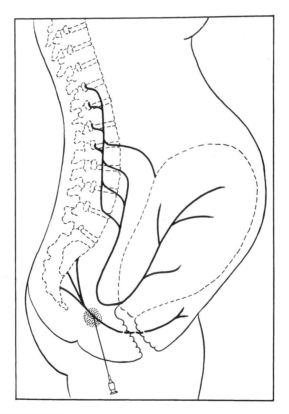

Figure 20–7

The pudendal nerve block involves only S3–S5 for the pain associated with the second stage of labor. (From Bonica JJ, McDonald JS: Principles and Practice of Obstetric Analgesia and Anesthesia, ed 2. Baltimore: Williams & Wilkins, 1994.)

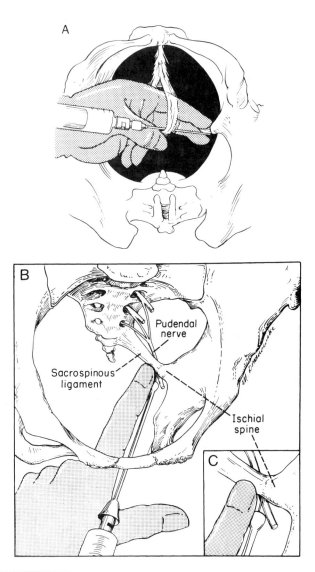

Figure 20–8

The transvaginal approach to pudendal neuroblockade. This technique is performed bilaterally. The needle passes behind the sacrospinous ligament and posterior to the ischial spine. Before injection of the local anesthetic drug, aspiration is prudent to avoid inadvertent intravascular administration. (From Bonica JJ, McDonald JS: Principles and Practice of Obstetric Analgesia and Anesthesia, ed 2. Baltimore: Williams & Wilkins, 1994.)

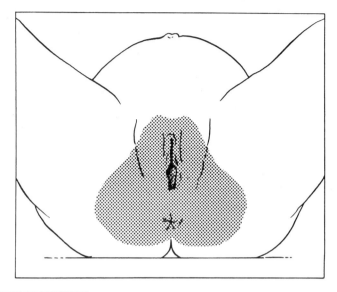

Figure 20–9

Stippled area illustrates the extent of analgesia/anesthesia provided by
pudendal neuroblockade. This is sufficient for the second stage of labor pain.
(From Bonica JJ, McDonald JS: Principles and Practice of Obstetric Analgesia
and Anesthesia, ed 2. Baltimore: Williams & Wilkins, 1994.)

5 mg/kg of lidocaine (1% solution with or without 1:200,000
epinephrine) total dose, provides relief of perineal pain within
3 to 5 minutes (Figs. 20–8 and 20–9).

■ Bilateral Paracervical Block

Paracervical block interrupts uterine nociceptive pain pathways
T10 through L1, effecting complete relief of pain of the first
stage of labor (Fig. 20–10). This does not, however, relieve
perineal pain of the second and third stages of labor. Using up
to 5 mg/kg of lidocaine in a 1% solution total dose gives good
pain relief for approximately 2 hours. Associated transient fetal
bradycardia has been reported with the use of paracervical
blockade and thus should be used with caution. Local anesthetics with epinephrine should not be used, since the fetal head is
so close to the injection site and the proximate location of

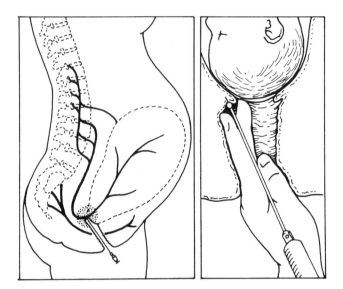

Figure 20–10

A technique for bilateral paracervical block. Neuroblockade involving T10–L1, when accomplished, is adequate for the pain associated with the first stage of labor. Injections are made into the bilateral fornices of the vagina. Note the proximity of the presenting part, as well as the deeper pelvic plexus with uterine arteries and ureters. (From Bonica JJ, McDonald JS: Principles and Practice of Obstetric Analgesia and Anesthesia, ed 2. Baltimore: Williams & Wilkins, 1994.)

the uterine artery and venous plexus may increase the risk of epinephrine uptake by mother or fetus.

■
Anesthesia for Cesarean Section

Spinal Anesthesia

The advantages of spinal anesthesia that are responsible for its current popularity include relative simplicity, rapidity, certainty, duration, low failure rate, and minimal side effects. It also offers the lowest drug exposure, since local anesthetic is being exposed directly to nerve fibers with minimal systemic drug uptake. The primary disadvantages of spinal anesthesia are the effects of high T2–T4 blockade—maternal hypotension and postdural puncture headaches (Table 20–8).

The risks of the "high spinal" include sympathectomy with

resultant unopposed parasympathetic stimulation. This leads to hypotension, increased gastric motility, increased nausea and vomiting, and instability of uterine perfusion. In parturients with severe asthma or reactive airway disease this may precipitate bronchospasm. Also, the high motor blockade may inhibit motor fibers of the respiratory muscles, impeding normal ventilation.

The postdural puncture headache risks are related directly to the size and type of the needle. With the 24- or 26-gauge Sprotte (blunted) needles now used, the risk is <1% in patients of this age group.

An important factor in the dispersion of local anesthetic is the position of the patient. As Figure 20–11 shows, the lowest point of the recumbent spine is T_5; care should therefore be taken to raise the patient's head, in an effort to reduce the inadvertent cephalad spread of drug.

Complications of subarachnoid block include these:

- *Physiologic:* Hypotension, bradycardia, or possible cardiac arrest
- *Nonphysiologic:* Respiratory arrest and toxicity reactions
- *Neurologic:* Paraplegia, arachnoiditis, or postdural puncture headache

---

Table 20–8

The Principal Disadvantages of the Use of Spinal Anesthesia and the Contraindications

Primary Disadvantages
Frequency of hypotension
Postdural puncture headaches

Contraindications
Infection at the site of puncture
CNS disease
Severe hypovolemia secondary to hemorrhage, dehydration, or malnutrition
Parturient's refusal or fear of the procedure or emotional unsuitability for regional anesthesia
Severe hypotension or hypertension
Lack of skilled anesthetist
Lack of resuscitation equipment in the immediate area

From Bonica JJ, McDonald JS: Principles and Practice of Obstetric Analgesia and Anesthesia, ed 2. Baltimore: Williams & Wilkins, 1994.

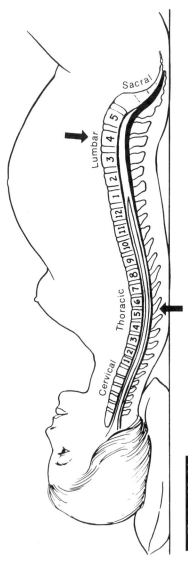

Figure 20-11

The natural curves of the female spine in the supine position. Gravity tends to extend the level of anesthetic spread to T3–T5; therefore, early head-up tilt would ensure a lower level of blockade. (From Bonica JJ, McDonald JS: Principles and Practice of Obstetric Analgesia and Anesthesia, ed 2. Baltimore: Williams & Wilkins, 1994.)

Cervical

Thoracic

Lumbar

Sacral

General Anesthesia for Cesarean Section

General anesthesia is reserved for life-threatening situations, including severe "fetal distress," cord prolapse, shoulder dystocia, intrauterine exploration for retained placenta or a twin, and repositioning of an inverted uterus. In obstetric anesthesia, the anesthesiologist is responsible for two lives: the mother's and the baby's.

Preanesthesia preparation includes a history and physical examination with emphasis on cardiac and pulmonary disease, evaluation of the airway, height-weight comparison, allergies, current medications, intravenous access, and blood product availability. Every pregnant woman beyond the first trimester is considered to have a full stomach and is at risk for aspiration of gastric contents. This demands prophylaxis with a nonparticulate antacid, an H_2 blocker, and metoclopramide. The most common cause of maternal death related to general anesthesia is aspiration pneumonia secondary to inability to secure the airway with an endotracheal tube.

Induction of Anesthesia

The patient should be placed on the operating table with a leftward pelvic tilt to prevent aortocaval compression with monitors applied. She should receive a 500- to 1000-mL bolus of lactated Ringer's while preoxygenation is performed. Cricoid pressure should be applied as Sellick's maneuver is performed, to prevent regurgitation of stomach contents into the lungs. Intravenous induction with thiopental (3 to 5 mg/kg), propofol (1 to 2 mg/kg), ketamine (1 mg/kg), or etomidate (0.2 to 0.3 mg/kg) may be used. Succinylcholine, 1 mg/kg intravenously, is given to achieve muscle relaxation to facilitate endotracheal intubation. Maintenance of balanced general anesthesia with both inhalational agents and intravenous muscle relaxants is performed until the baby is delivered. At this time, narcotics may be given to reduce the concentration of inhalational drugs needed.

Before extubation the patient should be completely awake and in control of her airway-protective reflexes. It is important to understand that the risk of aspiration is just as great at the end of surgery (extubation) as at the start (intubation). Figure 20–12 is a guide to failed intubation events.

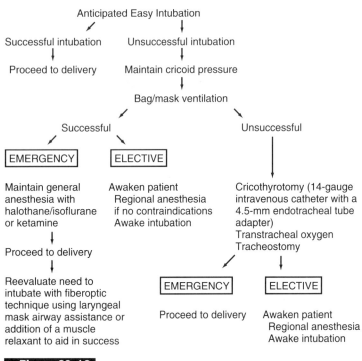

Figure 20-12

Guide for failed intubation.

■ Special Considerations

Preeclampsia

Preeclampsia is a multisystem disease. Although its hallmarks are hypertension and proteinuria, patients may develop renal failure, thrombocytopenia, hemolysis, liver dysfunction, and CNS involvement. For labor, epidural or epidural/spinal with narcotic/local anesthetic combinations are optimal to reduce the added stress related to pain. Whether epidural or general anesthesia is best for cesarean delivery remains controversial. Epidural anesthesia for cesarean section requires a high block (T4), with the associated risk of maternal hypotension. General anesthesia requires intubation, which with tracheal stimulation may result in dangerous hemodynamic aberrations, including hypertension, increased mean pulmonary artery pressure, and increased pulmonary capillary wedge pressure. With adequate invasive monitors such as an arterial line (with or without a pulmonary artery catheter), careful hydration, use of ephedrine, and slow onset of the block, epidural blockade can be safely conducted. Also, the use of beta-blocker agents (preinduction) or lidocaine to blunt the tracheal stimulation of intubation can also be safe. Close monitoring of the patient and open discussion with the obstetrician of the patient's preoperative status is helpful in determining the optimal anesthetic plan for mother and baby (see Chapter 5).

Preterm Birth

Patients with preterm labor, whatever the cause, most likely have been taking tocolytic drugs. If beta-adrenergic drugs were used to secure uterine relaxation, care must be taken to prevent cardiac irritability, which could be exaggerated by general anesthetics. In parturients receiving intravenous magnesium sulfate as a tocolytic agent, potentiation of muscle relaxant drug activity should be anticipated. Since preterm fetuses often have low birth weight and with diminished compensatory reserve, special attention should be directed at maintaining uteroplacental perfusion (see Chapters 22 and 24).

Parturients Infected with Human Immunodeficiency Virus

Concern has been voiced in the literature that HIV-positive parturients may not be candidates for regional anesthesia. The fear of spreading the infection to the central nervous system, adverse neurologic sequelae, or attenuation of the immune status of the patient has been questioned. To date, the data support the use of epidural anesthesia in these patients, and there is no substantiated evidence that these concerns are valid (see Chapter 28).

Coagulopathies

The preoperative laboratory tests recommended in a parturient with a suspected coagulopathy include hemoglobin, hematocrit, platelet count, prothrombin time (PT), partial thromboplastin time (PTT), and bleeding time. There is no one source (authority) that specifies the best test or laboratory value for determining risk for epidural hematoma. In the following situations epidural anesthesia is not recommended:

- Elevated PTT in a parturient on heparin therapy
- Parturient with known factor deficiency (e.g., von Willebrand's with low factor 8 levels)
- Parturient with severe HELLP syndrome with low platelets, elevated PT, elevated liver function tests, and an anticoagulated profile
- Parturient with disseminated intravascular coagulopathy
- Parturient actively bleeding and hemodynamically unstable

Many examples of stable, but abnormal laboratory values may be amenable to an epidural technique; however, discussion with the obstetrician about whether active bleeding is occurring and an overall risks-benefits discussion of general versus conduction anesthesia, in a given high-risk circumstance, may help determine the parturient's best overall anesthesia management.

Cardiac Disease or Congenital Heart Disease

The degree of shunting of blood in women with intracardiac defects is determined principally by the balance of resistances in the systemic (systemic vascular resistance) and pulmonary vascular beds (pulmonary vascular resistance). During pregnancy, these resistances decline proportionally during the various stages of pregnancy. With atrial septal defect (ASD), ventricular septal defect (VSD), or patent ductus arteriosus (PDA) with a left-right shunt, these parturients usually tolerate pregnancy, anesthesia, and delivery well. Reminders are to be aware of arrhythmias, systemic embolism, right ventricular hypertrophy and failure, and pulmonary hypertension. These concerns are especially problematic in the postpartum period, when placental shunting is gone (increased blood volume), resulting in an increased preload that places a strain on the shunt balance. In parturients with right-to-left shunts, such as uncorrected tetralogy of Fallot or Eisenmenger's syndrome, the conditions can be exacerbated by hypoxemia, hypercarbia, and decreased systemic vascular resistance.

In right or left ventricular outflow obstruction such as valvular stenosis or coarctation of the aorta, volume depletion, or decreased systemic vascular resistance can significantly exacerbate symptoms. With careful monitoring and attention to the specifics of the cardiac lesion and resultant cardiopulmonary pathophysiology, anesthesia and analgesia can be safely conducted in high-risk parturients (see Chapter 8).

Pulmonary Disease and Pulmonary Edema

When pulmonary edema occurs during pregnancy, invariably there is a predisposing cause (Table 20–9). Basic management of this condition includes establishing the cause and reversing the effects of hypoxemia. Hemodynamic monitoring—in the form of a pulmonary artery catheter and arterial line—can be extremely useful in elucidating the cause and the most appropriate treatment for pulmonary edema (see Chapter 12).

In most circumstances, anesthetic management for delivery of the baby may be conduction anesthesia; however, the parturient with severe respiratory failure may require general anesthesia with endotracheal intubation to achieve stability.

Table 20–9

Causes of Pulmonary Edema

Cardiogenic (high pressure)

Cardiac dysfunction:	Decreased left ventricular contractility, mitral stenosis, mitral regurgitation, intravascular volume overload, dysrhythmias
Pulmonary venous dysfunction:	Venous occlusive disease, neurogenic pulmonary vasoconstriction
Pulmonary embolization:	Amniotic fluid, thrombus, fat, air
Airway obstruction:	Edema, asthma, foreign body
Preeclampsia:	Pulmonary hypertension
Miscellaneous:	Pneumothorax, tumor, one lung anesthesia (down lung syndrome)

Noncardiogenic (permeability)

Adult respiratory distress syndrome
Aspiration syndromes
Pulmonary embolization
Abruptio placentae
Dead fetus syndrome
Sepsis

From Bonica JJ, McDonald JS: Principles and Practice of Obstetric Analgesia and Anesthesia, ed 2. Baltimore: Williams & Wilkins, 1994.

■ Conclusion

In conclusion, once an understanding of the nature of the parturient's pain is gained with techniques available to the anesthesiologist and obstetrician, an optimal care plan can be attained, even for high-risk parturients.

■ Bibliography

Bonica JJ, McDonald JS: Principles and Practice of Obstetric Analgesia and Anesthesia, ed 2. Baltimore: Williams & Wilkins, 1994.

Collis RE: Randomized comparison of combined spinal-epidural and standard epidural analgesia in labour. Lancet 1995; 345(8962):1413–1416.

Fanaroff AA: Neonatal-Perinatal Medicine: Diseases of the Fetus and Infant, ed 5. St. Louis: CV Mosby, 1992.

Guyton AC, Hall JE: Textbook of Medical Physiology, ed 9. Philadelphia: WB Saunders, 1996.

Hughes S: Parturients infected with human immunodeficiency virus and regional anesthesia. Anesthesiology 1995; 82(1):32–37.

Norris MC: Spinal opioid analgesia for labor. Int Anesthesiol Clin 1994; 32(2):69–81.

Shnider SM: Anesthesia for Obstetrics, ed 3. Baltimore: Williams & Wilkins, 1993.

Wallace D: Randomized comparison of general and regional anesthesia for cesarean delivery in pregnancies complicated by severe preeclampsia. Obstet Gynecol 1995; 86(2):193–199.

21

JOHN P. ELLIOTT

Special Considerations for the Patient with a Multifetal Gestation

Human reproduction is most efficient when the mother carries one fetus. Additional fetuses increase reproductive wastage and the likelihood of complications for the mother and the fetuses. The incidence of multiple gestations is given in Table 21–1. As reproductive technologies improve, the complications of infertility treatment also increase; namely, the incidence of multiple gestations. Multiple gestations are complex pregnancies that need special consideration.

■ Important Physiologic Adaptations of Multiple Gestation

- Cardiac output increases 30% to 50%—both stroke volume and heart rate. (Twin gestations are associated with an

Table 21–1
Incidence of Multifetal Gestations

| | Spontaneous | Induced | | |
		Clomiphene	Menotropins	GIFT*
Twins	1.2/100	8%	18%	22%
Monozygotic	40/10,000			
Dizygotic	80/10,000			
Triplets	1/6,889	0.5%	3%	4%
Quadruplets	1/575,000	0.3%	1.2%	1.2%
≥Quintuplets	$1/47 \times 10^6$	0.13%		

*Gamete intrafallopian tube transfer procedure

even more dramatic increase, to approximately a 70% increase in cardiac output over the nonpregnant state.)
- Systemic vascular resistance is decreased (although presumably not significantly more with twins than with a singleton).
- Renal plasma flow in pregnancy is 35% to 40% above non-pregnant levels and probably is further increased in multiple gestations.

■ The Importance of Placentation

Twin, triplet, and quadruplet pregnancies can result from the splitting of one zygote into two or more embryos, from fertilization of several eggs, or from a combination of the two processes. It is important to determine the number of amnions and chorions in a multiple gestation because this affects pregnancy risk and management. Real-time ultrasonography is invaluable for classifying the placentation. Separate placentas or different sex fetuses identify dichorionic/diamniotic placentas. When the placentas are fused, a thin, wispy membrane suggests monochorionic placentation, whereas a thicker, more "echodense" membrane indicates dichorionic placentas (Fig. 21–1). Placental tissue extending between the amnions ("twin peak sign") also indicates two chorions. Monochorionic placentation is associated with a higher rate of fetal loss and places that pregnancy at risk for twin-twin transfusion syndrome (TTTS).

Two thirds of twins are diamniotic/dichorionic, one third are diamniotic/monochorionic, and 1% are monoamniotic/monochorionic. Triplets and quadruplets are most often the result of multiple ovulations, so monochorionic placentas are rare in high-order multiples.

■ Complications of Multiple Gestations

Table 21–2 summarizes findings of several pertinent studies in the literature regarding complications associated with multifetal gestations. This table illustrates that, as each extra fetus is added, complications tend to increase dramatically.

■ Critical Care Environment for Multiple Gestations

Prevention of prematurity is the single most important aspect of the obstetric management of multiple gestations. Efforts to pre-

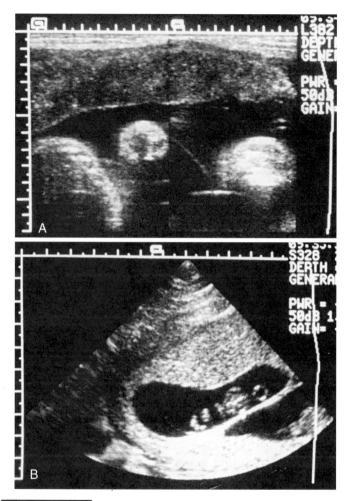

Figure 21-1

A, Ultrasound image depicts a thin, wispy dividing membrane suggesting monochorionic placentation. *B,* Image reveals a thicker, more echodense membrane with placental tissue extending between amnions ("twin peak sign"), indicating dichorionic placentation.

vent prematurity may place the mother in critical care situations. Twins deliver at a mean gestational age of 36.5 weeks, triplets at 33 weeks, quadruplets at 30 weeks, and quintuplets at 26.5 weeks. Preterm labor occurs in more than 40% of twin pregnan-

Table 21-2

Prevalence of Complications of Multifetal Gestations

Complication	Prevalence (%)			
	Singleton	Twins	Triplets	Quadruplets
SGA	4.6	17.4	30	10
Antepartum hemorrhage	2.0	2.8	6.7	10
PIH	8.2	23	28	75
Anemia	3.5	2.5	19	40
Preterm labor	8.4	42.7	84	80
IUFD >20 wk	0.98	3.7	6.7	0

Data from Phoenix Perinatal Associates.

Key: SGA, small for gestational age; IUFD, intrauterine fetal demise.

cies and in 80% of those with triplets and quadruplets. Preterm labor is a more formidable event in multiple gestations than in a singleton pregnancy. The obstetrician must be prepared to use multiple tocolytic drugs, often in maximum doses, for 3 to 4 days before the labor process is finally halted. Magnesium sulfate, the tocolytic drug of choice, is administered intravenously in a bolus dose (over 20 minutes) of 6 gm, followed by maintenance infusion of 3 to 5 gm/hour. Owing to the increased creatinine clearance with multiple gestations, higher infusion rates are often necessary to achieve therapeutic serum levels of magnesium (6.5 to 8.0 mg/dL). When treating preterm labor with triplets and quadruplets it is very important to be aggressive and continue to fight against delivery. It may be necessary to add terbutaline, 0.25 mg, administered subcuticularly every 3 hours and/or indomethacin, 25-50 mg, orally or rectally every 6 hours.

Corticosteroids are often administered to the mother to enhance fetal pulmonary function should premature delivery occur. Elliott and Radin demonstrated that steroids can initiate labor when administered in triplet and quadruplet pregnancies. Labor begins and the risk of delivery is statistically increased when the steroids are given when uterine contractions are occurring at the rate of 3.5 or more per hour. When the baseline uterine activity was no more than 3.0 contractions/hour, steroids produced no cervical changes and no deliveries occurred.

Pregnancy-induced hypertension (PIH) is more common with multiple gestations, and the consequences can contribute to obstetric critical care situations. Preeclampsia in multifetal pregnancies tends to become more severe because the effort to avoid prematurity prompts the clinician to delay delivery as long as possible.

The physiology of multiple gestations, the greater prevalence of complications (abruptio placentae, PIH, anemia), and therapeutic interventions (tocolysis, corticosteroids) place these pregnancies at high risk for potentially disastrous complications. Disseminated intravascular coagulopathy (DIC); (see Chapter 4) can occur when a dead fetus from a multiple gestation is retained. Abruptio placentae can also cause DIC and hemorrhagic shock. Bleeding complications can occur after delivery because of the increased risk of uterine atony because of the overdistended uterus associated with high-order multiple gestations.

Triplets and quadruplets are at increased risk for pulmonary edema. In our series, 3 of 14 women with quadruplets developed pulmonary edema. All three patients had the combination of PIH with anemia, low colloid osmotic pressure (COP), and tocolytic therapy. Pulmonary edema in these patients should be treated as follows (see Chapter 12):

- Oxygen is administered and titrated by pulse oximetry and arterial blood gases. Continuous positive airway pressure (CPAP) by mask is frequently utilized to assist with oxygenation.
- The patient is placed in an upright tilted position.
- Diuretic therapy should be vigorous: 40 to 80 mg IV furosemide. Significant hypertension is controlled with intravenous hydralazine or labetalol, as needed.
- Pulmonary artery catheterization should be used to evaluate left heart filling pressures should the conservative methods, described above, fail.

Another complication of multiple gestations that may place the pregnancy in the intensive care setting is twin-twin transfusion syndrome (TTTS). Virtually all monochorionic placentas have vascular communications between the placentas. Artery-artery or vein-vein anastomoses do not result in hemodynamic changes since the pressure in each vessel is equal; however, an arteriovenous anastomosis can potentially pump blood from one twin ("donor") into the placenta and circulation of the other twin ("recipient"). If the effect of this anastomosis is not balanced by an equal shunt in the opposite direction, volume overload in the recipient leads to polyuria and polyhydramnios. The donor

Table 21–3

Criteria for Diagnosis of Severe TTTS

Early onset (16–18 wk)
Same sex/monochorionic placenta
Difference in fetal size ≥1.5 wk
Difference in size of umbilical cord
Disparity in echogenicity of placental cotyledons supplying two fetuses
Presence of polyhydramnios in one sac
Presence of severe oligohydramnios in the "stuck twin"
Hemoglobin concentrations not affected

twin becomes hypovolemic and, retaining its fluid, develops severe oligohydramnios ("stuck twin"); (Table 21–3).

Severe TTTS or stuck twin syndrome is a critical care situation for the babies rather than the mother. Untreated, this syndrome has approximately 100% mortality (Table 21–4). Massive polyhydramnios leads to preterm labor or premature rupture of membranes (PROM) at 22 to 26 weeks with neonatal death; alternatively, continued volume shifting can eventually cause the death of one baby. The surviving twin remains at extreme risk of death and organ compromise owing to volume shifts through persistent anastomoses, since the dead baby now offers no resistance to the blood pumped by the survivor.

Table 21–4

Outcome in Severe TTTS* with No Therapy

Investigator	Patients (No.)	Survival (%)	Intrauterine Death (1)
Urig	12	3/24 (12.5)	4 (2 donors, 2 recipients)
Mahony	5	2/10 (20)	1 (donor)
Chescheir	5	0/10 (0)	
Weir	6	0/12 (0)	
Bebbington	14†	4/28 (14)	Not given
Pretorius	5	1/10 (10)	Not given
Saunders	4	0/8 (0)	
Mahony	2	0/4 (0)	
Total	**53**	**10/106 (9.4)**	**Survivors (5)**

*Diagnosis: <26 weeks; polyhydramnios/oligohydramnios.

†50% of survivors associated with one intrauterine death and eventual survival of other twin.

Table 21–5

Outcome in Severe TTTS* with Intervention

Investigator	Patients (No.)	Intervention	Survival (No.; %)
Elliott	16	Therapeutic amniocentesis	25/32 (78)
Mahony	7	Therapeutic amniocentesis	9/14 (64)
Schneider	7	Therapeutic amniocentesis	6/14 (43)
De Lia	3	Laser and therapeutic amniocentesis	4/6 (66)
Total	**33**		**44/66 (66)**

*Diagnosis: <26 weeks; polyhydramnios/oligohydramnios.

Therapy for severe TTTS appears to be most successful when therapeutic amniocentesis is used. Elliott and colleagues and Mahony and colleagues reported excellent results in treating TTTS with aggressive removal of large volumes of amniotic fluid (therapeutic amniocentesis). Survival was 78% in the Elliott study and 64% in the Mahony study (Table 21–5).

AMNIOTIC FLUID DRAINAGE

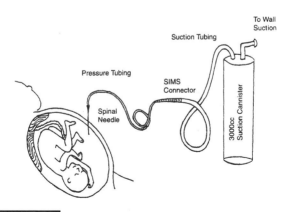

Figure 21–2

Amniotic fluid drainage equipment set-up.

Table 21-6

Technique of Therapeutic Amniocentesis

Sedate mother with narcotic drugs.
Infiltrate skin and subcuticular tissue with local anesthetic.
Use 18-gauge spinal needle.
Extension tubing with a Sims adapter allows connection to wall suction.
Adjust the wall suction to remove 1 L of amniotic fluid over 20 min.
Remove as much fluid as possible. (See Fig. 21–2.)

Amniocentesis is performed as soon as the diagnosis is made. An 18-gauge spinal needle is used after local anesthesia of the skin and underlying dermis. Pressure-resistant extension tubing is attached to the needle, followed by a Sim's adapter that is then connected to wall suction tubing and is attached to the wall suction (Fig. 21–2). Amniotic fluid is withdrawn at a rate of about 1 L every 20 minutes. As much fluid as possible is removed with one needle stick, with the goal of reducing the volume of fluid in the hydramniotic sac to normal or low normal. The procedure is repeated as soon as the fluid in the recipient twin's sac exceeds 8 cm as the largest pocket (Table 21–6).

Antibiotics are not used routinely. Tocolytics may be necessary to control preterm labor either before or after the procedure.

Approximately 75% of fetuses survive but there are several potential complications. In the donor, hypovolemia can lead to hypoxic injury to the brain or kidney, with resultant hypoxic-ischemic encephalopathy or renal infarcts. Cardiomyopathy may result in the large baby from prolonged hypervolemia.

Multiple gestations are special pregnancies that are at higher risk for developing conditions that need intensive treatment. Both mother and babies can be at risk from various complications. Treating multiple gestations requires understanding of the underlying physiology of pregnancy and the changes associated with multiple gestations.

■
Bibliography

Elliott JP: Twin-twin transfusion syndrome: Role of therapeutic amniocentesis. Cont Obstet Gynecol 1992; 37:30–47.
Elliott JP, Radin TG: Serum magnesium levels during magnesium

sulfate tocolysis in high order multiple gestations. J Reprod Med 1995; 40:450–459.

Elliott JP, Radin TG: The effect of corticosteroid administration on uterine activity and preterm labor in high order multiple gestations. Obstet Gynecol 1995; 85:250–254.

Elliott JP, Urig MA, Clewell WH: Aggressive therapeutic amniocentesis in the treatment of acute twin-twin transfusion syndrome. Obstet Gynecol 1991; 77:537.

Finberg HJ, Clewell WH: Definitive prenatal diagnosis of monoamniotic twins: Swallowed contrast agent detected in both twins on sonographically selected CT images. J Ultrasound Med 1991; 10:513.

Kovacs BW, Kirschbaum TH, Paul RH: Twin gestations, I. Antenatal care and complications. Obstet Gynecol 1989; 74:313.

Mahony BS, Petty CN, Nyberg DA, et al: The "stuck twin" phenomenon: Ultrasonographic findings, pregnancy outcome, and management with serial amniocenteses. Am J Obstet Gynecol 1990; 163:1513–1522.

Veille JC, Morton MJ, Burry KJ: Maternal cardiovascular adaptation to twin pregnancy. Am J Obstet 1985; 153:261.

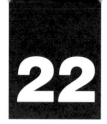

MICHAEL C. McQUEEN

Fetal Considerations in the Obstetric Intensive Care Patient

Virtually any pathologic condition in a pregnant patient has some effect on the fetus. The purpose of this chapter is to focus on the acutely ill intensive care obstetrics patients, with regard to effects and fetal responses to maternal physiologic derangements.

■ Pathophysiology

Maternal Shock and the Fetus

The clinical syndrome of shock occurs when the peripheral delivery of oxygen is insufficient to meet the demands of all organs and tissues. In the gravid patient, the peripheral dependents include the uterus, the placenta, and the fetus, and in a critically ill perinatal patient the status of the fetus is largely dependent on the maintenance of uterine blood flow and maternal oxygenation.

In adults, delivery of oxygen (Do_2) is the product of cardiac output (CO) and arterial oxygen content (Cao_2):

$$Do_2 = CO \times Cao_2$$
$$Cao_2 = (Hgb \times 1.34 \times Sao_2^*) + (Pao_2^\dagger \times .003)$$

Similarly, delivery of oxygen to the fetus is the product of umbilical blood flow and the oxygen content of umbilical venous blood. Subsequently, any maternal condition that compromises either of these two factors impairs delivery of oxygen to the fetus, resulting in fetal hypoxia and acidosis. The fetus has several homeostatic mechanisms, including blood and tissue buffers for regulation of acid-base balance, an ability to excrete

---

*Percentage of arterial oxygen hemoglobin saturation.
†Partial pressure of oxygen in arterial blood.

Table 22–1
Maternal Causes of Decreased Umbilical Blood Flow
Hypotension
Hypovolemia
Hypertension
Increased uterine vascular resistance

acidified urine in response to an acid load, redistribution of blood flow to vital organs, and the ability via increased heart rate to increase cardiac output. In addition, fetal well-being may be compromised by maternal compensatory mechanisms, which act to preserve maternal systemic arterial blood pressure at the expense of uterine blood flow. Because of this, alarming fetal heart rate (FHR) patterns may be present even when the mother's status is apparently stabilized.

Hypoxia

Under normal circumstances, fetal oxygen delivery is approximately 22 mL/kg/min, and umbilical venous Po_2 is about 30 to 35 mm Hg. Because of the tight affinity of fetal hemoglobin for oxygen, umbilical venous oxyhemoglobin saturation is 85% to 95%. Umbilical blood flow or umbilical venous oxygen content may be decreased by maternal, placental, or fetal factors. Complications that impair oxygen delivery to the fetus are listed in Tables 22–1 through 22–4.

Independent of the cause of hypoxia, several fetal responses to *acute* hypoxia have been identified:

- Increased arterial blood pressure and bradycardia
- Redistribution of cardiac output to brain and heart

Table 22–2
Maternal Causes of Decreased Umbilical Venous Oxygen Content
Anemia
Cigarette smoking
Hemoglobinopathies
Maternal hypoxemia from any cause

Table 22-3

Placental Causes of Decreased Umbilical Venous Oxygen Content

Placental infarction
Abruption
Placental edema
Villitis (idiopathic or infectious)
Fetoplacental vasoconstriction
Impaired transplacental diffusion of oxygen from infarction, abruption, edema, villitis

---

- Increased catecholamine and increased renin release
- Increased vasopressin and erythropoietin levels
- Decreased fetal breathing movements
- Increased glucose, lactate, and free fatty acids

In addition, rapid fetoplacental vasoconstriction has been seen in response to maternal hypoxia. This vasoconstriction is reversible with normalization of the maternal Pao_2.

Fetal responses to *chronic* hypoxia (2 weeks' duration) in a sheep model showed decreased fetal Pao_2, a compensatory increase in hemoglobin, increased arterial pressure, minimal change in resting FHR, and transient decrease in cardiac function which recovered in approximately 1 week. In studies of populations at high altitude, relative chronic hypoxia has been documented to result in decreased birth weights, although persistent fetal cerebral blood flow redistribution has been documented,

---

Table 22-4

Fetal Causes of Decreased Umbilical Venous Oxygen Content

Cord anomalies
Fetal hypertension
Hydrops
Congestive heart failure
Arrhythmias, especially fetal bradycardia
Fetal hemoglobin replaced with adult hemoglobin from repeated exchange transfusion secondary to Rh incompatibility
Anemia
Hemoglobinopathy

---

providing a "brain-sparing" effect. There is evidence, however, that during labor, contractions with FHR decelerations are associated with desaturation of fetal cerebral hemoglobin. It is not known if FHR decelerations resulting from either acute or chronic hypoxia are associated with the same phenomenon. Because of the characteristics of the fetal oxygen-hemoglobin dissociation curve, supplemental maternal oxygen may benefit the hypoxic fetus. Oxygen-hemoglobin dissociation curves for fetal and adult blood at normal pH and temperature are shown in Figure 22–1.

Note that because of the tight affinity of fetal hemoglobin for oxygen, fetal hemoglobin saturation is at least 85% when maternal Pao_2 is above 60 mm Hg. When maternal Pao_2 is less than 60 mm Hg, however, fetal hemoglobin may be rapidly

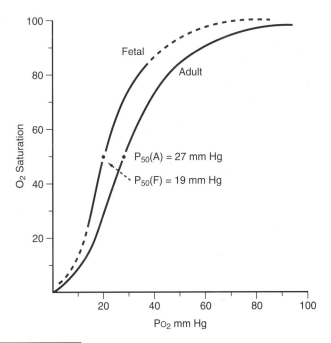

Figure 22–1

Oxygen dissociation curves for human adult and fetal blood at pH 7.4 and 37°C. Note the higher oxygen affinity of fetal blood compared with adult blood (P_{50} = Po_2 required for 50% saturation of hemoglobin with oxygen). (From Sacks LM, Delivoria-Papadopoulos M: Hemoglobin–oxygen interactions. Semin Perinatol 1984; 8(3):168.)

desaturated. Similarly, because of the steepness of the fetal curve, incremental increases in fetal Pao_2 may significantly improve fetal oxygen saturation and greatly benefit fetal oxygen delivery. One study reported that when supplemental oxygen raised maternal Pao_2 from 91 to 583 mm Hg, fetal umbilical vein Po_2 increased only from 32 to 40 mm Hg, but that increase in Po_2 resulted in a rise in oxygen saturation of approximately 15%.

Recall the fetal oxygen delivery equation (umbilical venous flow $\times$ umbilical O_2 content), and recognize that improving fetal oxygen delivery via increased blood oxygen content depends on maintaining adequate uterine and placental blood flow. Uterine blood flow (UBF) is determined by uterine artery pressure (UAP), uterine venous pressures (UVP), and uterine vascular resistance (UVR):

$$UBF = \frac{UAP - UVP}{UVR}$$

Maternal and Fetal Acidosis

Respiratory Acidosis

The respiratory alkalosis of pregnancy serves to accentuate the fetal-maternal carbon dioxide gradient. Maternal respiratory compromise therefore decreases that gradient, resulting in fetal accumulation of carbon dioxide and fetal acidosis. Increased maternal and fetal $PaCo_2$ causes an immediate increase in fetal breathing movements. Significantly, there is evidence that the respiratory response to hypercarbia of fetuses exposed to chronic hypoxia is blunted or absent. If maternal respiratory compromise persists, the fetal status may be further compromised by hypoxia (with fetal responses as described) and/or concomitant metabolic acidosis, with potentially severe consequences for the fetus.

Table 22–5
Normal Anion Gap ($<$12)
Bicarbonate loss
Renal tubular acidosis
Hyperchloremic states

Table 22-6
Increased Anion Gap (>12)

Ketoacidosis
Uremia
Salicylates
Methanol intoxication
Alcoholic ketoacidosis
Lactic acidosis
(Memory aid: KUSMAL)

Metabolic Acidosis

Maternal (and, subsequently, fetal) metabolic acidosis may be a prominent feature of the obstetric intensive care patient. A partial list of potential causes of maternal metabolic acidosis is presented in Tables 22–5 and 22–6. Even acute maternal glucose infusion may result in fetal metabolic acidosis, with maternal and fetal hyperglycemia, hyperinsulinism, and increases in blood lactate levels, with significant decreases in umbilical artery and vein pH values.

Fetal homeostatic mechanisms to adapt to acidosis are limited. There is obviously no pulmonary route of increased carbon dioxide excretion through hyperventilation. The fetal kidneys can increase acid excretion when presented with an increased acid load, but it is likely that this mechanism is of limited value in the face of severe maternal acidosis. The fetus does have blood and tissue acid buffers similar to adults', but there is good evidence that an important source for buffering the fetus against maternal acidosis is the placental tissue bicarbonate pool. This may explain reports of either negligible or delayed effects on fetal pH in response to maternal metabolic acidosis.

Prolonged or severe acidosis has been associated with impaired fetal cardiac function, severe periventricular leukomalacia, and sudden demise in utero. Treatment consists of identifying the cause of the maternal acidosis and correcting it.

Management: Algorithm for Fetal Oxygen Delivery

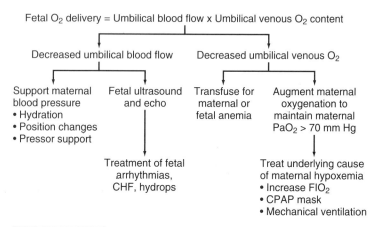

Fetal O_2 delivery = Umbilical blood flow x Umbilical venous O_2 content

Decreased umbilical blood flow

Decreased umbilical venous O_2

Support maternal blood pressure
• Hydration
• Position changes
• Pressor support

Fetal ultrasound and echo

Transfuse for maternal or fetal anemia

Augment maternal oxygenation to maintain maternal $PaO_2 > 70$ mm Hg

Treatment of fetal arrhythmias, CHF, hydrops

Treat underlying cause of maternal hypoxemia
• Increase FIO_2
• CPAP mask
• Mechanical ventilation

Figure 22–2

Algorithm for fetal oxygen delivery.

Conclusion

Well-defined fetal responses to maternal physiologic derangements have been described. Monitoring of intensive care obstetric patients should include aggressive fetal monitoring, both for the benefit of early corrective intervention for the distressed fetus and for early detection of potential impending changes in the mother's condition.

Bibliography

Acute Hypoxia and the Fetus

Ashwal S, Majcher JS, Longo LD: Patterns of fetal lamb regional cerebral blood flow during and after prolonged hypoxia. Pediatr Res 1980; 14:1104–1110.

Clark SL: Shock in the pregnant patient. Semin Perinatol 1990; 14(1):52–58.

Cohn HE, Sacks EJ, Heymann MA, et al.: Cardiovascular responses to hypoxemia and acidemia in fetal lambs. Am J Obstet Gynecol 1974; 120:817–824.

Howard RB, Hosokawa T, Maquire MH: Hypoxia-induced fetoplacental vasoconstriction in perfused human placental cotyledons. Am J Obstet Gynecol 1987; 157:1261–1266.

Jones CT, Richie JWK: Endocrine metabolic changes associated with periods of spontaneous hypoxia in fetal sheep. Biol Neonate 1976; 29:286–293.

Koos BJ, Sameshima H, Power GG: Fetal breathing, sleep state, and cardiovascular responses to graded hypoxia in sheep. J Appl Physiol 1987; 62:1033–1039.

Peebles DM, Edwards AD, Wyatt JS, et al: Changes in human fetal cerebral hemoglobin concentration and oxygenation during labor measured by near-infrared spectroscopy. Am J Obstet Gynecol 1992; 166:1369–1373.

Rudolph AM: Distribution and regulation of blood flow in the fetal and neonatal lamb. Circ Res 1985; 57:811–821.

Rudolph AM: Fetal circulatory responses to stress. In Hawkins DF, DiRenzo GC, Cosmi EV (eds): Progress in Perinatal Medicine. Cooper Station, NY: Harwood, 1990.

Sacks LM, et al: Hemoglobin-oxygen interactions. Semin Perinatol 1984; 8(3):168.

Wulf KH, Kunzel W, Lehmann V: Clinical aspects of placental gas exchange. In Respiratory Gas Exchange and Blood Flow in the Placenta. XXV International Congress of Physiological Sciences Symposium. 1971, Hannover, Germany: DHEW Publication No. (NIH) 73-361.

Chronic Hypoxia and the Fetus

Alonso JG, Kitanaka T, Gilbert RD, et al.: Fetal sheep cardiovascular responses to long-term hypoxemia. In Hawkins DF, DiRenzo GC, Cosmi EV (eds): Progress in Perinatal Medicine. Cooper Station, NY: Harwood, 1990.

Lichty JA, Ting RY, Bruns PD, et al: Studies of babies born at high altitude. I. Relation of altitude to birth weight. J Dis Child 1957; 93:666–669.

McClung J: Effects of High Altitude on Human Birth. Observations on Mothers, Placentas and the Newborn in Two Peruvian Populations. Cambridge: Harvard University Press, 1969.

Wladimiroff JW, Tonge HM, Stewart PA: Doppler ultrasound assessment of cerebral blood flow in the human fetus. Br J Obstet Gynaecol 1986; 93:471–475.

Fetal Response to Acidosis

Aarnoudse JG, Illsley NP, Penfold P, et al: Permeability of the human placenta to placenta to bicarbonate: In-vitro perfusion studies. Br J Obstet Gynaecol 1984; 91:1096–1102.

Low JA, Froese AF, Galbraith RS, et al: The association of fetal and newborn metabolic acidosis with severe periventricular leukomalacia in the preterm newborn. Am J Obstet Gynecol 1990; 162:977–982.

Miodornik M, Lavin JP, Harrington DJ, et al: Effect of maternal ketoacidemia on the pregnant ewe and the fetus. Am J Obstet Gynecol 1982; 144:585–593.

Philipson EH, Kalhan SC, Riha MM, et al: Effects of maternal glucose infusion on fetal acid-base status in human pregnancy. Am J Obstet Gynecol 1987; 157:866–873.

Van Weering HR, Wladimiroff JW: The effect of maternal hypercapnia and hyperoxia on breathing movements in the normal and growth retarded fetus. Acta Obstet Gynecol Scand 1982; 61:69–74.

Wladimiroff JW, VanWeering HK, Roodenburg PJ: The effect of changes in blood gases on fetal breathing movements. In Beard RW, Campbell S (eds): The Current Status of Fetal Heart Rate Monitoring and Ultrasound in Obstetrics. London: Royal College of Obstetricians and Gynaecologists, 1977.

HARRIS J. FINBERG

Role of Sonography in the Obstetric Intensive Care Setting

Certain observations on an obstetric sonogram imply imminent risk of fetal or maternal death or deterioration. These findings may be of the fetus, umbilical cord, amniotic space, cervix, placenta, adnexa, or maternal abdomen. When such an acute problem is identified, the sonographer should immediately involve the physician interpreting the study, who, in turn, should give an urgent verbal report directly to the referring obstetrician. A written report transmitted by routine channels is not sufficient. The obligation implied by the recognition of any of these high-risk conditions is not fulfilled until an appropriate management plan for the problem has been established.

■ Pathophysiologic Findings

Fetal Hydrops

Presence of fetal hydrops must be considered as strongly indicative of impending fetal demise. Sonographic findings in the fetus may include ascites, pericardial and/or pleural effusion, and scalp or generalized skin edema (Fig. 23–1). The placenta may be abnormally thickened. Alternatively, isolated ascites may be seen as a result of perforation of an obstructed urinary or intestinal tract. Although serious, these anomalies do not, in general, carry the risk of imminent fetal death associated with hydrops.

The etiology of hydrops must be sought, in hope of finding a treatable cause (Table 23–1). When possible, it is clearly preferable to give therapy in utero to reverse hydrops (permitting later elective delivery of a well-compensated, older fetus) than to perform emergent delivery of an extremely ill, premature fetus.

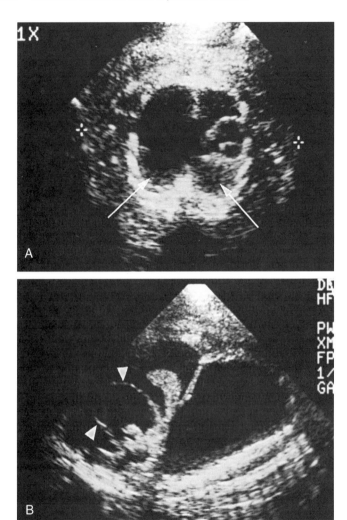

Fetal hydrops due to high-pressure left pleural effusion. *A,* Transverse thorax. A large left pleural effusion shifts the heart far to the right, compressing the lungs *(arrows).* There is marked skin edema (skin surface marked by cursors). *B,* Sagittal left thorax and abdomen. The effusion depresses and inverts the left hemidiaphragm. Ascites outlines the left lobe of the liver, and fluid is trapped between the folds of the omentum *(arrowheads).* (From Finberg HJ: Ultrasound guided interventions in pregnancy. Ultrasound Q 8:3:217, 1990.)

Table 23–1

Causes and Therapies for Fetal Hydrops

Treatable Causes

Anemia—Fetal transfusion via cordocentesis
  Immunoincompatibility (e.g., Rh, Kell)
  Fetal-maternal hemorrhage—(Diagnostic test: Kleihauer-Betke test for
    nucleated fetal red blood cells in maternal blood)
  Parvovirus (can cause reversible bone marrow suppression)
Cardiac arrhythmias
  Tachyarrhythmia—pharmacologic agents
  Heart block—systemic lupus erythematosus. Delivery and postnatal
    cardiac pacemaker
High-pressure thoracic fluid collections—In utero thoracocentesis and
    possible thoracoamniotic shunt placement
  Primary pleural effusion (lymphatic discontinuity)
  Pericardial effusion (association with intrapericardial teratoma)
Twin-Twin Transfusion Syndrome—volume reduction amniocentesis from sac
    of hydropic recipient twin
Maternal causes
  Severe anemia
  Hypoproteinemia
  Severe diabetes mellitus

Potentially Treatable Causes—in Utero Surgery

Diaphragmatic hernia
Solid thoracic masses
  Cystic adenomatoid malformation
  Intrapericardial teratoma or intracardiac tumor
Vascular tumor—Sacrococcygeal teratoma, hemangioma

Natural History Only—No Available Therapy

Viral and other infections
  Cytomegalic inclusion virus
  Toxoplasmosis
  Other
Lymphatic malformation/discontinuity sequence
  Cystic hygroma as in Turner syndrome
Cardiomyopathies, valvular and other cardiac malformations
Restrictive skeletal dysplasias
Homozygous α thalassemia
Numerous additional specific chromosomal aneuploidies, anatomic
  anomalies, malformation syndromes, and metabolic disorders

Intrauterine Growth Retardation

The concern in intrauterine growth retardation (IUGR) is not specifically the reduced size of the fetus but the risk that the underlying cause, especially uteroplacental circulatory inadequacy, may lead to fetal hypoxic distress with its dangers of neurologic damage or death. When IUGR is suggested on a sonogram, the examination should be extended to evaluate fetal well-being. Evidence of fetal compromise requires an urgent management plan.

Umbilical Cord Abnormalities

The umbilical cord is the lifeline of the fetus. Obstruction or interruption of blood flow through the cord may cause extremely rapid fetal death.

Umbilical Cord Prolapse or Presentation. Prolapse or herniation of the umbilical cord into or through the dilated cervix in advance of the fetus is an extreme emergency that requires immediate cesarean delivery. Pressure by the fetal presenting part, as it descends with uterine contraction or rupture of membranes, compresses the cord, occluding fetal blood flow.

   Cord presentation, also referred to as "funic presentation," implies the probability of prolapse if the cervix dilates, as well as the risk of cord compression by the fetus with uterine contractions (Fig. 23–2). Nonstandard fetal lie such as transverse lie, contracted maternal pelvis, and lower uterine or intra-pelvic adnexal masses such as leiomyomas or ovarian cystic lesions may all predispose to cord presentation. The cord may transiently present and spontaneously reduce before the fetus becomes engaged. A marginal cord insertion into the caudal aspect of a low-lying placenta may produce an obligate cord presentation. Cord presentation should be treated as an urgent problem when identified in the latter half of the third trimester. Cesarean delivery will be necessary unless the condition can be reduced. Recognition earlier in pregnancy should prompt a search for irreversible causes of cord presentation such as those described above. These also require cesarean delivery with prenatal surveillance for signs of impending labor.

Vasa Previa. The presence of placental blood vessels from the fetal circulation crossing the internal os of the cervix is referred to as vasa previa (Fig. 23–3). Cervical dilatation can tear these

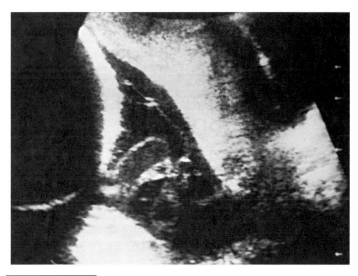

Figure 23-2

Obligate cord presentation. Sagittal midline scan of lower uterine segment. There is an anterior low-lying placenta with a marginal cord insertion just beyond the internal cervical os. With cervical dilatation, cord prolapse can be anticipated. Note that, with a low-lying marginal cord insertion, aberrant chorionic surface vessels could cross the cervix, producing vasa previa. (From McGahan JP, Porto M: Obstetrical Ultrasound—A Systemic Approach. Philadelphia: J.B. Lippincott, 1994.)

vessels, causing rapid exsanguination of the fetus. This condition may occur in three circumstances:

1. Vessels connecting a succenturiate lobe of a placenta to the main portion of the placenta may cross the cervix.
2. There may be a velamentous (membranous) insertion of the umbilical cord into the placenta. In this condition, the chorionic surface fetal vessels extend under the chorion for some distance beyond the margin of the placenta before forming the umbilical cord. These unprotected vessels may cross the cervix.
3. With a marginal cord insertion into the caudal end of a low-lying placenta, aberrant chorionic surface vessels may extend beyond the placental edge and cross the cervix.

Duplex Doppler and color flow imaging using endovaginal transducers may help establish the diagnosis of vasa previa; however, when the location and configuration of the placenta

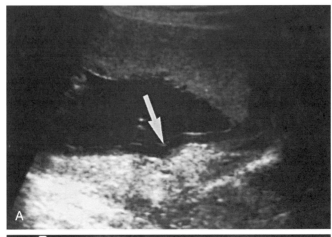

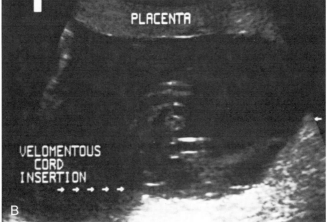

Figure 23–3

Vasa previa from velamentous cord insertion. *A*, Midline sagittal scan shows an anterior placenta with a prominent chorionic vessel extending from its caudal margin and coursing over the internal os of the cervix *(arrow)*. *B*, The vessel(s) continue onto the posterior uterine wall, where the actual umbilical cord originates.

and cord raise the possibility of vasa previa, it may be most prudent to manage the pregnancy as if the condition is present unless it can convincingly be excluded by the imaging studies. Surveillance of a patient with vasa previa should be at least as intensive as for the one with placenta previa. Such a patient should not be allowed to labor.

Cord Lesion, Cord Knot. Focal lesions of the umbilical cord, including cyst, hemangioma, teratoma, arterial aneurysm, venous varix, and true cord knot may all infrequently be encountered. Each has been reported as a cause of fetal demise, but in many cases no fetal compromise occurs. All such cases should receive close fetal monitoring with appropriate intervention if signs of deterioration are detected. If the fetus remains well-compensated, routine vaginal delivery is not contraindicated.

Nuchal Cord. The presence of a circumferential nuchal cord is found in nearly one quarter of all deliveries without significant impact on perinatal outcome. No special management is indicated. If, however, the nuchal loops are tight enough to indent the skin of the fetal neck, it is advisable to keep the pregnancy under surveillance for fetal well-being (Fig. 23–4).

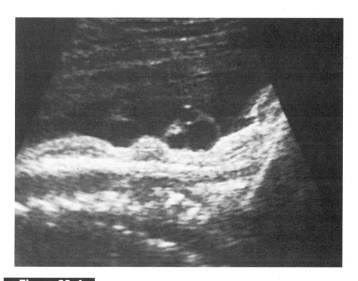

Figure 23–4

Tight nuchal cord. Two cross-sections of the umbilical cord are seen in this scan longitudinally oriented along the fetal neck, indicating that the cord encircles the neck. The skin of the neck is indented, implying that the nuchal cord is tight.

Oligohydramnios

Oligohydramnios may occur in the following circumstances: (1) premature rupture of membranes; (2) severe intrauterine growth retardation; (3) nonsteroidal antiinflammatory drugs utilized for tocolysis in premature labor (i.e., indomethacin); (4) fetal urinary tract obstruction or nonfunction. Regardless of the cause, oligohydramnios subjects the fetus to significant risks and may, by itself, be an indication for delivery. The risks include these:

1. Cord compression between the uterine wall and fetus, especially with contractions, can impair fetal blood flow and cause hypoxemia and acidosis.
2. Fetal compromise—or even demise—may occur from the effects of cord compression or from underlying deterioration of uteroplacental function that has become severe enough to cause oligohydramnios.
3. Pulmonary hypoplasia can be anticipated if there has been longstanding severe oligohydramnios regardless of cause. Complete oligohydramnios developing before 20 to 22 weeks is very likely to cause lethal pulmonary hypoplasia, whereas those cases beginning in the third trimester are rarely associated with critically severe pulmonary hypoplasia.
4. Intrauterine sepsis may complicate any ongoing pregnancy after rupture of membranes. Persistent oligohydramnios implies ongoing loss of newly produced amniotic fluid owing to disrupted membranes, and the likelihood of the development of sepsis is greater than with transient amniotic leakage with subsequent sealing of the membranes.

Oligohydramnios should be reported expeditiously to permit appropriate management planning.

◼ Monitoring of Fetal Well-Being

When there is concern for possible fetal compromise, as in all the conditions discussed above, a program of ongoing fetal surveillance becomes an important aspect of pregnancy management. Specific tests used include (1) daily fetal movement counting, (2) biophysical profile, and (3) umbilical artery (and other fetal vessel) Doppler waveform analysis. The full biophysical profile consists of evaluation of five separate parameters most often scored on a 10-point scale according to specific criteria establish by Manning and coworkers. The parameters are non-stress fetal cardiac monitoring (NST), fetal breathing movement (FBM), limb/body movement (FM), fetal tone (FT), and adequacy of amniotic fluid volume (AFV).

Frequently, subsets of these tests are analyzed and the full biophysical profile is reserved for cases when results of the subset initially tested are nonreassuring. The two most often used modifications are the ultrasound imaging criteria only—FBM, FM, FT, and AFV, without the NST—or the NST and AFV only. A complete biophysical profile scoring less than 8 points, or a biophysical subset in which any criterion is not successfully fulfilled, should be called to the referring obstetrician's attention.

The role of umbilical artery Doppler evaluation in assessing fetal compromise is still under investigation. Currently, abnormally high resistance patterns (abnormally low diastolic velocities as compared to systolic velocity) are further evaluated by biophysical profile testing before intervention or pregnancy interruption is contemplated. Nonetheless, severely abnormal umbilical artery waveforms (i.e., those with absence or reversal of direction of diastolic flow) should be called to the attention of the referring obstetrician even when the biophysical profile is normal.

Abnormalities of the Cervix

Cervical findings during ultrasound assessment may indicate increased risk for cervical incompetence or incipient premature labor (Fig. 23–5). These findings include (1) dilatation of the internal cervical os; (2) cervical effacement resulting in a residual measured length less than 3 cm; (3) bulging of the membranes through the endocervical canal into the vagina; and (4) "beaking" or "funneling" of the endocervical canal as an early sign. Other phenomena may affect the ultrasound study of the cervix. Overdistention of the urinary bladder or a postvoiding concentric lower uterine segment contraction may each mask significant cervical changes. Spontaneous uterine/cervical muscle contractions may also mask cervical change. In all cases, the greatest demonstrated extent of cervical dilatation and effacement should be taken as the degree of severity of cervical change and of risk for preterm delivery.

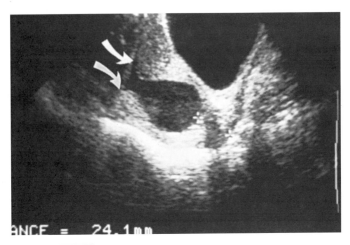

Figure 23–5

Cervical effacement and dilatation. Amniotic fluid extends through the dilated internal os, with residual closed length of the endocervical canal only 24 mm (lower limit of normal, 30 mm). Note anterior and posterior bulging of the lower uterine segment *(arrows),* indicative of a ring of contraction, as part of the patient's preterm labor. One minute earlier the contraction had been more distal, and the cervix looked completely closed and normal in length.

■ Placental Abnormalities: Previa, Accreta, Abruption

Placenta Previa. It is well recognized that placenta previa appears to be present in many late first or second trimester pregnancies that will have clinically proven absence of placenta previa at delivery. This observation can be explained by the concept of "trophotropism," preferential proliferation of placental trophoblastic villi into regions of the uterus with richer blood supply along with atrophy of villi in areas of poorer blood supply. The pericervical lower uterine segment has less adequate circulation than the uterine corpus and fundus, so a placenta that implants low in the uterus is likely to migrate with advancing pregnancy due to differential growth and atrophy.

Resolution of placenta previa is more likely if the initial appearance of the previa is marginal, partial, or even complete but only by a small peripheral portion of the placenta than it is if the placenta is positioned centrally over the internal cervical os. Until and unless placenta previa resolves, it is still true previa, with the attendant risks of bleeding and harm to the pregnancy. Findings of placenta previa should be reported no matter when during the pregnancy it is diagnosed. The majority of cases of placenta previa diagnosed in the second trimester resolve by the time of delivery, particularly if they are positioned asymmetrically, rather than centrally, relative to the internal cervical os. The appropriate clinical assessment of placenta previa should be maintained, with periodic sonographic surveillance to check for regression. If the placenta previa resolves, management precautions may be lifted. Note that bleeding episodes may still occur from marginal abruptions of a residually low-lying placenta, even after resolution of placenta previa. A trial of labor for a vaginal delivery may still be warranted in this setting, depending on the clinical judgment of the obstetrician.

Placenta Accreta. The decidua of the endometrium serves as a barrier, preventing the invasion of placental villi into the uterine myometrium. Scarring of the endometrium may damage this decidual barrier. A common cause of scarring in the lower uterine segment is cesarean section. According to Clark and coworkers, prior cesarean sections predispose to increased frequency of placenta previa and to considerably greater risk of placenta accreta (abnormally adherent or invasive placenta) when placenta previa has occurred (Table 23–2).

Placenta accreta is defined as presence of chorionic villi in

Table 23–2

Risk of Placenta Previa/Accreta and Cesarean Sections

Risk of Placenta Previa after Cesarean Section

# of Prior C-sections	Risk of Previa
0	0.26%
1	0.65%
2	1.8%
3	3.0%
4	10.0%

Risk of Placenta Accreta When There is Previa and Prior C-section

Previa and 0 C-section	5%
Previa and 1 C-section	24%
Previa and 2 or more C-sections	48%

Data from Clark SL, Koonings PP, Phelan JP: Placenta previa/accreta and prior cesarean section. Obstet Gynecol 1985; 66:89–91.

direct contact with myometrium without intervening decidua. More deeply invasive variants include placenta increta (villi invading the myometrium) and placenta percreta (villi invading to the uterine serosa or beyond it into adjacent organs such as the urinary bladder). This group of conditions, collectively called "placenta accreta," is associated with severe maternal morbidity and real risks of maternal death, all due to severe bleeding. Most often, immediate hysterectomy is required to achieve hemostasis.

Historically, placenta accreta has not been recognized until the third stage of labor, when the placenta fails to detach completely and profuse hemorrhage occurs. There are ultrasound findings that can predict or exclude the presence of placenta accreta with much—although not perfect—reliability in the setting of placenta previa crossing the operative area of the lower anterior uterine segment in a patient with a history of one or more cesarean sections.

The ultrasound signs of placenta accreta include these (Fig. 23–6):

1. Loss of the normal hypoechoic myometrial zone between the anterior placenta previa and the uterine serosa.
2. Focal areas of thinning or interruption of the echodense boundary representing the anterior uterine serosa and posterior bladder wall.
3. Nodular masses of placental echotexture extending beyond the uterine serosa.
4. Numerous, oddly shaped vascular lakes within the parenchyma of the placenta.

If criteria 1, 2, and 3 or 1 and 2 are seen, the probability of placenta accreta is very high. If alone, criterion 1 is false positives in a quarter to half of such cases. If neither 1 nor 2 nor 3 is present, accreta is very unlikely. Intraparenchymal vascularity is a separate risk criterion that need not be present but that increases the likelihood of accreta relative to that predicted by the presence or absence of the first three criteria.

Sonographic diagnosis of placenta accreta requires urgent and intensive management appropriate to the associated placenta previa, but it also permits detailed planning for a carefully controlled elective operative delivery, likely with significant blood loss and, in many cases, with hysterectomy. Placenta accreta has not been diagnosed reliably in patients without placenta previa and history of cesarean sections, but if similar

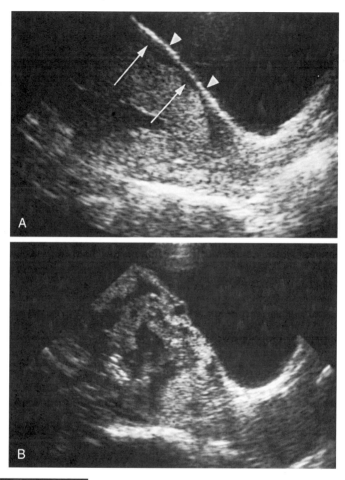

Figure 23-6

Findings for placenta accreta with placenta previa in patients with prior
cesarean sections. *A,* Uncomplicated placenta previa. A hypoechoic myometrial
zone *(arrows)* is present. The echodense uterine serosa–bladder wall interface
(arrowheads) is uniformly thick and intact. The placental parenchyma has no
prominent venous lakes. *B,* Placenta previa accreta. The myometrial zone is
obliterated, and the serosal boundary is regionally effaced. Large and bizarrely
shaped venous spaces are interspersed within the placental parenchyma.
(From Finberg HJ, Benirschke K: Recent Observations on the Ultrasound
Diagnosis of Placenta Previa and Placenta Accreta with Correlation to the
Principles of Placental Pathophysiology. State of the Art Ob/Gyn Imaging
Course Syllabus. American Institute of Ultrasound in Medicine, Laurel,
Maryland, 1992.)

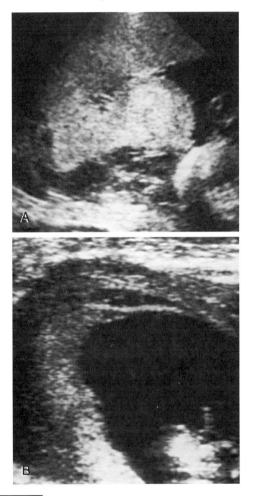

Figure 23-7

Placental abruption. *A*, A large subplacental abruption elevates the posterior third of the fundal placenta. Increased echogenicity in this portion of the placenta is consistent with infarction. The fetus was unstable, and urgent delivery (successful) was required. *B*, Marginal abruption is seen at the anterior edge of this fundal placenta, with little disruption of the placental attachment to the uterine wall. The bleeding episode ceased, the fetus remained stable, and the pregnancy continued uneventfully.

findings were identified in other pregnancy situations, it would certainly be appropriate to organize a similar management plan.

Placental Abruption. Most often, placental abruption is suspected clinically because of vaginal bleeding, sometimes associated with localized uterine tenderness or uterine irritability. In such cases clinical management will be guided by the presentation, even if ultrasonography fails to detect a specific site of abruption. In fact, sonographic evidence of abruption can be anticipated in fewer than half the cases of clinically suspected abruption. Positive sonographic findings should still be reported expeditiously. Subplacental abruptions detected by ultrasound tend to be the more extensive lesions with interruption of maternal arteries into the placenta and have significant risk of fetal compromise. Cases in which a submembrane blood collection is found adjacent to or at some distance from the placenta without dissection under it are more likely to be due to venous bleeds from the placental marginal sinus and tend to have a better prognosis (Fig. 23–7).

Acute Pain with an Adnexal Lesion

The differential diagnosis for an adnexal lesion found by sonography in a pregnant patient who presents with acute onset of pelvic pain includes four entities, which should be specifically considered or excluded. *Hemorrhage in a corpus luteum cyst* may stretch the ovarian capsule, and leakage of blood from it may cause peritoneal signs (Fig. 23–8). The condition is usually self-limited, and if the sonogram is sufficiently suggestive, close observation and comfort care may be appropriate. *Acute degeneration of a uterine leiomyoma* may cause severe pain. If the leiomyoma is pedunculated, the lesion may simulate an adnexal lesion. If the pedicle is identified by ultrasound, observation and comfort care can be considered (Fig. 23–9). *Ovarian torsion,* more often than not of an ovary containing a preexisting cystic or other lesion, presents with sudden severe pain and is an indication for emergency surgery (Figs. 23–9, 23–10). Unlike the pedunculated leiomyoma, stalklike attachment to the uterus is seen only in the relatively rare case of torsion of the entire adnexa at the cornual origin. *Coexistent ectopic and intrauterine pregnancies,* although exceedingly rare in the general population, must be considered when acute pain with an adnexal mass

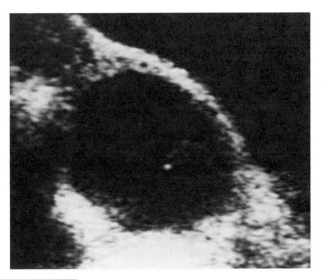

Figure 23-8

Hemorrhagic corpus luteum cyst. Clumplike echoes and debris are seen within this 4-cm thin-walled cyst found on a 14-week obstetric sonogram. A repeat scan 3 weeks later showed reduced internal echoes and partial shrinkage of the cyst, which resolved without intervention.

develops in a patient who has undergone fertility induction, especially techniques involving intrafallopian introduction of multiple gametes. This, too, must be considered a surgical emergency.

Acute Abnormalities of the Maternal Abdomen

Acute abnormalities that might require surgical intervention may affect other organ systems during pregnancy. These include, but are not limited to, acute cholecystis, urinary tract calculi and obstruction (Fig. 23–11), intestinal obstruction (Fig. 23–12), and local or systemic infection (Fig. 23–13). An important concept of patient care is that diagnostic tests and therapeutic interventions necessary to prevent maternal morbidity and mortality should not be delayed because of the pregnancy. This principle applies to radiography during pregnancy, as well.

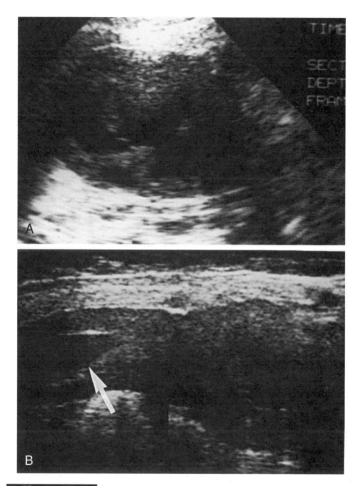

Figure 23–9

Degenerating uterine leiomyoma. Acute left pelvic pain led to sonographic evaluation of this patient, who was in the eighth week of pregnancy. *A,* A scan through the left adnexa shows a thick-walled complex cystic mass containing thick and thin septa. This image, taken alone, could easily represent a serous cystadenocarcinoma. *B,* A transverse scan demonstrates the gestational sac *(arrow)* within the uterus and a broad pedicle connecting the lesion to the uterus, indicating it to be a degenerating leiomyoma.

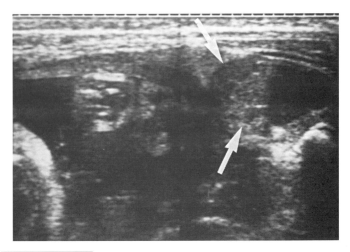

Figure 23-10

Torsion of a left ovary containing a dermoid cyst in a patient at 28 weeks of pregnancy. The patient presented with left-side abdominal pain, centered over the area of the lesion, adjacent to the left upper aspect of the gravid uterus. The ovary *(arrows)* is enlarged by a complex cystic mass. Urgent surgical resection was required.

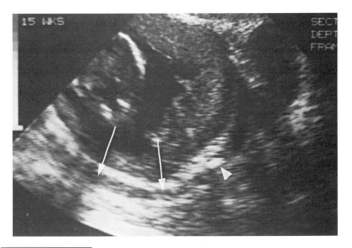

Figure 23-11

Obstructing right distal ureteral calculus in a 17-week pregnant patient with right flank pain. The gravid uterus pushes intestine aside, permitting visualization of the urine-distended right ureter *(arrows)* and the obstructing calculus *(arrowhead)*.

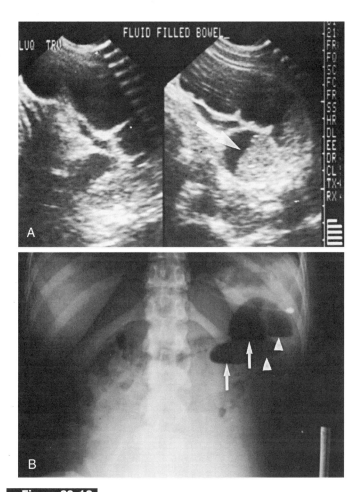

Figure 23–12

Intestinal obstruction at 25 weeks' pregnancy. The patient presented with
nausea and vomiting. *A,* Sonogram of the left upper quadrant shows distended
loops of intestine, with fluid-material level *(arrow).* The level is not horizontal
in the image, obtained with the patient in a left decubitus lie, but it is
horizontal to the direction of gravity. *B,* A single upright radiograph, centered
on the upper abdomen, obtained with shielding of the lower abdomen and
pelvis, confirms differential air-fluid levels in the distended small intestine.
(Compare the height of the arrow and arrowhead in each of the two loops.)
This confirmed obstruction as opposed to ileus. At surgical exploration,
obstructing adhesions were lysed.

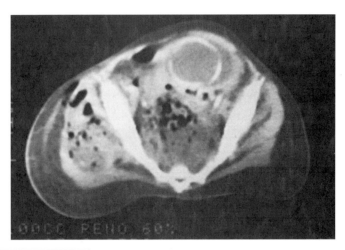

Figure 23–13

Gluteal extension of perirectal abscess from gas-forming organisms in 16-weeks pregnant patient with known inflammatory bowel disease. The patient was admitted for right hip pain. She had taken prednisone intermittently for her bowel disease and was afebrile with a normal white blood cell count. Imaging studies were deferred because of the pregnancy. On day 6, the patient spiked a high fever, becoming obviously septic, and the fetus died. This CT scan confirmed a right gluteal abscess tracking through the sciatic notch from a perirectal abscess. Despite wide débridement, the patient died.

If a radiographic procedure is needed for appropriate diagnosis during pregnancy, the following guidelines apply:

1. Do the examination when it is needed. It is not reasonable to wait until later in the pregnancy. This would unnecessarily jeopardize the mother's health.
2. Shield the pregnancy, but only to the extent that it does not interfere with the diagnostic requirements of the examination.
3. Tailor the examination, paring it to the minimum number of exposures that will permit accurate diagnosis. Analyze each image as it is obtained, ordering an additional view as needed and stopping when the diagnostic information has been acquired.
4. In the second or third trimester, consider using magnetic resonance imaging (MRI), which does not use ionizing radiation. MRI can cause heating of internal tissues and has theoretical risks to the embryo during the first trimester. MRI should, in general, be avoided during the first trimester

unless there is no alternative way of obtaining necessary diagnostic information.

■ Bibliography

Anderson JC, Rayburn WF: Cervical incompetence. In Chervenak FA, Isaacson GC, Campbell S (Eds): Ultrasound in Obstetrics and Gynecology. Boston: Little, Brown, 1993.

Clark SL, Koonings PP, Phelan JP: Placenta previa/accreta and prior cesarean section. Obstet Gynecol 1985; 66:89–91.

Finberg HJ, Kurtz AB, Johnson RL, et al: The biophysical profile: A literature review and reassessment of its usefulness in the evaluation of fetal well being. J Ultrasound Med 1990; 9:583–591.

Finberg HJ, Williams JW: Placenta accreta: Prospective sonographic diagnosis in patients with placenta previa and prior cesarean section. J Ultrasound Med 1992; 11:333–343.

Finberg HJ: Umbilical cord and amniotic membranes. In McGahan JP, Porto M (eds): Obstetrical Ultrasound—A Systematic Approach. Philadelphia: J.B. Lippincott, 1994.

Hansman M, Arabin B: Nonimmune hydrops fetalis. In Chervenak FA, Isaacson GC, Campbell S (eds): Ultrasound in Obstetrics and Gynecology. Boston: Little, Brown, 1993.

Kier R, McCarthy SM, Scoutt LM, et al: Pelvic masses in pregnancy: MR imaging. Radiology 1990; 176:709–713.

Nyberg DA, Finberg HJ: The placenta, placental membranes, and umbilical cord. In Diagnostic Ultrasound of Fetal Anomalies: Text and Atlas. In Nyberg DA, Mahoney BS, Pretorius DH (eds): Diagnostic Ultrasound of Fetal Anomalies: Text and Atlas. Chicago: Year Book, 1990.

Sassone AM, Timor-Tritsch IE, Artner A, et al: Transvaginal sonographic characterization of ovarian disease: Evaluation of a new scoring system to predict ovarian malignancy. Obstet Gynecol 1991; 78:70–76.

Stabile I: Clinical and ultrasound aspects of ectopic pregnancy. In Chervenak FA, Isaacson GC, Campbell S (Eds): Ultrasound in Obstetrics and Gynecology. Boston: Little, Brown, 1993.

Zelop CC, Bromley B, Frigoletto FD, et al: Second trimester sonographically diagnosed placenta previa: Prediction of persistent previa at birth. Int J Obstet Gynaecol 1994; 44:207–210.

JOHN P. ELLIOTT

Management of Complications Associated with Administration of Tocolytic Agents

Pharmacologic inhibition of preterm uterine contractions is a medical strategy that has been used for more than 30 years. In this chapter I discuss the side effects and complications of currently used tocolytic medications.

■ Beta-Adrenergic Agonists

Ritodrine and terbutaline are the beta-adrenergic (i.e., beta-agonist) drugs most widely used in the United States for treatment of preterm labor. These medications exert their effect by stimulating beta-adrenergic receptors, of which there are two types: β_1 receptors are located in the heart and small intestine whereas β_2 receptors predominate in blood vessels, bronchioles, and myometrium. Beta$_2$-receptor stimulation is desired for tocolysis; β_1 activity is generally associated with unwanted cardiovascular side effects. Unfortunately, all beta-adrenergic drugs possess some degree of β_1 activity. The important physiologic effects of β_1 and β_2 adrenergic stimulation are outlined in Figure 24–1. Tachycardia results from direct stimulation of the myocardium in concert with diminished systemic vascular resistance due to peripheral vasodilatation. As a consequence, systolic blood pressure falls and cardiac output increases; however, most serious complications occur during prolonged, continuous intravenous treatment.

The most frequent serious complication of beta agonists is pulmonary edema, developing in as many as 5% of patients and occasionally resulting in maternal death (Table 24–1). Most cases of pulmonary edema develop after 24 hours of intravenous beta agonist infusion and are heralded by dyspnea, tachypnea, hemoptysis, rales, or radiographic evidence of bilateral alveolar

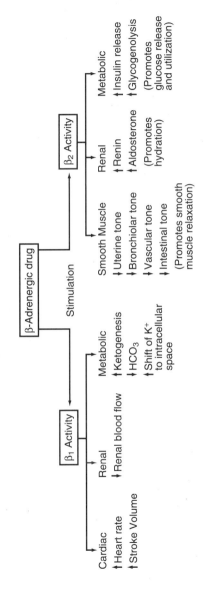

Figure 24–1

Physiology of beta-adrenergic stimulation.

337

Table 24–1

Side Effects of Beta Agonist Tocolytics

Common
- Antidiuresis
- Anxiety, agitation
- Chest pain
- Headache
- Hyperglycemia
- Hypokalemia
- Jitteriness
- Nausea/vomiting
- Reduced uterine blood flow
- Shortness of breath
- Tachycardia

Uncommon

Cardiac dysrhythmias	Hypocalcemia*
Cardiac failure*	Hypotension*
Death	Ileus
Diabetic ketoacidosis*	Myocardial ischemia*
Electrocardiographic changes	Pulmonary edema*
Fever	Rash
Hyperlactacidemia	Transaminase elevation

*Acutely life-threatening conditions

---

infiltrates. Arterial blood gas analysis demonstrates an increased alveolar-arterial oxygen gradient. Factors ascribed to the development of pulmonary edema include anemia, multiple gestation, low colloid oncotic pressure, chronic hypertension, pregnancy-induced hypertension, fluid overload, and corticosteroid administration. Beta agonist–induced pulmonary edema is of the non-cardiogenic variety, generally occurring in the presence of capillary permeability defects. Maternal bacterial infections (e.g., chorio-amnionitis, pyelonephritis) are the most common causes of capillary injury.

The impact of beta agonists upon other maternal systems must also be considered before treatment with this class of tocolytics is initiated (Table 24–2). For example, intravenous beta agonist administration reduces blood flow to the kidneys, reducing urine production, increasing sodium retention, and increasing plasma volume sufficiently to reduce the maternal hematocrit and colloid oncotic pressure by as much as 15%. Beta agonists may also produce considerable maternal hyperglycemia by augmenting glucagon and hepatic glucose production.

Table 24–2

Contraindications to Beta Agonist Tocolysis

Cardiac disease	Growth-retarded fetus
Chorioamnionitis	Hyperthyroidism
Cocaine exposure	Preeclampsia
Diabetes (poorly controlled)	Pyelonephritis
Fetal demise	Third trimester bleeding
Fetal distress*	

*Relative contraindication

Diabetic ketoacidosis has been reported among insulin dependent diabetics given beta agonists to combat preterm labor. Hypokalemia may occur during intravenous administration of beta mimetics by forcing extracellular potassium into the intracellular space. This generally does not need to be treated, as it is a minor, transient effect; however, serum potassium levels less than 2 mEq/L should prompt replacement to avoid cardiac dysrhythmias. Treatment of severe beta agonist complications is noted in Table 24–3.

■
Magnesium Sulfate

Contraindications to magnesium sulfate tocolysis are listed in Table 24–4. Frequent side effects include nausea, vomiting,

---

Table 24–3

Treatment of Severe Beta Agonist Complications

Immediate care*
1. Discontinue beta agonist
2. Blood pressure support
3. Continuous electrocardiography
4. Beta blockade (propranolol, 1–2 mg IV)
5. Treat pulmonary edema (see Chapter 12)
6. Treat diabetic ketoacidosis (see Chapter 11)

Subsequent care*
7. Pulse oximetry
8. Potassium supplementation
9. Calcium supplementation
10. Supplemental oxygen
11. Substitute other tocolytic

*As clinically indicated

Table 24–4

Contraindications to Magnesium Sulfate Tocolysis

Concomitant use of calcium channel–blocking drugs*
Hypocalcemia
Impaired renal function*
Myasthenia gravis (absolute contraindication)

*Relative contraindication

blurred vision, diplopia, weakness, headache, and chest heaviness (Table 24–5). Patients usually adapt to these effects over time. A slight reduction in the rate of magnesium infusion usually reduces symptoms once the patient's preterm labor has been stabilized. Serious side effects occur in about 2% to 5% of patients and include pulmonary edema, although this complication is more frequent with beta agonists. As renal excretion is the principal mechanism of magnesium excretion, close monitoring of urine output is recommended for patients receiving this tocolytic. Reflexes are lost at serum magnesium levels of 8 to 10 mg/dL. Therefore, it can generally be assumed that a patient with normal reflexes has a serum concentration below this level. If reflexes are absent, serum magnesium levels should be assessed every 6 hours. Serum levels of 12 mg/dL are associated with respiratory depression. Cardiac arrest occurs at serum

Table 24–5

Side Effects of Magnesium Sulfate Tocolysis

Common	Uncommon
Blurred vision, diplopia	Death
Constipation	Decreased bone density
Decreased baseline fetal heart rate	Diminished reflexes
Drowsiness	Hypotension (mild)
Dry mouth	Neuromuscular blockade* (with
Flushing	concomitant use of calcium
Headaches	channel blockers)
Hypocalcemia	Nystagmus
Muscle weakness	Pulmonary edema*
Nausea/vomiting	Respiratory depression*
	Urinary retention

*Acutely life-threatening conditions

Table 24–6

Treatment of Severe Magnesium-Associated Complications

Immediate care*
1. Discontinue magnesium infusion
2. Ventilatory support
3. Calcium gluconate (1 gm IV, infused over 3 min)
4. Diuresis (furosemide, 20–40 mg, IV)
5. Treat pulmonary edema (see Chapter 12)

Subsequent care*
6. Discontinue concomitant use of calcium channel–blocking drugs
7. Pulse oximetry
8. Substitute another tocolytic

*As clinically indicated

---

levels of 20 to 24 mg/dL. Treatment of magnesium intoxication is outlined in Table 24–6. Close monitoring and support of the patient are paramount until excess magnesium is excreted by the kidneys.

Prostaglandin Synthetase Inhibitors

Prostaglandin synthetase inhibitors inhibit conversion of arachidonic acid into prostaglandin E_2, the agent involved in the initiation of myometrial contractions. These compounds also have antiinflammatory, antipyretic, and analgesic properties.

Table 24 –7

Side Effects of Prostaglandin Synthetase Inhibitor Tocolytics

Common	Uncommon
Gastrointestinal complaints	Acute renal failure*
Oligohydramnios	Hypertension
Premature closure of ductus arteriosus	Interstitial nephritis
Prolonged bleeding time	Peptic ulcer disease
	Proctitis/rectal bleeding (with suppository use)
	Pulmonary edema*

*Acutely life-threatening conditons

Table 24–8

Contraindications to Prostaglandin Synthetase Inhibitor Tocolytics

Active peptic ulcer disease
Aspirin-induced asthma
Bleeding
Coagulation disorders
Concurrent use of aminoglycosides
Ductus-dependent fetal cardiac defects
Gestational age >32–34 wk
Hypertensive disease
Intrauterine growth retardation
Liver dysfunction
Oligohydramnios
Pyelonephritis
Twin-twin transfusion syndrome

Side effects of these drugs are listed in Table 24–7. Prostaglandin synthetase inhibitors may also affect renal blood flow in mother and fetus, oligohydramnios being a worrisome side effect. Therefore, weekly amniotic fluid volume assessment during ongoing therapy is warranted. Discontinuation of the drug generally reverses oligohydramnios. Owing to maternal and fetal platelet inhibition, mother and child may be at risk for hemorrhagic sequelae if delivery occurs during administration of these agents. Perinates may also suffer from premature closure of the

---

Table 24–9

Treatment of Severe Prostaglandin Synthetase Inhibitor–Associated Complications

Immediate care*
  1. Discontinue prostaglandin synthetase inhibitor
  2. Treat pulmonary edema (see Chapter 12)
Subsequent care*
  3. Antacids, H_2 blockers
  4. Monitor liver and kidney function
  5. Platelet transfusion
  6. Gastroenterology and/or nephrology consultation
  7. In setting of oligohydramnios, careful monitoring of fetal heart rate
  8. Substitute other tocolytic

*As clinically indicated

Table 24–10
Side Effects of Calcium Channel Blocking Tocolytics

Common	Uncommon
Dizziness	Hepatotoxicity*
Flushing	Hypotension
Headache	Impaired platelet aggregation (mild)
Nausea/vomiting	Neuromuscular blockade* with
Palpitations	concomitant use of magnesium
Tachycardia	sulfate

*Acutely life-threatening conditions

ductus arteriosus. As a result, most authorities advise discontinuation of these drugs between 32 and 34 weeks' gestation. There are also reports that necrotizing enterocolitis may occur more frequently among premature infants exposed to these drugs before delivery. Contraindications to the use of these medications are listed in Table 24–8. Treatment of severe complications of these drugs is listed in Table 24–9.

■ Calcium Channel Blockers

Calcium channel–blocking agents act by inhibiting the influx of calcium ions into myometrial cells. Side effects include vasodila-

Table 24–11
Treatment of Severe Calcium Channel Blocker–Associated Complications

Immediate care*
1. Discontinue calcium channel–blocking medication
2. Ventilatory support
3. Calcium gluconate (1 gm, IV infused over 3 min)
4. Blood pressure support

Subsequent care*
5. Discontinue concomitant use of magnesium
6. Gastroenterology consultation as needed
7. Substitute other tocolytic

*As clinically indicated

Table 24–12

Contraindications to Calcium Channel–Blocking Tocolytics

Concomitant use of magnesium sulfate*
Liver disease

*Relative contraindication

tation with resultant decreased peripheral vascular resistance and hypotension (Table 24–10). Nifedipine, the most selective inhibitor of myometrial contraction in this class, may theoretically potentiate the effect of magnesium and result in neuromuscular blockade. Hepatotoxicity has also been reported with this agent. Although this occurs infrequently, baseline and periodic evaluations of liver function are recommended when prolonged use is anticipated. Treatment of severe complications of calcium channel–blocking medications is listed in Table 24–11. Contraindications to the use of these drugs are listed in Table 24–12.

■
Bibliography

Brazy JE, Pupkin MJ: Effects of maternal isoxsuprine administration on preterm infants. J Pediatr 1979; 94:444.

Caritis SN, Darby MJ, Chan L: Pharmacologic treatment of preterm labor. Clin Obstet Gynecol 1988; 31:635–651.

Caritis SN, Toig G, Heddinger LA, et al: A double-blind study comparing ritodrine and terbutaline in the treatment of preterm labor. Am J Obstet Gynecol 1984; 150:7–14.

Elliott JP: Magnesium sulfate as a tocolytic agent. Am J Obstet Gynecol 1983; 147:277–284.

Elliott JP, O'Keeffe DF, Greenberg P, et al: Pulmonary edema associated with magnesium sulfate and betamethasone administration. Am J Obstet Gynecol 1979; 134:717.

Hall DG, McGaughey HS, Corey EL, et al: The effects of magnesium therapy on the duration of labor. Am J Obstet Gynecol 1959; 78:27.

Harbert GM, Cornell GW, Thornton WN: Effect of toxemia therapy on uterine dynamics. Am J Obstet Gynecol 1969; 105:94.

Hatjis CG, Swain M: Systemic tocolysis for premature labor is associated with an increased incidence of pulmonary edema in the presence of maternal infection. Am J Obstet Gynecol 1988; 159:723–728.

Hickok DE, Hollenbach KA, Reilley SF, et al: The association between decreased amniotic fluid volume and treatment with nonsteroidal anti-inflammatory agents for preterm labor. Am J Obstet Gynecol 1989; 160:1525–1531.

Jacobs MM, Knight AB, Arias F: Maternal pulmonary edema resulting from beta mimetics and glucocorticoid therapy. Obstet Gynecol 1980; 56:56–59.

Katz M, Robertson PA, Creasy RK: Cardiovascular complications associated with terbutaline treatment for preterm labor. Am J Obstet Gynecol 1981; 139:605–608.

Katz VL, Seeds JW: Fetal and neonatal cardiovascular complications from β-sympathomimetic therapy for tocolysis. Am J Obstet Gynecol 1989; 161:1–4.

Kirshon B, Mari G, Moise KJ: Indomethacin therapy in the treatment of symptomatic polyhydramnios. Obstet Gynecol 1990; 75:202–205.

Kirshon B, Moise KJ, Wasserstrum N, et al: Influence of short-term indomethacin therapy on fetal urine output. Obstet Gynecol 1988; 72:51.

Leveno KJ, Little BB, Cunningham FG: The national import of ritodrine hydrochloride for inhibition of preterm labor. Obstet Gynecol 1990; 76:12–15.

Moise KJ: Effect of advancing gestational age on the frequency of fetal ductal constriction in association with maternal indomethacin use. Am J Obstet Gynecol 1993; 168:1350–1353.

Moise KJ, Huhta JC, Sharif DS, et al: Indomethacin in the treatment of premature labor. Effects on the fetal ductus arteriosus. N Engl J Med 1988; 319:327–331.

Murray C, Haverkamp AD, Orleans M, et al: Nifedipine for treatment of preterm labor: A historic prospective study. Am J Obstet Gynecol 1992; 167:52–56.

Ogburn PL, Julian TM, Williams PP, et al: The use of magnesium sulfate for tocolysis in preterm labor complicated by twin gestation and beta mimetic-induced pulmonary edema. Acta Obstet Gynecol Scand 1986; 65:793–794.

Parisi VM, Salinas J, Stockmar EJ: Fetal vascular responses to maternal nicardipine administration in the hypertensive ewe. Am J Obstet Gynecol 1989; 161:1035–1039.

Pisani RJ, Rosenow EC: Pulmonary edema associated with tocolytic therapy. Ann Intern Med 1989; 110:714–718.

Sherer DM, Cialone PR, Abramowicz JS, et al: Transient symptomatic subendocardial ischemia during intravenous magnesium sulfate tocolytic therapy. Am J Obstet Gynecol 1992; 66:33–35.

Thorp JM, Spielman FJ, Valea FA, et al: Nifedipine enhances the cardiac toxicity of magnesium sulfate in the isolated perfused Sprague-Dawley rat heart. Am J Obstet Gynecol 1990; 163:655–656.

Vanhaesebrouck P, Thierz M: Oligohydramnios, renal insufficiency, and ileal perforation in preterm infants after intrauterine exposure to indomethacin. J Pediatr 1988; 113:738–743.

Wiggins D, Elliott JP: Oligohydramnios in each sac of a triplet gestation casued by Motrin—fulfilling Koch's postulates. Am J Obstet Gynecol 1990; 162:460.

Wilkins IA, Lynch L, Mehalek KE, et al: Efficacy and side effects of magnesium sulfate and ritodrine as tocolytic agents. Am J Obstet Gynecol 1988; 159:685–689.

Wurtzel D: Prenatal administration of indomethacin as a tocolytic agent: Effect on neonatal renal function. Obstet Gynecol 1990; 76:689–692.

STEVEN C. CURRY

GEORGE BRAITBERG

25

Poisoning in Pregnancy

Many emotional, clinical, and ethical issues surface immediately when a physician is confronted with a pregnant patient who suffers from acute or chronic poisoning. Fortunately, however, with rare exceptions the proper management of pregnant patients differs little from that for other women who are "poisoned."

Two general principles should be kept in mind when treating pregnant women who are poisoned:

1. With rare exception, we save the baby by saving the mother.
2. More harm and damage usually result from withholding needed therapy because of concerns for the fetus than from immediately providing such therapy.

Excluding drugs of abuse, the three most common intentional poisonings during pregnancy are those by *acetaminophen* (APAP), *iron,* or *aspirin.* This chapter specifically addresses the perinatal concerns and management of these poisonings.

■ Specific Agents

Acetaminophen

APAP is the most common drug taken in overdose during pregnancy.

Maternal Concerns
Pathophysiology. Most APAP is metabolized in the liver by being conjugated with sulfate or glucuronide to form nontoxic metabolites that are excreted in the urine (Fig. 25–1). Approximately 7% of APAP, however, is metabolized in liver and kidneys by cytochrome P_{450} to form a toxic metabolite, N-acetyl-p-benzoquinoneimine (NAPQI). NAPQI is an extremely reactive molecule that covalently binds to macromolecules, leading to cell death.

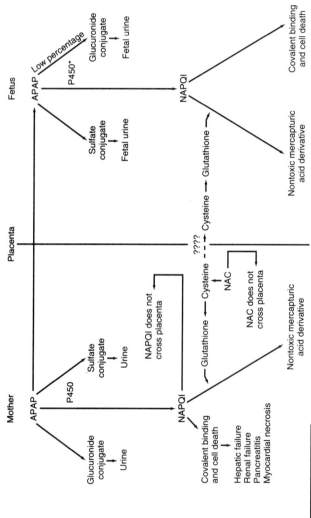

Figure 25-1

Pathophysiology of acetaminophen poisoning. APAP, acetaminophen; NAC, *N*-acetylcysteine; NAPQI, *N*-acetyl-*p*-benzoquinoneimine; *P450 steadily increases after 14 weeks of life.

This concept explains why APAP poisoning principally affects the liver (and, to a lesser extent, the kidneys).

NAPQI normally undergoes detoxification by combining with glutathione, forming a nontoxic mercapturic acid metabolite that is excreted in the urine. With APAP overdose, however, so much NAPQI is formed that glutathione stores become depleted; the result is NAPQI-induced cytotoxicity.

Toxic Doses and Clinical Course. Patients *acutely* ingesting >140 mg/kg of acetaminophen are at risk for hepatotoxicity. One can predict which patients are at risk for developing hepatotoxicity after *acute, single* ingestion by obtaining a serum APAP concentration at least 4 hours after ingestion and plotting the result on a standard nomogram (Fig. 25–2). If an antidote is not given promptly, hepatotoxicity is associated with elevation of liver enzymes (commonly into the thousands), preceded by a prolonged prothrombin time. Enzyme values usually peak between 36 and 72 hours after ingestion. Jaundice rarely appears unless fulminant hepatic failure occurs and attendant complications are present (e.g., coagulopathy, hypoglycemia, metabolic acidosis).

While nausea and vomiting commonly develop early in APAP poisoning, patients who ingest fatal doses may suffer no symptoms or no abnormal physical findings until the onset of symptomatic liver failure 1 to 3 days later. Therefore, a serum APAP value must be obtained from both symptomatic and asymptomatic patients so as to gauge the severity of overdose.

Patients who habitually take excessive doses of acetaminophen are more likely to develop renal failure along with hepatotoxicity. What doses can produce chronic toxicity remain ill-defined, and serum APAP concentrations in these patients cannot be correlated with severity of illness or risk for hepatotoxicity. Seriously poisoned patients occasionally suffer pancreatitis and myocardial necrosis or heart failure. For reasons that are not understood, persons who take a massive overdose may present in the first few hours (before the onset of liver failure) with coma and severe metabolic acidosis (elevated lactate levels).

Treatment. The antidote for APAP poisoning is *N*-acetylcysteine (NAC, Mucomyst). NAC undergoes conversion to cysteine, which, in turn, is metabolized to glutathione. NAC's main effect, then, is to maintain glutathione stores so that NAPQI can be detoxified. Started within 8 hours after APAP ingestion, NAC prevents maternal hepatic and renal toxicity from APAP. To

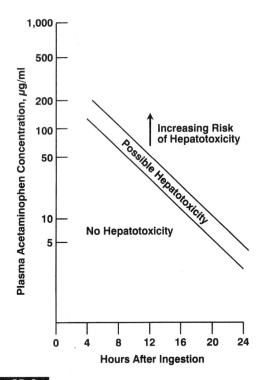

Figure 25–2

Acetaminophen nomogram. For use only after a single, acute ingestion in a patient who was not recently taking acetaminophen prior to ingestion. A level should not be plotted on the nomogram unless it was obtained at least 4 hours after ingestion. If a level falls above the lower line, N-acetylcysteine should be continued (if already started) or begun immediately.

ensure that NAC is not started too late, it is generally most prudent to begin NAC therapy immediately and discontinue it only if serum APAP concentrations are found to be in the non-toxic range on the nomogram. NAC therapy benefits the mother, despite a prolonged delay in administration. The efficacy, however, begins to fall the longer therapy is delayed beyond 8 hours.

If the serum APAP level measured at least 4 hours after ingestion falls above the lower line of the nomogram, a full course of NAC therapy is delivered. It is vital that NAC therapy not be stopped prematurely simply because, on repeat serum APAP test, the level has fallen to zero or to below the lower line on the nomogram.

Because APAP-induced vomiting is common and NAC delivered intravenously produces much higher blood levels than when taken by mouth, potentially increasing the transplacental movement of NAC (see evidence *against* this below) or secondarily formed cysteine, NAC is best administered intravenously. An intravenous formulation is prepared in the pharmacy by aseptically passing oral NAC solution through a 0.2-μm filter and diluting it in 5% dextrose in water, to create an intravenous solution. An intravenous protocol commonly used in the United States is described in Figure 25–3. Occasionally, patients suffer symptomatic histamine release from intravenous NAC and require treatment with antihistamines. On rare occasion, patients suffer life-threatening anaphylactoid reactions requiring fluids, epinephrine, antihistamines, and corticosteroids. If the pharmacy cannot timely prepare intravenous NAC, oral NAC therapy should be started immediately. Treatment for adjunctive complications (e.g., liver failure, renal failure) is entirely supportive and identical to that for other pregnant patients.

Fetal Concerns

Fetal death from APAP overdose has been reported in all trimesters. To our knowledge, it has not occurred after an *acute, single* maternal APAP ingestion of less than 140 mg/kg. We are also unaware of APAP-induced fetal demise when the mother habitually ingested excessive amounts of APAP unless maternal toxicity was also present.

Maternal NAPQI does not cross the placenta. Maternal APAP, however, *does* cross and has the potential to produce toxic fetal concentrations. The fetus's ability to produce NAPQI from APAP begins as early as 14 weeks' intrauterine life and increases until term. The fetus's ability to detoxify APAP by conjugation to sulfate and glucuronide remains impaired until after birth, possibly shunting more APAP through cytochrome P$_{450}$. The third trimester fetus, therefore, appears to be at greatest risk for *direct* toxicity from APAP. Nevertheless, fetal loss appears to be most common in the first trimester: not because the fetus is necessarily poisoned, but because any maternal illness is more likely to lead to fetal loss at that time.

Unfortunately, because NAC does not cross the ovine placenta or that of a living, perfused human placenta, it is not known whether maternal NAC therapy directly benefits the fetus. Investigators can only speculate whether maternal cysteine produced from NAC crosses in amounts large enough to maintain fetal glutathione stores. At least one authority has recom-

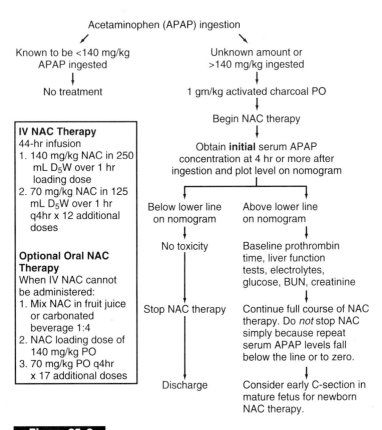

Acetaminophen (APAP) ingestion

Known to be <140 mg/kg APAP ingested → No treatment

Unknown amount or >140 mg/kg ingested → 1 gm/kg activated charcoal PO → Begin NAC therapy → Obtain **initial** serum APAP concentration at 4 hr or more after ingestion and plot level on nomogram

Below lower line on nomogram → No toxicity → Stop NAC therapy → Discharge

Above lower line on nomogram → Baseline prothrombin time, liver function tests, electrolytes, glucose, BUN, creatinine → Continue full course of NAC therapy. Do *not* stop NAC simply because repeat serum APAP levels fall below the line or to zero. → Consider early C-section in mature fetus for newborn NAC therapy.

IV NAC Therapy
44-hr infusion
1. 140 mg/kg NAC in 250 mL D$_5$W over 1 hr loading dose
2. 70 mg/kg NAC in 125 mL D$_5$W over 1 hr q4hr x 12 additional doses

Optional Oral NAC Therapy
When IV NAC cannot be administered:
1. Mix NAC in fruit juice or carbonated beverage 1:4
2. NAC loading dose of 140 mg/kg PO
3. 70 mg/kg PO q4hr x 17 additional doses

Figure 25–3

General guidelines in managing acetaminophen poisoning. IV NAC therapy is preferred because it produces higher blood levels. Oral NAC should be used when IV NAC cannot be prepared by pharmacy and promptly administered. NAC, *N*-acetylcysteine; APAP, acetaminophen. See text for discussion on role of C-section.

mended that the mature fetus be delivered by cesarean section, so that NAC therapy can be administered directly to the baby at risk (i.e., when maternal serum APAP concentrations are toxic), assuming the mother is not at undue risk for the procedure (e.g., because of coagulopathy). Advocates of immediate delivery argue that the maternal and fetal risk of a late third trimester cesarean section are extremely low as compared to data from the several case reports describing fetal death from APAP. Unfortunately, no animal or human studies directly examine the benefits of immediate delivery followed by direct newborn NAC therapy. Currently, there is no consensus or standard of care to guide clinicians who face this dilemma; the decision, therefore, lies with the treating physician.

Iron

For pregnant women the second most common overdose is from prenatal vitamins with iron. Large doses of iron are extremely toxic and may lead to multiorgan system dysfunction and death. Strong evidence indicates that the fetus is protected from elevated maternal iron levels. Iron poisoning is almost entirely a situation in which fetal survival depends on saving the mother. Table 25–1 reviews the pathophysiology of iron toxicity.

Maternal Concerns

Toxic Doses. To determine how much iron was ingested, the elemental iron content must be calculated. On a milligram basis, ferrous sulfate is 20% iron; ferrous fumarate, 33% iron; and ferrous gluconate, 12% iron. *Any patient who ingests more than 20 mg/kg elemental iron, any patient with symptoms, and any patient in whom the amount of ingested iron is not known requires evaluation.*

Clinical Effects. Traditionally, clinical effects are considered in four stages, although the distinctions between stages are not always clear. Death can occur at any stage.

Table 25–1

Pathophysiology of Iron Toxicity

A. Iron is corrosive to the gastrointestinal tract, producing nausea, vomiting, diarrhea, abdominal pain, gastrointestinal bleeding, and rare perforations.

B. Systemically absorbed iron causes venodilatation and increased capillary permeability with associated third-spacing of fluid.

C. Iron causes cell dysfunction and death by disrupting ATP formation in mitochondria and by catalyzing the formation of oxygen-free radicals that destroy cell membranes. The liver takes the brunt of the injury with potential for fulminant hepatic failure, but in massive iron poisoning, any organ can be affected.

D. Early after ingestion, high serum iron concentrations directly inhibit serine proteases (thrombin) and lengthen the prothrombin time, even in the absence of hepatic failure.

Stage 1. Onset of effects occurs 1 to 6 hours after ingestion. Stage 1 effects result from corrosive action of iron on the gut, resulting in gastroenteritis, abdominal pain, and gastrointestinal bleeding. Hypotension and metabolic acidosis may result from hypovolemia and occasional severe anemia. Serum iron levels may be normal or elevated.

Stage 2. Stage 2 is not always seen (e.g., in particularly severe poisonings the disorder may progress from stage 1 to stage 3) and it may last through the 24th hour after ingestion. It is characterized by resolution of gastroenteritis and elevated tissue iron levels. Physicians may be falsely reassured by the resolution of gastroenteritis. Metabolic acidosis and hypotension result from uncorrected hypovolemia, venodilation, "third-spacing" of fluid, and cytotoxic effects of iron. Serum iron concentration may be elevated, and metabolic acidosis may be present. Liver enzyme values are normal. Prothrombin time may be elevated if serum iron concentrations are high.

Stage 3. Stage 3 represents systemic organ damage or failure from cytotoxic effects of iron. Its onset is observed at any time from ingestion through 48 hours. Stage 3 is characterized by hepatic failure, lethargy/coma/convulsions, renal failure, and, occasionally, heart failure. Hypoglycemia and coagulopathy reflect liver damage. In this setting metabolic acidosis has numerous causes, including liver failure, low cardiac output, and impaired oxidative phosphorylation. The liver is the first organ to be "assaulted" by the iron load and typically is the first organ to fail.

Stage 4. Stage 4 is characterized by gastric outlet or small bowel obstruction from gastrointestinal scarring several weeks after the poisoning.

Evaluation and Treatment. Serum Iron Concentrations. While most patients who suffer iron poisoning of stage II or greater are thought to have *peak* serum iron concentrations >350 mg/dL, the actual peak level is seldom accurately revealed, as a consequence of mistiming. Serum iron levels reach their peak sometime between 2 and 6 hours after ingestion. Normal or mildly elevated serum iron concentrations can be misleading, since they do not always reflect the tissue iron burden. That is, the serum iron concentration may be low, approaching or following the nadir, leaving a toxic amount of iron in tissues to produce toxicity in the latter case. Therefore, as an isolated finding, a normal serum iron concentration cannot always be used to exclude iron poisoning in the symptomatic patient.

Asymptomatic Patients. Generally, patients who remain completely asymptomatic for 6 hours after ingestion and have a normal physical examination do not require treatment for iron poisoning (Figs. 25–4, 25–5). Asymptomatic patients who have ingested >20 mg/kg of elemental iron but are seen within 6 hours may benefit from gastric lavage with saline. If vomiting has already occurred, it is not thought that gastric lavage would be of further benefit. We advise *against lavage* with bicarbonate, phosphate, or deferoxamine solutions. A single dose of milk of magnesia (60 mL/gm ingested elemental iron) is thought to significantly reduce iron absorption.

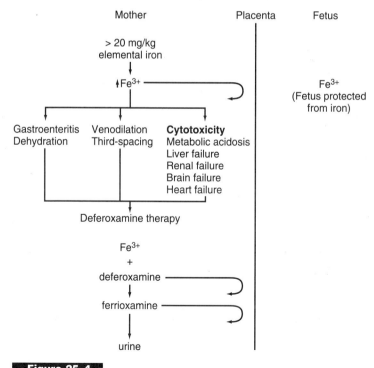

Figure 25–4

Pathophysiology of iron poisoning and rationale for treatment.

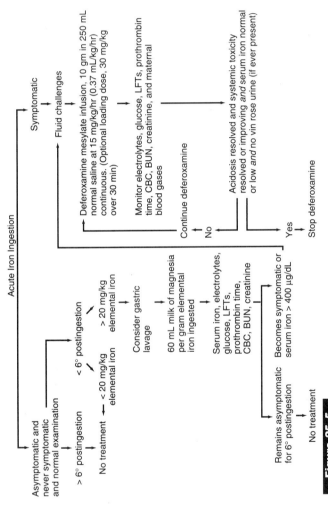

Figure 25–5

Algorithm for acute iron ingestion.

Symptomatic Patients. Patients are considered symptomatic when they present with more than minimal symptoms (e.g., more than one emesis). These patients require treatment with fluids and deferoxamine mesylate, in addition to milk of magnesia, with or without lavage. When a patient has significant clinical symptoms, it is *never* prudent to wait for results of a serum iron concentration before beginning therapy (including deferoxamine) (Table 25–2).

Fetal Concerns

The placenta selectively transports maternal transferrin-bound iron only when it is required by the fetus. Studies of animal models of iron poisoning in pregnancy, along with human experience, lead to the conclusion that the fetus does not develop elevated iron burdens in the face of maternal iron poisoning. Fetal demise appears to be due entirely to maternal illness or death. In addition, deferoxamine and ferrioxamine do not appear to cross the placenta (despite information in the package insert). As fetal outcome depends on the well-being of the mother, it is in the interest of both mother and child that significant poisoning be treated promptly with deferoxamine. *Pregnancy or fetal concerns are never reasons to withhold deferoxamine therapy.*

Salicylate

Sources of salicylate include aspirin (acetylsalicylic acid), oil of wintergreen (methylsalicylate), salicylic acid, and salsalate. All of these compounds are converted to salicylate after absorption. With the exception of aspirin's ability to inhibit platelet function, salicylate is responsible for most of the observed effects.

Salicylate poisoning remains one of the most misunderstood, misdiagnosed, and mismanaged poisonings. This problem is further compounded by pregnancy, when only moderate maternal toxicity may result in fetal demise secondary to the propensity of the drug to concentrate in the fetus. Few intoxications require as much effort on the physician's part for a successful outcome.

Maternal Concerns

Kinetics and Toxic Doses. Generally, significant salicylate toxicity is said to develop after the ingestion of at least 150 mg/kg aspirin (or its equivalent). However, given the fetus's ability to

---

Table 25–2

Management: Symptomatic Iron Overdose

A. With rare exceptions, all symptomatic patients are hypovolemic. Administering 500–1000 mL fluid challenges (Ringer's lactate or normal saline) to restore fluid volume and ensure urine output of 1–2 mL/kg/hr is therapeutic. Patients commonly require maintenance infusions at twice normal rates to keep up with gastrointestinal losses and third spacing.

B. A complete blood count, prothrombin time, electrolytes, serum glucose, liver function studies, arterial blood gases, and blood urea nitrogen/creatinine and serum iron concentration should be obtained. Do not order a total iron binding capacity, as it does not assist in treatment and is frequently falsely elevated in iron poisoning.

C. Deferoxamine mesylate is an iron-chelating agent that is given to remove iron from tissues. Deferoxamine binds to iron to form ferrioxamine, which is excreted in the urine over days to weeks. Ferrioxamine occasionally produces a *vin rose* color to the urine. *This color change is unreliable and inconsistent; it should not be used to determine need for deferoxamine.* Deferoxamine mesylate can be mixed in the crystalloid of choice and should be infused continuously at 15 mg/kg/hr after an optional loading dose of 30 mg/kg over 30 min (Fig. 25–5).

Note: Many statements in the package insert for deferoxamine do not reflect common practice and are misleading or incorrect. Deferoxamine is not *contraindicated in pregnancy for the treatment of acute iron poisoning (see below). At 15 mg/kg/hr, most patients will receive well over 6 gm deferoxamine mesylate per day and this dose is safe for short-term treatment of iron poisoning. Intramuscular deferoxamine is* not *recommended.*

Deferoxamine should be continued until the serum iron concentration is normal or low *and* systemic toxicity is resolved (e.g., resolved acidosis, liver function studies normal or improving) *and* if it was present, obvious vin rose–colored urine disappears. Most patients require 12 to 24 hr of deferoxamine infusion. Occasional patients taking very large overdoses require a longer duration of therapy.

If renal failure develops, deferoxamine should be continued, but at much lower infusion rates. Assuming that therapeutic deferoxamine levels have been obtained, anuric patients should continue to receive infusions at about 1.5 mg/kg/hr, based on the known prolonged half-life in renal failure.

D. General supportive care for attendant complications (e.g., liver failure, gastrointestinal bleeding) is the same as that for any other pregnant patient.

concentrate salicylate, concern arises when acute, single maternal ingestions exceed 75 mg/kg. Salicylate levels may not peak until 24 hours after the drug is absorbed. Enteric coated aspirin may not produce toxic serum concentrations for many hours after ingestion.

Salicylate exists in blood in an equilibrium between the ionized and the un-ionized form (Fig. 25–6). The un-ionized, non–protein bound fraction of salicylate is in equilibrium with tissue stores and easily moves into body compartments because of its lipophilic nature. As serum salicylate levels rise, protein binding becomes saturated, producing a higher free fraction of the drug; and as pH falls, the un-ionized fraction of salicylate rises. Therefore, as serum salicylate concentrations rise and/or as pH decreases, the free, un-ionized fraction increases and moves across cell membranes into target organs. This important concept is critical in understanding both the pathophysiology and the management of salicylate toxicity, since the serum salicylate concentrations can fall while tissue concentrations and severity of toxicity increase. In salicylate poisoning, most salicylate is eliminated unchanged by the kidneys. Elimination half-lives can be as long as 1½ to 2 days, because of saturable elimination kinetics.

Pathophysiology and Clinical Effects. Salicylate has numerous metabolic actions that may result in variable end-organ effects. Diverse clinical manifestations result, in part, from impaired adenosine triphosphate (ATP) formation from salicylate's actions on cellular metabolism.

Gastrointestinal Irritation. Direct corrosive injury to the gut is responsible for abdominal pain, nausea, vomiting, gastrointestinal bleeding, and rare reports of perforation.

Respiratory Alkalosis. Salicylate directly stimulates the brain stem to cause hyperventilation; however, onset of coma or co-ingestion of sedatives commonly masks hyperventilation, and can even produce hypercapnia.

Metabolic Acidosis. Salicylate affects numerous metabolic pathways to inhibit ATP formation. Salicylate inhibits the Krebs cycle, uncouples oxidative phosphorylation, and enhances lipolysis. All of these actions serve to produce metabolic acidosis. Ketonuria is almost always present, and lactate levels are usually normal. The anion gap can be normal or elevated.

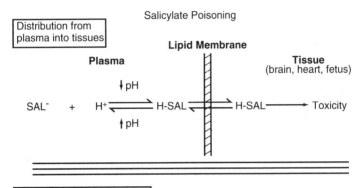

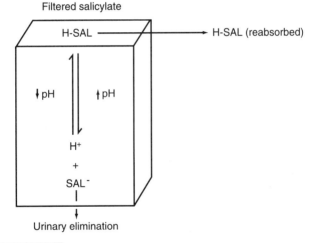

Figure 25–6

Salicylate distribution between blood and tissues and in urine. A smaller fraction of salicylate is protein bound at higher concentrations. A fall in pH increases the fraction of un-ionized salicylate. Therefore, falls in pH or rises in salicylate concentrations result in a greater fraction of drug that can move into tissues, including the brain and the fetus. Alkalinization of blood helps prevent movement of salicylate into tissue. Alkalinization of urine traps salicylate in an ionized form so it cannot be reabsorbed, enhancing urinary elimination. H-SAL, undissociated salicylate acid; SAL⁻, salicylate ion.

Glucose Metabolism. Increased glucose demand accompanied by glycogenolysis explains occasional hyperglycemia seen early in poisoning. However, salicylate inhibits gluconeogenesis so that, when glycogen stores become depleted, hypoglycemia is possible.

Fluid and Electrolytes. Dehydration from gastrointestinal losses and hyperventilation is common. Both hypokalemia and hyperkalemia may be observed. Hypokalemia results from gastrointestinal losses and obligatory urinary excretion of potassium with organic acids (e.g., salicylate). Hyperkalemia usually reflects severe dehydration and prerenal azotemia.

Pulmonary. Low-pressure pulmonary edema can develop with salicylate poisoning; however, hydrostatic (high-pressure) pulmonary edema may also occur in persons with chronic heart disease or salicylate-induced heart failure, or in those whose fluid therapy has not been carefully monitored for fluid balance.

Cardiovascular. The metabolic insult to the myocardium induced by salicylate results in tachycardia, ventricular arrhythmias, heart failure or hypotension, and sudden death. In the absence of heart disease, metabolic acidosis and neurotoxicity almost always precede severe cardiac dysfunction and shock.

Central Nervous System. Impaired ATP production produces neurotoxicity, which is manifested by hallucinations, agitation, delirium, lethargy, coma, convulsions, malignant cerebral edema, and brain death. Patients who die despite supportive care usually die from cerebral failure.

Coagulation and Platelets. Salicylate impairs vitamin K–dependent coagulation factors to prolong prothrombin time. Aspirin also inhibits platelet function.

Miscellaneous. Hyperthermia may be observed, but usually it is mild. Acute tubular necrosis has been reported. Rhabdomyolysis contributes to hyperkalemia, coagulopathy, and renal failure. Tinnitus is common.

Clinical Presentation
Acute Salicylate Poisoning. Patients who present shortly after an overdose are awake and complain of tinnitus, abdominal pain, nausea, and vomiting. Other abnormalities include tachy-

pnea, tachycardia, respiratory alkalosis with alkalemia, hypovolemia, hypokalemia, and gastrointestinal bleeding.

Progression of the poisoning is characterized by metabolic acidosis and acidemia, progressively severe neurotoxicity, alterations of glucose homeostasis, elevated prothrombin time, pulmonary edema, and cardiotoxicity. The combination of acidemia and neurotoxicity carries a grave prognosis unless aggressive treatment is initiated promptly.

Chronic Salicylate Poisoning. Chronic salicylate poisoning is best described as a syndrome resulting from repeated doses of salicylate. Patients are brought in by friends or family because of altered mental status, including lethargy, hallucinations, agitation, seizures, and coma. Occasionally, hypoglycemia contributes to encephalopathy. Prothrombin times are typically elevated, and acidemia from metabolic acidosis is more common than alkalemia. Pulmonary edema leading to adult respiratory distress syndrome (low pressure) occurs more often than with acute poisoning. As compared with acute salicylate poisoning, serum salicylate concentrations are lower for any given degree of toxicity in chronic poisoning because of larger tissue burdens of salicylate, reflecting a larger volume of distribution.

Serum Salicylate Concentrations

Interpretation of serum salicylate concentrations can be difficult because of changing tissue burdens of the drug for identical serum levels, depending on pH, protein binding, and other factors. Because of these factors, tissue concentrations of salicylate can actually rise while serum levels are falling, causing the patient's condition to deteriorate while the physician is falsely reassured by falling serum drug concentrations. It is always more important to treat the patient than the serum salicylate concentration.

Furthermore, because of delayed or prolonged absorption, basing treatment and disposition on a single serum salicylate concentration can be misleading and is to be discouraged. We are generally reassured that the *mother* is out of danger only when serum salicylate concentrations are <25 mg/dL *and* are known to be falling, *and* the patient exhibits no laboratory or clinical evidence of toxicity. Because the fetus develops higher serum and tissue concentrations of salicylate than the mother, it is possible for a mother to have become asymptomatic after overdose (with low serum salicylate levels) but to have suffered fetal loss or to still carry a fetus with significant toxicity.

Management

General Principles. All patients with salicylate poisoning should be admitted to an intensive care setting, whether in labor and delivery or in a medical intensive care unit. Successful maternal management of acute salicylate poisoning hinges on compulsive, attentive medical care. Specifically, frequent attention to fluid balance, electrolyte and acid-base status, bedside examination, and rapid institution of hemodialysis at the earliest signs of central nervous system (CNS) deterioration, especially in the presence of acidemia, is important. As noted below, we also recommend that hemodialysis be performed earlier than in nonpregnant patients, given the ability of the fetus to concentrate salicylate (Fig. 25–7).

The rationale for sodium bicarbonate therapy outlined below has two principal purposes (see Fig. 25–6):

1. Most important, alkalinization of blood helps prevent movement of salicylate out of the serum into target organs. Of prime concern is minimization of movement into the CNS and the fetus. Blood pH should be kept between 7.45 and 7.50. A drop in blood pH from 7.4 to only 7.20 can almost double the concentration of un-ionized salicylate that is able to move into the brain and fetus.
2. Alkalinization of urine promotes ionic trapping of salicylate in urine, preventing reabsorption and enhancing elimination. Urine pH should be greater than 7.0, to lessen salicylate reabsorption.

Airway. As with any patient, immediate attention to airway and adequate oxygenation are mandatory.

Glucose Abnormalities. Hypoglycemia must be sought immediately and treated, especially in any patient with altered mental status.

Gastrointestinal Decontamination. Most patients suffering from acute salicylate poisoning vomit repeatedly, rendering further attempts at gastric emptying (lavage and ipecac) unnecessary. A single dose of 1 gm/kg activated charcoal should be given. If salicylate levels continue to rise, repeated doses of 0.25 gm/kg activated charcoal every 4 to 6 hours should be considered if the patient has normal gastrointestinal motility. Compazine is to be discouraged, as it is usually ineffective and lowers the seizure threshold.

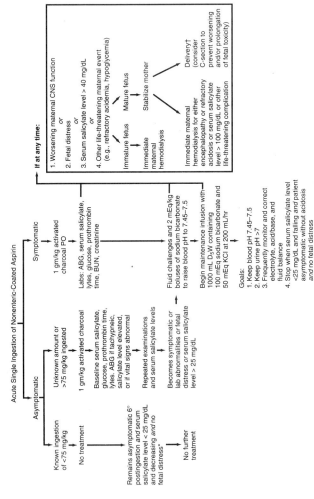

Figure 25-7

Treatment guidelines for salicylate poisoning. *Enteric-coated aspirin may not produce toxic serum salicylate concentrations until well after 6 hours postingestion. †See text for discussion.

Fluid and Electrolyte Therapy. Most patients suffer moderate to severe dehydration and require immediate fluid challenges with normal saline or Ringer's lactate until urine output is 2 to 3 mL/kg/hr. Initial sodium bicarbonate boluses of 2 mEq/kg are given, if needed, to raise arterial blood pH to 7.45 to 7.5.

A recommended *initial* regimen for maintenance fluid therapy *after* fluid resuscitation is a continuous infusion of 1000 mL of 5% dextrose in water to which is added 100 mEq sodium bicarbonate and 50 mEq potassium chloride to run at 150 to 200 mL/hr. Obviously, irreversible impairment of renal function demands potassium and fluid restriction.

Hypokalemia must be treated aggressively. Urine alkalinity cannot be achieved in the setting of hypokalemia because the kidneys secrete hydrogen ions rather than potassium ions when reabsorbing sodium. Additionally, for the reasons outlined above, the patient usually presents with a total body potassium debt, and ongoing losses continue as salicylate anions combine with potassium cations in the urine during elimination.

Fine-Tuning Therapy. In moderately to severely ill patients, arterial blood gases, urine pH, electrolytes, and serum glucose should be measured every 1 to 2 hours, at which time fluid balance is also reassessed. Fluid and electrolyte infusions are modified as needed to prevent fluid overload, normalize electrolytes, ensure adequate urine output, and prevent acidemia and hypoglycemia. Serum salicylate concentrations should be obtained every 1 to 2 hours until it is clear that they are falling, and findings should be interpreted in the context of the patient's condition. Efforts are directed at preventing drops in arterial pH below 7.45 and at keeping urine pH elevated. Aciduria in the face of alkalemia is treated with further doses of potassium, as long as hyperkalemia is not present. Any deterioration in neurologic function, especially if associated with acidemia, is an indication for immediate hemodialysis.

Noncardiogenic Pulmonary Edema. Adult respiratory distress syndrome (ARDS) is more common in chronic toxicity and should be treated with oxygen and continuous positive airway pressure (CPAP) or positive end-expiratory pressure (PEEP), if required. Only cautious use of diuretics is recommended, as these patients are usually volume depleted.

Miscellaneous. A 20-mg parenteral dose of vitamin K_1 reverses elevated prothrombin times produced by salicylate over several hours. In an emergency, fresh-frozen plasma rapidly corrects coagulopathy (but not platelet dysfunction). Serial blood hemoglobin values should be followed to determine if gastrointestinal bleeding becomes severe enough to require transfusions. Oral antacids are recommended. Serial serum creatine kinase (CK) activity should be evaluated to rule out rhabdomyolysis, which, if present, will require specific therapy (e.g., mannitol, urinary alkalinization).

Hemodialysis. Hemodialysis is effective and life saving in that it removes salicylate and corrects acid-base-electrolyte abnormalities. It is best performed using high-flux hemodialysis with the largest–surface area cartridge available. It is indicated immediately in the following situations:

- Patients with renal insufficiency.
- Onset of significant or worsening neurotoxicity, even if serum salicylate concentrations are falling.
- Other life-threatening complications accompanied by elevated serum salicylate concentrations.
- To ensure fetal survival (see below).

Fetal Concerns
Salicylate crosses the placenta and concentrates in the fetus at higher levels than in the mother. The relative acidemia of the fetus ensures higher *tissue* salicylate levels for its already elevated serum concentrations. In addition, the fetus has less capacity to buffer the acidemic stress imposed by salicylate and, relative to the mother, a reduced capacity to excrete the toxin. Collectively, this places the fetus at greater risk for death and forms the basis for the subsequent recommendation of hemodialysis and cesarean section.

The Premature Fetus. Given that the fetus concentrates salicylate and suffers greater toxicity than the mother, it seems wise to institute hemodialysis for lesser degrees of maternal toxicity than would be done in nonpregnant patients. Unfortunately, there are no studies to guide clinicians in this setting. From our experience, we recommend immediate hemodialysis in the face of any signs of fetal distress, in the face of maternal chronic salicylate poisoning (where high tissue levels predominate), or whenever maternal serum salicylate concentrations exceed 40 mg/dL.

The Mature Fetus. Using the rationale for premature fetuses, it makes sense that delivery by cesarean section, when safe for the mother, should be undertaken in the presence of chronic salicylate poisoning or whenever maternal serum salicylate concentrations exceed 40 mg/dL. Again, there are no studies outside of our clinical experience to guide us in making this recommendation. In fact, some suggest that immediate maternal hemodialysis might more rapidly and safely reverse elevated fetal salicylate levels than direct care of the poisoned newborn following emergent delivery. If cesarean section is not performed, hemodialysis should be instituted immediately.

■
Bibliography

Acetaminophen

Riggs BS, Bronstein AC, Kulig K, et al: Acute acetaminophen overdose during pregnancy. Obstet Gynecol 1986; 74:247–253.

Selden BS, Curry SC, Clark RF, et al: Transplacental transport of *N*-acetylcysteine in an ovine model. Ann Emerg Med 1991; 20:1069–1072.

Smilkstein MJ, Bronstein AC, Linden C, et al: Acetaminophen overdose: A 48-hour intravenous *N*-acetylcysteine treatment protocol. Ann Emerg Med 1991; 20:1058–1063.

Iron

Curry SC, Bond GR, Raschke R, et al: An ovine model of maternal iron poisoning in pregnancy. Ann Emerg Med 1990; 19:632–638.

Mills KC, Curry SC: Acute iron poisoning. Emerg Med Clin North Am 1994; 12:397–413.

Salicylate

Buck ML, Grebe TA, Bond GR: Toxic reaction to salicylate in a newborn infant: similarities to neonatal sepsis. J Pediatr 1993; 122:955–958.

Curry SC: Salicylates. In Reisdorff EJ, Roberts MR, Wiegenstein JG (eds): Pediatric Emergency Medicine. Philadelphia: W.B. Saunders, 1993; pp 667–673.

Tennenbein M: Poisoning in pregnancy. In Koren G (ed): Maternal-Fetal Toxicology. A Clinician's Guide, ed 2. New York: Marcel Dekker, 1994.

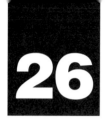

26

CRISTINA CARBALLO

Neonatal Evaluation, Resuscitation, and Survival

It becomes evident after reviewing the previous chapters that maintaining physiologic stability during a high-risk obstetric situation is paramount to ensuring a healthy outcome for both mother and fetus. The culmination of the carefully managed high-risk pregnancy, ideally, is the birth of a physiologically intact, although perhaps premature, newborn.

This chapter will serve the reader by giving him or her the tools to assess, stabilize, and resuscitate, if required, a newborn. Part of the decision to resuscitate involves having a knowledge base about survival of certain populations.

■ Initial Evaluation of the Newborn

The best scenario possible is knowing the clinical status of the mother and fetus before delivery. This information facilitates the formation of two critically important mental checklists. The first should highlight the probable physiologic state of that particular newborn at birth. The second should highlight the possible neonatal complications that would need to be managed quickly and efficiently. Both are important to maximize the outcome for that infant.

Before we embark on the evaluation and management of each different clinical scenario, let us first briefly review the pathophysiology of asphyxia (Fig. 26–1). Probably the most frightening experience is to encounter an apneic infant with a heart rate slower than 100 bpm. All apneic infants have had some degree of asphyxia that may have been preceded by hypoxic spells, which often are documented as "fetal distress." In the rhesus monkey model, rapid gasps accompanied by muscular thrashing of extremities precedes the onset of asphyxia. When asphyxia occurs, the first clinical sign is primary apnea (responsive to stimulation alone), which lasts approximately 1

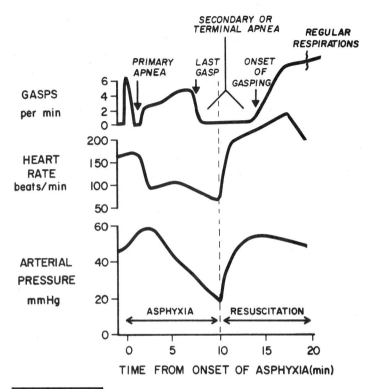

GASPS per min

HEART RATE beats/min

ARTERIAL PRESSURE mmHg

TIME FROM ONSET OF ASPHYXIA(min)

SECONDARY OR TERMINAL APNEA

REGULAR RESPIRATIONS

PRIMARY APNEA LAST GASP ONSET OF GASPING

ASPHYXIA RESUSCITATION

Figure 26–1

Pathophysiology of asphyxia. (From Fisher DE, Paton JB: Resuscitation of the Newborn Infant. In Klaus MH, Fanaroff AA (eds): Care of the High-Risk Neonate, ed 4. Philadelphia: WB Saunders, 1993.)

minute. After 4 to 5 minutes of gasping, a final gasp occurs at approximately 8 minutes. This heralds the onset of secondary or terminal apnea (unresponsive to stimulation alone) and requires respiratory intervention. It is especially important to remember that an apneic infant encountered in the delivery room may have either primary or secondary apnea, and resuscitation efforts should be started immediately. Only after you note the baby's response to the resuscitative effort can you retrospectively speculate as to the duration of the asphyxia event. In an infant with secondary apnea, every minute's delay in the initiation of the resuscitation results in approximately 2 minutes (or more) before the first gasp is seen. In rhesus monkeys, death occurs after several minutes in the absence of resuscitation. A human new-

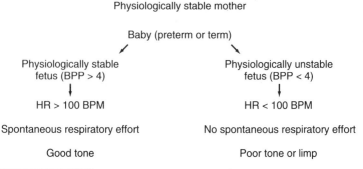

Figure 26–2

Neonatal effects of a physiologically stable maternal state.

born, however, may have more tolerance for apnea, owing to the presence of mechanisms that provide for greater anaerobic compensation. It should be noted, however, that each baby responds differently and we cannot fully predict outcomes solely on the onset of the first gasp. For a more detailed description the reader is referred to Klaus and Fanaroff (see Bibliography).

As we now begin to review each separate clinical scenario, the above discussions will help you better understand the baby's needs and responses. First let us focus on the mother's health. Our mental checklist should initially include whether the mother is physiologically stable (i.e., in the cardiovascular system) or not. From there we look at whether the fetus is preterm or term and its physiologic condition. I refer the reader to Figures 26–2 and 26–3. Let us first consider the following scenario: A preterm

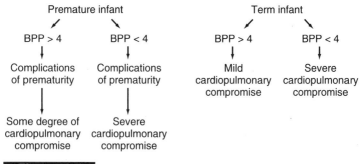

Figure 26–3

Neonatal effects of a physiologically unstable maternal state.

or term infant is about to be born and the mother has been physiologically stable. If there is fetal compromise, with a biophysical profile (BPP) less than 4, then we might anticipate, at the delivery, a neonatal heart rate less than 100 bpm, poor respiratory effort and poor tone. If the infant is premature as well as compromised, we must also anticipate the additional complications of respiratory distress, hypothermia, hypoglycemia, poor tone, and an immature autonomic nervous system. In the absence of fetal compromise (i.e., BPP greater than 4), then we might anticipate only the complications of prematurity as noted above.

Let us now review the scenario that involves a physiologically unstable maternal state. It is best with this maternal clinical presentation to think about each neonatal clinical situation separately. Let us start with the premature infant who was physiologically unstable as a fetus (BPP less than 4). This, of course, is the worst possible situation the baby and the resuscitative team can be in. Clinically, we must anticipate the complications of prematurity as noted above, along with severe cardiovascular compromise.

A slightly improved scenario is the premature infant that was physiologically stable as a fetus (BPP greater than 4). In this situation, we still need to consider the problems of prematurity, as listed above. The effects of the physiologically unstable mother, however, are not as devastating to the infant. We might anticipate persistent bradycardia despite adequate respiratory support. With further interventions (reviewed in Fig. 26–4) these infants respond (usually within 5 minutes) and demonstrate reversal of the initial shock-like symptoms.

In a term baby that was physiologically unstable as a fetus we should anticipate significant cardiovascular compromise, perhaps even collapse. This may be manifested by absence of tone, absent spontaneous respiratory effort, persistent bradycardia despite the institution of adequate respiratory support and possible shock with poor perfusion, requiring maximal cardiovascular support. As you can now recognize, this is what was described above as an asphyxiated infant. This will be delineated further. If the baby was physiologically stable as a fetus, then cardiovascular compromise is expected to be mild, demonstrated only by primary apnea, which typically responds to effective stimulation and/or initial respiratory resuscitation.

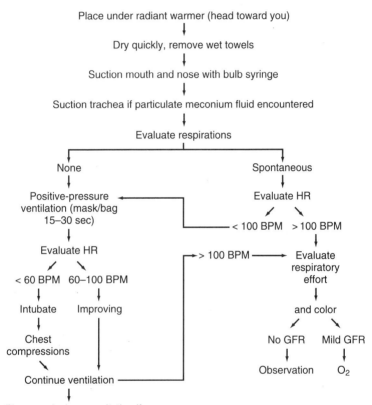

Place under radiant warmer (head toward you)
↓
Dry quickly, remove wet towels
↓
Suction mouth and nose with bulb syringe
↓
Suction trachea if particulate meconium fluid encountered
↓
Evaluate respirations

None → Positive-pressure ventilation (mask/bag 15–30 sec) → Evaluate HR

< 60 BPM → Intubate → Chest compressions

60–100 BPM → Improving → Continue ventilation

Spontaneous → Evaluate HR

< 100 BPM / > 100 BPM

> 100 BPM → Evaluate respiratory effort → and color

No GFR → Observation

Mild GFR → O₂

Pharmacologic resuscitation if:
 HR < 80 BPM after 30 sec
 PPV with 100% O₂
 Chest compressions
Consider:
 Thoracentesis and/or paracentesis and/or pericardiocentesis if hydrops
 present
 Pulmonary hypoplasia if small thorax and oligohydramnios present
 since < 20 weeks
 Hypovolemia: administer either O negative uncross-matched blood
 or albumin 5%, 100 mL/kg

Figure 26–4

Algorithm for resuscitation of the premature infant. GFR, Grunting, flaring, retracting.

■ Resuscitation of the Newborn

Once we have anticipated the potential clinical state of a baby in the delivery room, we can formulate a plan for responding to the different clinical scenarios that might present. Figure 26–4 outlines resuscitation for the premature infant, with or without cardiovascular collapse. Figure 26–5 outlines resuscitation for the term infant with cardiovascular compromise secondary to maternal instability.

Valuable points to remember when resuscitating an infant:

Keep the infant warm and dry.

Maintain an open airway through neck stabilization and suctioning of nose, mouth, and hypopharynx (tracheal suctioning if there is particulate meconium). Provide mask and bag ventilation or in more unstable infants, intubation/ventilation.

Maintain or restore cardiovascular stability. This is accomplished by initially maintaining or restoring respiratory stability followed by cardiac compression and pharmacologic therapy, if needed.

At minimum you will need a nurse to assist you. The more unstable and critical an infant becomes, the more likely you will need the resuscitative team on standby to provide assistance. Once the airway is stabilized, communicate with a family member and the mother, if awake, about the baby's condition, even if continued and/or additional support is needed. Unless the resuscitation is in another room, this can best be done by remaining at the baby's bedside and quickly informing the mother and/or family members across the room. If the resuscitation is in another room, you can have an assistant ask a family member to come to the baby's bedside. You should never leave the baby unless the resuscitation effort is failing and the only option is discontinuation of all support. In this situation, it has been my experience that it is best to go directly to the mother and speak quietly to her and any family members present.

The equipment you will need to provide adequate neonatal resuscitation is listed in Table 26–1. Medications used during resuscitation are listed in Table 26–2. The recommended order of administration during a resuscitation is outlined in Figure 26–6.

The goal, as noted before, is to restore and maintain physiologic stability as quickly as possible for the infant you are resuscitating. The ultimate goal, however, is to preserve intact

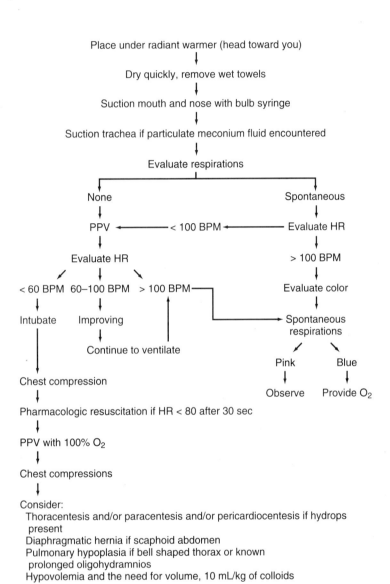

■ Figure 26–5

Algorithm for resuscitation of the term infant. PPV, Positive pressure ventilation.

Table 26–1

Neonatal Resuscitation Supplies and Equipment

Suction equipment
  Bulb syringe
  DeLee mucus trap with No. 10 Fr. catheter or mechanical suction
  Suction catheters, Nos. 5 or 6, 8, 10 Fr.
  No. 8 Fr. feeding tube and 20-mL syringe
Bag and mask equipment
  Infant resuscitation bag with pressure-release valve or pressure gauge
    (bag must be capable of delivering 90%–100% oxygen)
  Face masks, newborn and premature sizes (cushioned rim masks
    preferred)
  Oral airways, newborn and premature sizes
  Oxygen with flow meter and tubing
Intubation equipment
  Laryngoscope with straight blades, No. 0 (premature) and No. 1
    (newborn)
  Extra lightbulbs and batteries for laryngoscope
  Endotracheal tubes, sizes 2.5, 3.0, 3.5, 4.0 mm
  Stylet
  Scissors
  Gloves

Table 26–2

Neonatal Resuscitation Medications

Epinephrine 1:10,000–3-mL or 10-mL ampules
Naloxone hydrochloride (neonatal NARCAN) 0.02 mg/mL, 2-mL ampules
Volume expander: one or more of the following:
  Albumin 5% solution
  Normal saline
  Ringer's lactate
Sodium bicarbonate 4.2% (5 mEq/10 mL), 10-mL ampules
Dextrose 10%, 250 mL
Sterile water, 30 mL
Normal saline, 30 mL

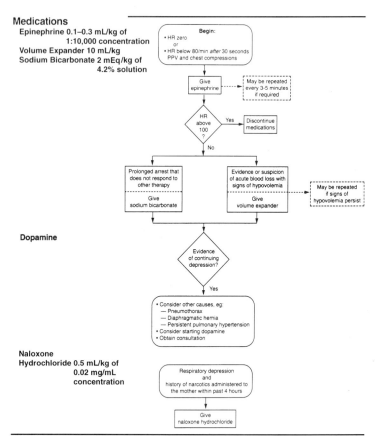

Medications
Epinephrine 0.1–0.3 mL/kg of
                1:10,000 concentration
Volume Expander 10 mL/kg
Sodium Bicarbonate 2 mEq/kg of
                4.2% solution

Dopamine

Naloxone
Hydrochloride 0.5 mL/kg of
                0.02 mg/mL
                concentration

Figure 26–6

Summary of key points related to the use of medications during neonatal resuscitation. (Reproduced with permission. Textbook of Neonatal Resuscitation, 1987, 1990, 1994. Copyright American Heart Association, Dallas.)

CNS survival. If the resuscitation is delayed or carried out poorly, consequences for the CNS and other organ functions can be devastating. Table 26–3 outlines the acute and long-term consequences of perinatal/neonatal asphyxia.

■
Survival

Knowing the survival rate for a specific group of patients allows the resuscitative effort to be tailored to that situation. When

Table 26-3
Consequences of Perinatal/Neonatal Asphyxia

System	Acute	Long-Term
Central nervous system	Cerebral edema Cerebral hemorrhage Hypoxic-ischemic encephalopathy (HIE) Seizures	Seizures 50% Cerebral palsy 12%–23%
Pulmonary	Respiratory depression Meconium aspiration	Bronchopulmonary dysplasia (BPD)
Cardiovascular	Myocardial failure Papillary muscle necrosis Persistent pulmonary hypertension (PPHN)	Permanent myocardial dysfunction
Renal	Cortical/tubular/ medullary necrosis	
Gastrointestinal	Necrotizing enterocolitis (NEC)	Consequences of NEC Short gut obstruction
Hematologic	Disseminated intravascular coagulation (DIC)	AIDS, hepatitis secondary to transfusions

discussing survival rates of different gestational groups, it is best that you investigate your own hospital's statistics and utilize these figures, since they are more specific to your region's ethnic and geographic characteristics.

Published articles describe outcome statistics for low birth weight infants. Table 26–4 outlines recent statistics for survival to 30 days and survival to discharge.

Consideration for quality of survival is also important when deciding on the extent of resuscitation efforts. More specifically, we shall focus on the incidence of chronic lung disease and grade III to IV intraventricular hemorrhage as the major contributors affecting expected quality of life. Table 26–5 outlines gestational age and birth weight–specific incidence of these morbidities. Additional points to keep in mind when formulating a plan of action on your way to the delivery room are outlined in Table 26–6.

Comment

It has been said that medicine is more art than science. So many of our decision processes rest on the previous experiences of a

Table 26–4

Survival 24–29 Weeks (Born 1986–1988)

Gestational Age (wk)	Birth Weight (gm)	Live-borns (No.)	Survival to 30 days	Survival to Discharge
24	645	10	2 (20%)	1 (10%)
25	780	21	11 (52%)	9 (43%)
26	892	30	25 (83%)	24 (80%)
27	1019	24	20 (83%)	20 (83%)
28	1126	24	22 (92%)	21 (88%)
29	1231	32	30 (94%)	29 (92%)
Total		141	110 (78%)	104 (74%)

From Wood B, et al: Survival and morbidity of extremely premature infants based on obstetric assessment of gestational age. Obstet Gynecol 1989; 74:889–892.

Table 26-5
Morbidity of Preterm Infants (Born 1986–1988) Morbidity 24–29 Weeks

Gestational Age (wk)	Birth Weight (gm)	Chronic Lung Disease		Intraventricular Hemorrhage GR 3/4*	Combined Morbidity at D/C
		30 D	D/C		
24	645	2 (100%)	0 (0%)	1 (100%)	1 (100%)
25	780	10 (91%)	2 (22%)	3 (33%)	5 (56%)
26	892	11 (44%)	5 (21%)	6 (25%)	11 (46%)
27	1019	17 (35%)	4 (20%)	4 (20%)	8 (40%)
28	1126	5 (23%)	3 (14%)	4 (19%)	7 (33%)
29	1231	4 (14%)	2 (7%)	2 (7%)	4 (14%)
Total		39 (35%)	16 (15%)	20 (19%)	36 (35%)

From Wood B, et al: Survival and morbidity of extremely premature infants based on obstetric assessment of gestational age. Obstet Gynecol 1989; 74:889–892.

*Grade III–IV is associated with a 64%–86% incidence of poor neurologic outcome.

Table 26–6

Important Considerations on the Way to the Delivery Room

1. Neonatology is an ever-changing and expanding field where new technologies afford better survival for smaller and smaller babies.
2. The limit of viability nationwide appears to be 23 wk. At this gestational age, we are still gathering data as to true survival and morbidity statistics. It seems that in this particular age group survival varies depending on where infants are born and what resources are available to them.
3. How a baby responds during resuscitation may actually be more indicative than gestational age of that infant's survival chances. An infant that is vigorous, attempting to breathe, crying, kicking, and overall active may have a better outcome than an infant whose initial presentation is depressed and requires vigorous resuscitation.
4. The best scenario, if at all possible, is to have all the information about the fetus before the delivery, not only so that you can make the best possible plans and decisions for that patient but so that you can empower the parents with all the information necessary to help the team make the appropriate decisions about the *aggressiveness of resuscitation efforts.*

---

similar situation; however, the social and ethical circumstances that envelop a baby and its family also influence these decisions.

Therefore, with each high-risk delivery that we attend we must quickly assess the perinatal, neonatal, social, and ethical factors involved, so that the emerging new life is given the best chance possible—not only for survival but for quality of life. Without this information at hand, medicine loses both its art and science and becomes nothing more than the evolutionary process of survival of the strongest.

■ Bibliography

American Heart Association: Textbook of Neonatal Resuscitation. Elk Grove Village, IL: American Academy of Pediatrics, 1994.

Fisher DE, Paton JB: Resuscitation of the newborn infant. In Klaus MH, Fanaroff AA (eds): Care of the High-Risk Neonate, ed 4. Philadelphia: W.B. Saunders, 1993, pp 38–61.

Horbar J, et al: Predicting mortality risk for infants weighing 501 to

1500 grams at birth: A National Institutes of Health Neonatal Research Network report. Crit Care Med 1993; 21:12–18.

Nishida H: Outcome of infants born preterm, with special emphasis on extremely low birth weight infants. Bailliere's Clin Obstet Gynecol 1993; 7:611–630.

Trautman M: Neonatal resuscitation. Contemp Ob/Gyn: 1994; 39:15–27.

Veelken N: Development of very low birth weight infants: A regional study of 371 survivors. Eur J Pediatr 1991; 150:815–820.

Wood B, et al: Survival and morbidity of extremely premature infants based on obstetric assessment of gestational age. Obstet Gynecol 1989; 74(6):889–892.

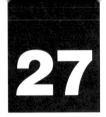

HOWARD S. SMITH

Fluids and Electrolytes for the Obstetric Intensive Care Patient

The ultimate goal of intravenous fluid and electrolyte therapy is to achieve appropriate volumes, tonicity, and salt balance in all intracellular and extracellular compartments. In this chapter I describe the basic principles pertaining to the dynamics of fluid and electrolyte physiology. Corrective interventions are highlighted to assist the clinician with appropriate management.

The human body is composed of extracellular fluid (ECF) and intracellular fluid (ICF) compartments. The extracellular compartment is most readily accessible for fluid sampling, monitoring, and administration. The ECF is composed of plasma and interstitial transudate.

$$\text{Total body water (TBW)} = 1/2 \, [\text{wt(kg)}].$$

Of this TBW, 66% is ICF and 34% ECF. The extracellular water is mostly interstitial (26% of TBW); this leaves only a small percentage as plasma (8% of TBW). Approximately three fourths of the ECF is interstitial and one fourth is plasma; therefore plasma is one twelfth of TBW.

It is important to remember that the majority of our fluid analysis and therapy is directed at the intravascular fluid compartment, which constitutes only 8% of TBW. This point is of paramount importance when attempting to correct total body fluid and electrolyte disturbances. A minor disturbance in the fluid and electrolyte balance of the extracellular compartment may represent a significant total body derangement.

By administering fluid into the intravascular compartment, we are essentially expanding the plasma volume. This can be done with electrolyte solutions that resemble the electrolyte contents of plasma. Conversely, a solution lacking or possessing a particular electrolyte can be chosen to correct an imbalance. Table 27–1 illustrates the contents of typical electrolyte solutions used in medical care.

The normovolemic fasting patient without electrolyte distur-

Table 27-1

Crystalloid Solution Composition

IV Solution	Na (mEq/L)	K (mEq/L)	Ca (mEq/L)	Cl (mEq/L)	Lactate (mEq/L)	Calories/L	mOsm/L
5% Dextrose injection, USP	0	0	0	0	0	170	252
10% Dextrose injection, USP	0	0	0	0	0	340	505
0.9% Sodium chloride injection, USP	154	0	0	154	0	0	308
Sodium lactate injection, USP (M/6 sodium lactate)	167	0	0	0	167	54	334
2.5% Dextrose & 0.45% sodium chloride injection, USP	77	0	0	77	0	85	280
5% Dextrose & 0.2% sodium chloride injection, USP	34	0	0	34	0	170	321
5% Dextrose & 0.33% sodium chloride injection, USP	56	0	0	56	0	170	365
5% Dextrose & 0.45% sodium chloride injection, USP	77	0	0	77	0	170	406
5% Dextrose & 0.9% sodium chloride injection, USP	154	0	0	154	0	170	560
10% Dextrose & 0.9% sodium chloride injection, USP	154	0	0	154	0	340	813
Ringer's injection, USP	147.5	4	4.5	156	0	0	309
Lactated Ringer's injection, USP	130	4	3	109	28	9	273
5% Dextrose in Ringer's injection	147.5	4	4.5	156	0	170	561
Lactated Ringer's with 5% dextrose	130	4	3	109	28	180	525

From McEntyre RL: Practical Guide to the Care of the Surgical Patient, 2nd ed. St Louis, MO, Mosby-Year Book, 1984, p. 260.

Table 27-2

Intravenous Maintenance Fluid Calculation

A rule of thumb frequently used to calculate intravenous fluid maintenance is the *4-2-1 Rule.*
  4 mL/kg for the first 10 kg
    plus
  2 mL/kg for the next 10 kg
    plus
  1 mL/kg for any additional kg
Usual adult maintenance is roughly 1.5–2 mL/kg/hr. For example, a 70 kg female patient will need:
  4 mL/kg for the first 10 kg → 40 mL/hr
  2 mL/kg for the next 10 kg → 20 mL/hr
  1 mL/kg for the remaining 50 kg → 50 mL/hr
Therefore her maintenance IV fluids are: 110 mL/hr

---

bances will need a parenteral solution that provides enough free water to replace losses from respiration, perspiration as well as electrolyte losses through the urine, feces, and sweat. Lactated Ringer's solution is an excellent choice for most obstetric circumstances.

The next question is, how much fluid to give. Table 27–2 reviews the replacement of maintenance fluids. One of the most important issues in assessing body fluid equilibrium is the evaluation of appropriate intravascular volume (euvolemia or normovolemia). Normal intravascular volume is important to ensure adequate delivery of oxygen and nutrients to the tissue level (i.e., adequate tissue perfusion). Table 27–3 addresses the assessment of hypovolemia.

■
"Invasive Monitors" and the Assessment of Volume Status

Central venous pressure (CVP) and pulmonary artery occlusion pressure (PAOP) (also referred to as the "wedge pressure") are used as rough approximations of the left ventricular filling pressure. Even the best clinicians have difficulty establishing the status of intravascular hydration in critically ill obstetric patients. This task is simplified by the judicious use of central pressure catheters. A CVP catheter can be extremely useful in helping to determine the filling status of the right heart chambers. CVP is,

---

Table 27–3

Clinical Assessment of Intravascular Volume Depletion (Hypovolemia)

History
  Nausea/vomiting, diarrhea, oral intake, urine output, drugs
Physical examination
  Pulse weak, thready, and >100 bpm
  Orthostatic vital signs
  Dry mucous membranes
  Poor skin turgor
  Flat neck veins
  Prolonged capillary refill time; "cold toes"
Laboratory
  Urine that looks and smells concentrated
  Urine specific gravity >1.025
  Urine sodium <10 mEq/L
  Elevated hematocrit (hemoconcentration)
  BUN/creatinine >20
  Elevated uric acid
  Fractional excretion of Na <1

---

however, a measurement of the pressure of the blood at the inflow tract of the heart. This may not reflect the true filling status of the left side of the heart. In my experience, if central venous access is recommended, a pulmonary artery catheter is utilized. Significantly more information on the hemodynamic variables can be obtained while offering risks comparative to those of a CVP catheter.

The Frank-Starling mechanism proposes that the length of a myocardial fiber (and therefore the filling volume) is proportional to the force and velocity of the ventricular contraction (and therefore the cardiac output). Therefore, the greater the volume in the left heart the higher the cardiac output. This, of course, is true only to a point. Once we exceed a critical fiber length cardiac output drops.

Left ventricular end-diastolic filling pressure (LVEDP) can be estimated by the use of a pulmonary artery catheter. The assumption we have to make is that myocardial fiber length correlates with left ventricular end-diastolic volume (LVEDV) and, thus, to LVEDP. LVEDP cannot be measured clinically by a pulmonary artery catheter. The closest clinically measurable parameter is PAOP.

At end diastole, with a normal mitral valve, the left atrial pressure is roughly equal to the left ventricular end-diastolic pressure. It is at this time that the pressure in the distal capillary bed of the lungs also equals left atrial pressure—and therefore LVEDP. This value is known as PAOP or "pulmonary capillary wedge pressure" (PCWP).

CVP often does not accurately reflect left ventricular filling in patients with preeclampsia, pulmonary processes, and cardiac disease. In these situations, utilizing a pulmonary artery catheter is extremely helpful in determining relative volume status. Unfortunately, the PAOP value does not always shed light on volume status. In these circumstances it may be helpful to use a "fluid challenge" technique to help obtain a "dynamic" picture of the patient's intravascular volume.

Although recommendations vary, the basic principle is as follows: A relatively small bolus of fluid (e.g., lactated Ringer's) is administered fairly rapidly (over 10 minutes) in an effort to attempt to determine the "reserve capacitance" of the cardiovascular system. A static value of PAOP that is normal may occasionally occur in hypovolemia, euvolemia, or hypervolemia. If additional intravascular volume is administered in the format outlined above (Table 27–4), further information may be obtained about the "effective intravascular volume" relative to the capacitance or distensibility of the cardiovascular system (i.e., a simplistic rough approximation of how "tanked up" or "filled" the cardiovascular system is).

Assuming that decreased distensibility is not a predominant feature of the patient's cardiovascular system, the following is true in response to a fluid bolus (Table 27–4):

When administering fluid to achieve euvolemia: Crystalloids are adequate for most clinical situations. In the clinical circumstance of a very low plasma colloid oncotic pressure (COP) or when the COP–PAOP gradient is ≤4 mm Hg, administering colloids may be optimal; however, this remains controversial in obstetric patients. Table 27–5 reviews the colloid oncotic pressure in the antepartum and postpartum periods in both normal and preeclamptic patients.

When administering colloids, it is important to remember that:

1. Less volume is needed (3 to 4 ml crystalloid to 1 ml colloid).
2. Colloids may trigger anaphylactoid reactions.
3. Colloids may alter hemostasis.
4. Colloids stay longer than crystalloids in the intravascular space.

Table 27–4		

The Effect of Volume Replacement on Ventricular Filling Pressures

"7-3 Rules" for Fluid Challenge

Start by measuring
  Baseline parameters
  Cardiac output (CO)
  Pulmonary artery occlusion pressure (wedge pressure; PAOP)
  Central venous pressure (CVP)
  Pulmonary artery pressure (PAP)
A fluid bolus of 200 mL lactated Ringer's solution is given. PAOP is measured after this fluid challenge. The following table summarizes the clinical decisions that follow.

PAOP after Fluid Bolus Clinical Action (Change from Baseline)

PAOP increase >7 mm Hg → → → Stop (i.e., no more fluid)
PAOP increase 3–7 mm Hg → → → Wait 10 min
If PAOP still >3 mm Hg → → → Stop
PAOP increase <3 mm Hg → → → Continue fluid administration

The two most common colloid solutions used in medical practice are 5% albumin and 6% hydroxymethyl starch (Hespan), (see Chapter 2). The latter is a synthetic polymer; the former, a product processed from blood.

■
Electrolytes

Fluid and electrolyte homeostasis is one of the most basic functions of life. The cell's internal and external milieus are carefully

Table 27–5		

Colloid Oncotic Pressure (COP)

Nonpregnant normal COP is 25 to 28 mm Hg
Normal PAOP is 7–13 mm Hg

	NL Pregnant	Preeclampsia
Antepartum COP	22 mm Hg	18 mm Hg
Postpartum COP	17 mm Hg	14 mm Hg

controlled. Perturbations of this environment may yield cellular dysfunctions that may be secondary to metabolic failure or impaired membrane integrity and function. Significant abnormalities, if not addressed, may result in major morbidity and mortality (i.e., malignant arrhythmias, seizures, coma, death).

Acute versus Chronic Disturbances

It is very important to distinguish acute electrolyte disturbances from chronic ones. With chronic electrolyte disturbances, homeostatic adjustments occur intracellularly to keep the relative transmembrane potential fairly constant. Acute electrolyte disturbances, however, may adversely alter the electrophysiologic milieu of the cell, resulting in relative hypo- or hyperpolarization. These dynamic changes in transmembrane potential may manifest clinically as seizures, cardiac arrhythmias, or even gross muscle dysfunction.

The cardiac tissue is particularly sensitive to electrolyte disturbances. The electrocardiogram (ECG) therefore serves as a very useful tool for alerting the clinician to significant electrolyte abnormality. ECG changes, however, tend to be most noticeable only when deviations from normal electrolyte values are large. Table 27–6 outlines the ECG aberrations associated with specific electrolyte abnormalities.

■
Assessment and Treatment of Electrolyte Abnormalities

The normal serum sodium concentration is 136–145 mEq/L. Normative reference ranges vary among laboratories. Serum sodium concentration (Na^+) is an approximate indicator of TBW. Table 27–7 reviews the normal sodium and water balance in pregnancy.

The primary signs and symptoms of hyponatremia (sodium <135 mEq/L) include nausea, vomiting, hypertension, increased intracranial pressure, convulsions with sodium <120 mEq/L, and oliguric renal failure. The development of cerebral edema (cellular edema) may occur with severe hyponatremia (<120 mEq/L). One of the most important early protective mechanisms to adapt to this cellular edema is extrusion of sodium from brain cells. Females appear less able to adapt to hyponatremia by limiting cellular edema. (They may be less able to extrude sodium to diminish brain cell osmolality.) Consequently, brain

---

Table 27–6

Electrocardiographic Aberrations Associated with Specific Electrolyte Abnormalities

Hypokalemia
  Flattened T waves
  Shortened PR interval/prolonged QT interval
  Prominent U waves
  ST segment depression
Hyperkalemia
  Tall, thin, and peaked T waves
  Prolonged PR interval
  Widened QRS interval
  ST elevation
Hypercalcemia
  Prolonged PR interval
  Short QT interval (T wave rapid upslope, gradual downslope)
  Widened QRS interval
Hypocalcemia
  Prolonged QT interval (long ST segment)
  Terminal T wave inversion

---

insult is more common in hyponatremic females than in hyponatremic males. In addition, the combination of hyponatremia and hypoxia is comparatively worse: hypoxia impairs brain adaptation to hyponatremia. It is therefore extremely important to limit hypoxemia in gravidas with hyponatremia. All symptomatic hyponatremic patients should have arterial blood gas measurements and continuous pulse oximetry. Intubation and mechanical ventilation may be required to achieve adequate oxygenation.

Table 27–7

Sodium and Water Balance in Pregnancy

Positive sodium balance (500–900 mEq)
Positive water balance (6–8 L H_2O)
Plasma volume increases (55%)
Expansion of extracellular fluid:
  Increased renin-angiotensin-aldosterone axis
  Increased natriuresis
Serum sodium decreases ~4 mEq/L
Plasma osmolarity decreases ~10 mOsm/kg
Plasma bicarbonate decreases ~20 mEq/L
Normal basal levels of arginine vasopressin

Important Clinical Note. The hyponatremic patient can go from alert and talkative to respiratory arrest and comatose in 20 minutes. Close clinical surveillance, therefore, is prudent.

Treatment of Hyponatremia

Establishing the cause of hyponatremia is an important first step in effecting appropriate treatment (Fig. 27–1). A common pitfall in the diagnosis is the concurrent presence of hyperglycemia. Glucose in the serum creates an osmotic gradient, forcing free water to move into the extracellular space and thus lowering plasma sodium. In the majority of clinical circumstances the correction of the hyperglycemia results in normalization of serum sodium.

NOTE: For every 110-mg/dL increase over the normal plasma glucose concentration, plasma sodium concentration decreases by 1.6 mEq/L.

Table 27–8 summarizes the treatment of hyponatremia. In

Table 27–8

Treatment of Hyponatremia

Calculate the Na deficit: Na deficit (mEq) = (0.5)(wt in kg) × (125 − Measured Na)

Sodium replacement: The calculated Na deficit in (mEq) = 2 × (volume of 3% NaCl in mL). To partially correct ($1/2$ total correction) the Na deficit, the volume of 3% NaCl in mL is the same as the calculated Na deficit in mEq.

Asymptomatic hyponatremia
  Generally doesn't require aggressive therapy.
  Hypertonic saline is usually not indicated.
  Fluid restriction usually suffices.
  Withdrawal of offending agents (if any).
  Achieve euvolemia.
  Pharmacologic therapy, if appropriate (e.g., hormone replacement)

Mild to moderate symptomatic hyponatremia
  Normal saline should be given intravenously.
  Consider using intravenous furosemide.

Severe symptomatic hyponatremia (e.g., seizures)
  Active therapy with hypertonic saline (regardless of duration, severity, acute or chronic) 3% NaCl (514 mEq/L) should be administered using an infusion pump increasing plasma sodium 1 mEq/L/hr until:
    1. The patient becomes alert and seizure free.
                  or
    2. The plasma sodium has increased by 20–25 mEq/L over 48 hr.
                  or
    3. Sodium concentration of 125–130 mEq/L is reached.

Monitor plasma electrolytes q 1–2 hr until patient is neurologically stable.

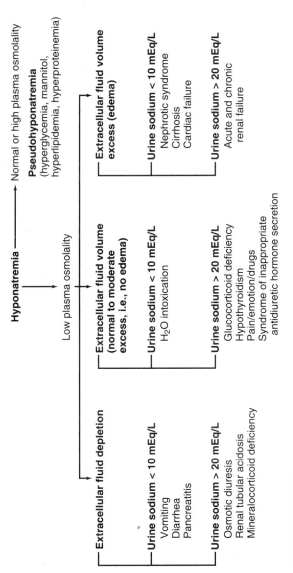

Hyponatremia

Normal or high plasma osmolality

Pseudohyponatremia
(hyperglycemia, mannitol,
hyperlipidemia, hyperproteinemia)

Low plasma osmolality

**Extracellular fluid volume
excess (edema)**

Urine sodium < 10 mEq/L
Nephrotic syndrome
Cirrhosis
Cardiac failure

Urine sodium > 20 mEq/L
Acute and chronic
renal failure

**Extracellular fluid volume
(normal to moderate
excess, i.e., no edema)**

Urine sodium < 10 mEq/L
H₂O intoxication

Urine sodium > 20 mEq/L
Glucocorticoid deficiency
Hypothyroidism
Pain/emotion/drugs
Syndrome of inappropriate
antidiuretic hormone secretion

Extracellular fluid depletion

Urine sodium < 10 mEq/L
Vomiting
Diarrhea
Pancreatitis

Urine sodium > 20 mEq/L
Osmotic diuresis
Renal tubular acidosis
Mineralocorticoid deficiency

Figure 27-1

Algorithm for the assessment of hyponatremia.

391

most cases hyponatremia can be treated by fluid restriction and corrections of the underlying abnormality.

Hypernatremia

Hypernatremia (sodium >150 mEq/L) is an excess of sodium in the extracellular compartment. The total body sodium, however, may be low, normal, or high. Symptoms include altered mental status, twitching, seizures, and coma. Acute severe increases of sodium greater than 160 mEq/L may lead to irreversible neurologic disease. Figure 27–2 summarizes the possible causes and therapeutic approaches to hypernatremia.

Potassium

Total body stores of potassium (normal range 3.5 to 5 mEq/L) are primarily stored intracellularly. Plasma potassium represents a small portion of total body potassium. A small drop in plasma potassium, therefore, may reflect a large total body deficit. Average individual total body potassium is 3500 to 4200 mEq. That in the ECF compartment is 50 to 60 mEq, whereas in the ICF compartment it is 3450 to 4140 mEq. Profound chronic hypokalemia may represent total body deficits of 500 to 1000 mEq.

Potassium is the most important intracellular cation. The potassium and sodium gradient between the extra- and intracellular spaces accounts for the negative intracellular transmembrane potential. This electrical potential is the result of different concentrations of these two ions at opposite sides of the cell membrane. It is no surprise that an imbalance in the potassium equilibrium leads to alterations in this potential. Neural and cardiac tissue are of primary concern and may be severely affected by any disturbances of potassium homeostasis. Figure 27–3 addresses the assessment and causes of hypokalemia.

Hypokalemia

Mild asymptomatic hypokalemia (3.0 to 3.4 mEq/L) can be treated with oral potassium salts. Generally these are well tolerated and very effective. A dose of 40 mEq of potassium chloride can be given by mouth, as needed every 6 hours.

Moderate severe asymptomatic hypokalemia (2.5 to 3.0 mEq/ L) should be treated with intravenous potassium salts administered at a rate no faster than 40 mEq/hr. Intravenous potassium preparations must be diluted and administered cautiously. Skin

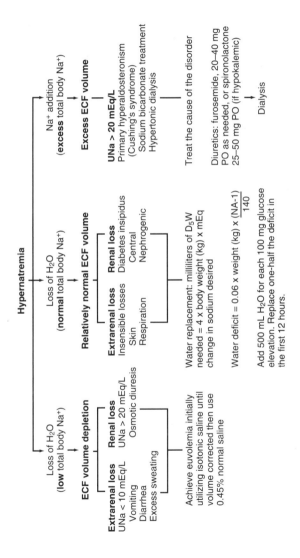

Hypernatremia

Loss of H₂O (low total body Na⁺)

ECF volume depletion

Extrarenal loss
UNa < 10 mEq/L
Vomiting
Diarrhea
Excess sweating

Renal loss
UNa > 20 mEq/L
Osmotic diuresis

Achieve euvolemia initially utilizing isotonic saline until volume corrected then use 0.45% normal saline

Loss of H₂O (normal total body Na⁺)

Relatively normal ECF volume

Extrarenal loss
Insensible losses
Skin
Respiration

Renal loss
Diabetes insipidus
Central
Nephrogenic

Water replacement: milliliters of D₅W needed = 4 × body weight (kg) × mEq change in sodium desired

Water deficit = $0.06 \times \text{weight (kg)} \times \frac{(NA-1)}{140}$

Add 500 mL H₂O for each 100 mg glucose elevation. Replace one-half the deficit in the first 12 hours.

Central diabetes insipidus 5–10 units vasopressin SC q4–6hr

Na⁺ addition (excess total body Na⁺)

Excess ECF volume

UNa > 20 mEq/L
Primary hyperaldosteronism (Cushing's syndrome)
Sodium bicarbonate treatment
Hypertonic dialysis

Treat the cause of the disorder

Diuretics: furosemide, 20–40 mg PO as needed, or spironolactone 25–50 mg PO (if hypokalemic)

Dialysis

Figure 27–2

Algorithm for the assessment and treatment of hypernatremia. ECF, extracellular fluid; UNa, Urine sodium; Na⁺, sodium.

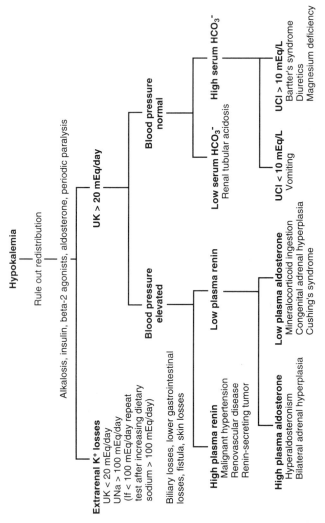

Figure 27–3

Algorithm for the assessment of hypokalemia. UK, urine potassium; UNa, urine sodium; UCl, urine chloride.

Hypokalemia

Rule out redistribution

Alkalosis, insulin, beta-2 agonists, aldosterone, periodic paralysis

UK < 20 mEq/day

Extrarenal K⁺ losses
UK < 20 mEq/day
UNa > 100 mEq/day
(If < 100 mEq/day repeat test after increasing dietary sodium > 100 mEq/day)

Biliary losses, lower gastrointestinal losses, fistula, skin losses

UK > 20 mEq/day

Blood pressure elevated

Low plasma renin

High plasma renin
Malignant hypertension
Renovascular disease
Renin-secreting tumor

High plasma aldosterone
Hyperaldosteronism
Bilateral adrenal hyperplasia

Low plasma aldosterone
Mineralocorticoid ingestion
Congenital adrenal hyperplasia
Cushing's syndrome

Blood pressure normal

Low serum HCO₃⁻
Renal tubular acidosis

High serum HCO₃⁻

UCl < 10 mEq/L
Vomiting

UCl > 10 mEq/L
Bartter's syndrome
Diuretics
Magnesium deficiency

394

sloughing may occur if subcutaneous infiltration occurs. ECG monitoring of these patients is also indicated.

Symptomatic hypokalemia (2.0 to 2.5 mEq/L) can be treated with potassium, 0.75 mEq/kg body weight (or 30 mEq/m² of surface area for obese persons) over 1 to 2 hours. This usually increases serum potassium by 1 to 1.5 mEq/L in normokalemic or mildly hypokalemic persons. With profound hypokalemia serum potassium will rise less, since a greater percentage of the administered potassium will move into the cells.

These patients should be carefully monitored in the intensive care unit. *Symptomatic hypokalemia (<2.0 mEq/L) associated with malignant cardiac arrhythmia* should be aggressively treated with 80 to 100 mEq infused over 1 hour. Two peripheral intravenous lines are usually adequate, 40 to 50 mEq/L infused in each over an hour. If a large volume load would create a problem, a more concentrated solution can be given through the central line.

Key Points

> Avoid hyperventilation.
> Avoid solutions containing glucose.
> Employ continuous electrocardiographic monitoring.
> Check serum potassium every 1 to 3 hours.
> Closely monitor urine output.

Hyperkalemia

Hyperkalemia is a disorder of normal or elevated total body potassium. Because of its ubiquitous nature, potassium can be redistributed across body compartments and create hyperkalemia only by virtue of redistribution. The end result is electrical tissue irritability and organ dysfunction. The clinician treating hyperkalemia should make an effort to find the etiology and treat the underlying cause. Figure 27–4 outlines the causes of hyperkalemia.

Assessment and Treatment

Hyperkalemia is not tolerated well, and corrective actions should be taken quickly. These actions are usually directed toward initiating redistribution of the ion back into the intracellular space. Short-term strategies are important first steps while arrangements for definitive potassium excretion are being made.

Avoidance of potassium redistribution is imperative; there-

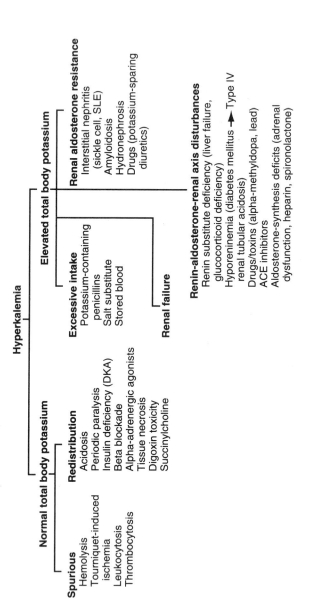

Hyperkalemia

Normal total body potassium

Spurious
Hemolysis
Tourniquet-induced ischemia
Leukocytosis
Thrombocytosis

Redistribution
Acidosis
Periodic paralysis
Insulin deficiency (DKA)
Beta blockade
Alpha-adrenergic agonists
Tissue necrosis
Digoxin toxicity
Succinylcholine

Elevated total body potassium

Excessive intake
Potassium-containing penicillins
Salt substitute
Stored blood

Renal failure

Renal aldosterone resistance
Interstitial nephritis (sickle cell, SLE)
Amyloidosis
Hydronephrosis
Drugs (potassium-sparing diuretics)

Renin-aldosterone-renal axis disturbances
Renin substitute deficiency (liver failure, glucocorticoid deficiency)
Hyporeninemia (diabetes mellitus ➞ Type IV renal tubular acidosis)
Drugs/toxins (alpha-methyldopa, lead)
ACE inhibitors
Aldosterone-synthesis deficits (adrenal dysfunction, heparin, spironolactone)

Figure 27–4

Algorithm for the assessment of hyperkalemia. SLE, systemic lupus erythematosus; DKA, diabetic ketoacidosis; ACE, angiotensin converting enzyme.

fore, drugs that release intracellular potassium, such as succinyl-choline, should be avoided. Efforts to correct hypoventilation and acidosis are prudent. Acidosis forces hydrogen ions intracellularly, and resultant extracellular shifts of potassium ions worsen the hyperkalemia. Hyperglycemia should be corrected with insulin, which will force potassium into the intracellular space along with glucose.

Certain drugs such as angiotensin-converting enzyme inhibitors have potassium-sparing ability. They are best avoided in the presence of hyperkalemia. Hemolysis and tissue hypoxia are carefully avoided, as these will release intracellular potassium. If the hyperkalemia is severe or symptomatic, corrective action must proceed quickly. While glucose and insulin are being initiated, intravenous calcium chloride, 300 mg over 10 minutes, protects the myocardium against potassium-induced arrhythmias. Figure 27–5 and Table 27–9 outline acute-phase management of hyperkalemia.

Potassium Redistribution Strategies. Treatment with insulin and glucose (10 units of regular insulin is given intravenously for each 25 gm of dextrose intravenously) forces the cells to transport glucose intracellularly and bring along potassium ions (cotransport). Hyperventilation and sodium bicarbonate administration also assist with the intracellular transport of potassium by cotransport.

Potassium Elimination Strategies. Kayexalate is an ion-binding resin that functions to eliminate serum potassium. It may be given orally or rectally. It is very effective though difficult to administer, usually takes hours to achieve effect, and subjects

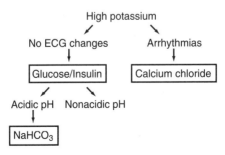

Figure 27–5

Algorithm for the initial treatment of acute hyperkalemia.

Table 27–9

Specific Treatment Modalities for Hyperkalemia

Therapy	Dose	Onset	Duration
Redistributive therapy			
Intravenous calcium chloride (check for ECG abnormalities)	7–14 mg/kg	Immediate	15–30 min (redistribution)
Intravenous glucose and regular insulin	25 gm + 10 U	15–30 min	3–6 hr (redistribution)
Sodium bicarbonate	0.7–1.4 mEq/kg	15–30 min	3–6 hr (redistribution)
Eliminative therapy			
Kayexalate	30 gm oral/rectal	1–3 hr	K$^+$ elimination
Peritoneal dialysis		1–3 hr	K$^+$ elimination
Hemodialysis		Rapid	K$^+$ elimination

the patient to a substantial sodium load. Peritoneal dialysis is highly effective but requires the placement of an invasive catheter in the peritoneal cavity. In addition, this procedure is time consuming and carries risks of surgical morbidity and mortality. Hemodialysis is also very effective but takes precious time to set up the complicated and cumbersome but necessary equipment. A large intravenous catheter or arteriovenous fistula is also needed. Utilizing potassium redistribution strategies in the acute setting followed by elimination strategies, if needed, appears to be a judicious approach to the care of hyperkalemic patients. Tables 27–10 through 27–19 systematically address additional, but less frequently encountered, electrolyte disturbances (e.g., calcium, magnesium, phosphate).

■ Summary

Table 27–20 summarizes the goals of appropriate fluid and electrolyte replacement in pregnant patients. The ultimate goal of restoring fluid and electrolyte balance is to provide tissues with adequate substrate necessary for cellular metabolism and integrity. Clinicians caring for a gravid patient are challenged with monitoring and correcting disturbances in fluid volumes, ion concentrations, pH imbalances, and oxygenation requirements on two patients who share a total fluid volume. The principles illustrated in this chapter attempt to address these problems in a systematic way.

Text continued on page 403

Table 27–10

Causes of Hypercalcemia

Increased gastrointestinal calcium absorption
   Vitamin D intoxication
   Granulomatous diseases (tuberculosis, sarcoidosis, coccidioidomycosis)
Increased calcium resorption from bone
   Primary hyperparathyroidism
   Hyperthyroidism
   Malignancy
   Chronic immobilization
Increased renal tubular calcium reabsorption
   Thiazide diuretics
Other
   Milk alkali syndrome
   Adrenal insufficiency
   Lithium administration

Table 27–11

Specific Treatment Modalities for Hypercalcemia

Treatment	Onset	Consideration
Saline & forced diuresis (furosemide 40 mg IV q 1–2 hr with indwelling Foley catheter)	Hours	Cardiac decompensation, hypokalemia, hypomagnesemia
Calcitonin	Hours	Lower calcium by 2–3 mg/dL; tachyphylaxis within 2–3 days
Plicamycin	24 hr	Toxicities: with repeat dosing, renal insufficiency, hepatic injury, qualitative & quantitative platelet abnormalities
Etidronate	24–48 hr	Hyperphosphatemia
Pamidronate	24–48 hr	Fever, hypophosphatemia, hypomagnesemia

Table 27–12

Causes of Hypomagnesemia

> Endocrine
>> Hyperthyroidism
>> Primary hyperparathyroidism
>> Hypoparathyroidism
>> Primary hyperaldosteronism
>> Diabetic ketoacidosis
>
> Gastrointestinal disorders
>> Malabsorption syndrome
>> Alcoholic cirrhosis
>> Pancreatitis
>> Fistulas
>> Chronic diarrhea/short bowel syndrome
>
> Renal magnesium wasting
>> Diuretics
>> Alcohol
>> Osmotic diuresis
>> Renal tubular disorder
>> Cisplatin
>
> Nutritional

Table 27–13

Specific Treatment Modalities for Hypomagnesemia

Mild Hypomagnesemia

Treat with diet and/or oral magnesium supplementation (oral magnesium oxide)

Symptomatic or Severe Hypomagnesemia ($Mg^{++} < 1.0$ mg/dL)

Treat with parenteral $MgSO_4$

> 1–2 gm (8–16 mEq) $MgSO_4$ IV bolus over 1 hr followed by continuous infusion of 2–4 mEq/hr. [$MgSO_4$: 1 gm = 8 mEq Mg^{++}; $MgCl_2$: 1 gm = 10 mEq Mg^{++}] If no intravenous access, 0.10 mEq IM $MgCl_2$
> (1 gm) q 4–6 hr until IV access is obtained.

Therapy should be guided by following serum Mg^{++} levels.

Infusion rate should not exceed 1 mEq/min.

Continuous cardiac monitoring (ECG), HR, BP q 5 min, and other indices of cardiac function as appropriate.

Frequently monitor patellar reflexes and respiratory rate.

Care must be taken when patients have impaired renal function.

Table 27–14

Causes of Hypermagnesemia

Increased magnesium administration (abuse of magnesium antacids or laxatives, $MgSO_4$ therapy)
Adrenal insufficiency
Hypothyroidism
Lithium therapy
Decreased renal excretion (renal insufficiency)

Table 27–15

Specific Treatment Modalities for Hypermagnesemia

A. Discontinue intake of all sources of magnesium.
B. Intravenous calcium if severe and symptomatic, initially 100–200 mg of elemental calcium [20 mL 10% calcium gluconate] over 5–10 min. If persistent or recurrent serious symptoms: repeat as necessary, 1 gm using ECG as a guide.
Calcium chloride is an acceptable substitute for calcium gluconate. Remember that 300 mg calcium chloride is roughly equivalent to 1 gm calcium gluconate.
C. Treat the underlying cause.
Infusion of 5% dextrose and 0.45% normal saline with IV furosemide, 40 mg intravenous q 1–2 hr enhances urinary magnesium excretion (diuresis with normal saline may lead to iatrogenic hypocalcemia, which may potentiate the effects of hypermagnesemia).
D. Consider the following:
Improve renal function
Dialysis if necessary
Close monitoring of blood pressure
Continuous ECG monitoring
Continuous pulse oximetry
Strict intake and output monitoring (with indwelling Foley catheter)
Follow serial measurements of calcium and magnesium

Table 27–16

Causes of Hypophosphatemia

Total body depletion or intercompartmental shifts
Trauma
Postoperative administration of IV glucose solutions, extended by
fasting; fluid losses secondary to trauma
Severe burns
Alcoholism
Parenteral hyperalimentation
Diabetic ketoacidosis and insulin therapy
Antacid consumption
Oncogenic osteomalacia
Prolonged respiratory alkalosis

Table 27–17

Specific Treatment Modalities for Hypophosphatemia

Oral phosphorus replacement is preferable to parenteral (because of risk of
hypocalcemia and metastatic calcification); however, if hypophosphatemia
is severe, symptomatic (CNS symptoms, hemolysis, cardiomyopathy,
rhabdomyolysis) or < 1 mg/dL, then parenteral therapy is indicated.
An initial infusion of 1000 mg P (elemental phosphorus) (as potassium or
sodium phosphate) in 1 L of fluid can be administered over 12 hr.
Avoid hyperglycemia
Avoid hyperventilation
Monitor closely, continuous ECG, continuous pulse oximetry
Check serum [PO_4] q 4–6 hr

Table 27–18

Causes of Hyperphosphatemia

Increased phosphate administration (e.g., phosphate laxative
abuse)
Redistribution (e.g., acidosis)
Increased tissue breakdown (e.g., massive tumor lysis following
chemotherapy)
Decreased renal excretion (e.g., renal insufficiency)

Table 27–19

Specific Treatment Modalities for Hyperphosphatemia

Phosphate restriction
Decrease gastrointestinal absorption by aluminum hydroxide
    therapy
Correct acidosis
Improve renal function/diuresis
Dialysis, if necessary

The basic principles of restoring oxygen delivery, addressing acid-base balance, and correcting electrolyte disturbances are accomplished systematically by supporting cardiopulmonary function. The steps involved invariably return to the principles of securing the airway, establishing ventilation, and supporting circulation of blood.

Once the circulation is established the process of oxygen delivery and carbon dioxide removal from the tissues allows acid-base problems to be managed successfully. Existing electrolyte disturbances are approached with caution and patience. The most severe disturbances are treated first, keeping in mind that the treatment should address the ultimate cause of the disturbance.

Table 27–20

Summary of Goals for Appropriate Fluid and Electrolyte Replacement in Pregnant Women

1. Ensure adequate oxygen delivery to peripheral tissues, including the fetus.
    Restore intravascular volume.
    Ensure adequate oxygenation.
    Maintain adequate cardiovascular function.
    Ensure adequate hemoglobin concentration.
2. Address pH and primary electrolyte disturbances (most severe) to allow "acid dumping" from the fetal compartment to the maternal compartment.
3. Correct remaining electrolyte disturbances.

■ Bibliography

Kassirer JP, Hricik DE, Cohen JJ: Repairing Body Fluids: Principles and Practice. Philadelphia: W.B. Saunders, 1989.

Maxwell MH, Kleeman CR, Narins RG: Clinical Disorders of Fluid and Electrolyte Metabolism, ed 4. New York: McGraw-Hill, 1987.

Pestana CC: Fluid and Electrolytes in the Surgical Patient, ed 4. Baltimore: Williams & Wilkins, 1989.

Pitts RF: Physiology of the Kidney and Body Fluids, ed 3. Chicago: Year Book, 1974.

Rose BD: Physiology of Acid Base and Electrolyte Disorders, ed 3. New York: McGraw-Hill, 1979.

Schrier RW: Renal and Electrolyte Disorders, ed 2. Boston: Little, Brown, 1980.

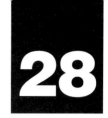

LINDA R. CHAMBLISS

Human Immunodeficiency Virus Infection and Pregnancy

Because patients infected with human immunodeficiency virus (HIV) present a formidable challenge to even the most experienced clinician, HIV-infected pregnant women should be managed by a team familiar with their problems and with the full range of ancillary and support services. It is also important to remember that, while the overwhelming majority of HIV-infected persons eventually develop the acquired immunodeficiency syndrome (AIDS), HIV infection is not *synonymous* with AIDS (see Appendix). Roughly 12% of HIV-infected persons are women, and 85% of them are between ages 15 and 44 years. Women comprise an increasing portion of the epidemic: the rate of increase of the disease is fourfold higher among women than among men. Three quarters of women with AIDS are black or Hispanic. The incidence of AIDS is 15 times greater for black women than for white women and 7 times greater for Hispanic women. Most women acquire the virus (directly or indirectly) via intravenous drug abuse; however, the rate of heterosexual transmission continues to increase. Except for those in the Northeastern United States, more women contract the disease heterosexually than through drug use.

■
Testing for HIV Infection

Patients may not admit to high-risk behavior or may be unaware of their partners'. Moreover, patients may have seroconverted since a previously negative screen. Therefore, all patients should be considered potentially infected. *HIV testing should be offered to all patients, particularly those who are pregnant* (Table 28 1). HIV testing consists of two analyses: enzyme-linked immunosorbent assay (ELISA) and Western blot test. A positive ELISA screen makes it necessary to perform the confirmatory Western

Table 28-1

Who Should Be Offered HIV Testing?

Patients with sexually-transmitted diseases
Patients who request HIV testing
Patients with clinical/laboratory findings suggestive of HIV
Patients aged 15 to 44 years admitted to hospitals that have seroprevalence rates >1% or where AIDS patients account for >1 in 1000 discharges
Patients with cervical dysplasia or evidence of human papillomavirus infection
Patients who engage in intravenous drug use, have sex with gay or bisexual men or have sex with partners who do
Patients with active tuberculosis
Patients from "endemic areas"
Those exposed to blood or body fluids
Donors of blood, semen, or organs
Health care workers who perform invasive procedures
Those transfused between 1978 and 1985

blot test. Both must be positive to designate seropositivity. A positive result indicates that the patient has antibodies against multiple HIV antigens. An indeterminate Western blot result may be due to recent exposure and may indicate that the patient is in the process of seroconversion. In this case, the Western blot will generally produce a positive result in 3 months. Indeterminate tests should be repeated in 6 to 12 months. As with all tests, both false-positive and false-negative results occur, the incidence of each being related to the prevalence of disease in the population studied. In low-risk populations, for example, the incidence of false-negative results is 0.001%, whereas among high-risk populations the incidence of false-negative results is 0.3%. Other methods of testing include viral culture and DNA polymerase chain reaction, neither yet widely available.

■
Pathogenesis

HIV is a retrovirus that binds to receptors on helper T lymphocytes, B lymphocytes, macrophages, lymph nodes, and brain cells. Retroviruses use reverse transcriptase to introduce their genome into the host's and thus take control of the cell. Since HIV replication kills the host cell, the population of cells is depleted over time.

HIV-Related Immune System Dysfunctions

- The thymus is destroyed.
- T lymphocytes malfunction:
  Fail to proliferate following antigen exposure
  Secrete inappropriate amounts of cytokines
- Macrophages fail to "present" antigens to T lymphocytes.
- Lymph node architecture is distorted: antigens are not trapped.
- B lymphocytes behave as if chronically activated:
  Spontaneous proliferation
  Polyclonal production of defective antibodies

■
Interpreting the CD4 Cell Count

The CD4 (helper T lymphocyte) cell count is the single most sensitive predictor of disease activity. Seropositive pregnant patients should have CD4 counts every trimester. Certain complications tend to be encountered at given CD4 counts. As a rule, threshold CD4 counts should be repeated 1 week before any therapeutic decision is made. The trend of CD4 counts is generally more useful than a single value. If a CD4 count is $<50/\mu L$ it is not repeated as results do not affect management. Multiple factors may depress the CD4 cell count (Table 28–2).

■
Signs and Symptoms Predictive of AIDS

Some clinical scenarios and laboratory findings are strongly predictive of AIDS (Table 28–3).

Table 28–2
Factors That Can Lower the CD4 Count

Pregnancy	Intra/inter assay variation
Recent steroid use*	Infections (tuberculosis, cytomegalovirus,
Antibiotics	hepatitis B, etc.)
Diurnal variation†	Seasonal/monthly variation
Major surgery	

*Chronic use has less impact.

†A 30% difference may be noted, depending on what time of day sample is obtained: nadir, 12:30 P.M.; peak, 8:30 P.M.

Table 28-3
Signs and Symptoms Predictive of Progression to AIDS
Oral *Candida* infection
Constitutional symptoms (weight loss, diarrhea, fever, sweats)
CD4 lymphocytes $<200/\mu L$
CD4 lymphocytes $<25\%$ of total lymphocytes
p24 antigenemia
Serum beta-2 microglobulin >3 $\mu gm/mL$
Hematocrit $<40\%$
Anti–p24 antibody
Thrombocytopenia

Immune System Changes in Pregnancy

The immune system changes of pregnancy are not completely understood, but one appears to be selective depression of cell-mediated immunity. Although overall cell-mediated immunity is generally preserved, poor maternal nutrition may impair immunoglobulin production.

Pregnancy and HIV Infection

Pregnancy does not appear to affect the progression of HIV infection.

A mother with AIDS may expose her fetus to serious risks. Common pregnancy complaints such as dyspnea, headache, low back pain, and fatigue should be investigated. In HIV-infected patients they should not be considered "part of normal pregnancy." Owing to polyclonal antibody production, HIV-seropositive patients may develop the anticardiolipin antibody or lupus anticoagulant. These do not appear to be associated with obstetric risk. If the patient requires blood products it is imperative that cytomegalovirus-negative blood be used.

Assessment of the Parturient with HIV

When an HIV-infected mother presents to the hospital, she and her fetus require comprehensive evaluation (Tables 28–4, 28–5).

Table 28-4

Assessment of HIV-Infected Mothers

Special attention should be given to:
History
    Medications, drug reactions, allergies
    Immunization status*
    Prior and current sexually transmitted diseases, drug use, alcohol use
    Mental health history (depression, domestic violence, dementia)
    Availability of support systems
    Contraception
Examination
    Vital signs
        Temperature, respiratory rate
    Skin
        Abscesses, dermatitis, rashes, vesicles, violaceous macules
    Head, eyes, ears, nose, and throat
        Dentition, funduscopic exam, oral thrush or ulcers, nuchal rigidity,
            visual fields
    Pulmonary
        Breath sounds, cough, sputum
    Cardiac
        Cardiomegaly, murmurs
    Abdomen
        Fetal heart tones, hepatosplenomegaly
    Genitourinary
        Genital lesions, vaginal discharge
    Neurologic
        Affect, confusion, ability to concentrate, focal neurologic deficits,
            memory deficits, mental status, neuropathy, weakness
Laboratories
    Baseline assessment of hematologic, renal, and liver functions
    Tuberculosis status
Miscellaneous
    Nutritional assessment
    Reduction of transmission risk (safe sex practices, abstinence from
        breast feeding, etc.)

---

*Immunize to optimize outcomes: hepatitis B (may require >3 doses), influenza, pneumococcus, *Haemophilus influenzae*, tetanus.

Prevention of Vertical Transmission

Almost all pediatric AIDS results from intrapartum transmission. Second-born twins may have lower rates of HIV infection, sug-

---

Table 28–5

Fetal Assessment in HIV Infection

Assess for factors that influence transmission risks:
↑ Risk: Maternal viral burden
↓ Risk: Antepartum zidovudine, second-born twin
Assess fetal well-being
Determine exposures (drugs, smoking, alcohol, cytomegalovirus, toxoplasmosis, syphilis)

---

gesting that cesarean delivery may reduce transmission. Infection has been documented in first and second trimester abortuses, however, implying that infection can antedate delivery. Antepartum zidovudine (AZT) may reduce the risk of intra-

---

Table 28–6

Administering Antepartum/Intrapartum Zidovudine

Who	When	Dose	Labs
All pregnant patients who are HIV positive	14–34 wk ante partum	100 mg PO 5 times/d	Baseline CBC, repeat q2wk Discontinue if: Hb <9 mg Platelets <10,000/mm³ Granulocytes <1000/mm³
	Intrapartum	2 mg/kg IV loading dose then 1 mg/kg/hr IV until delivery	Baseline serum creatinine Repeat monthly Baseline liver function tests. Repeat monthly. Discontinue if SGPT/SGOT values exceed normal by twofold or more.

*Unknown benefit for patients with prior zidovudine, CD4 cell counts <200/mm³, or if given after 34 wk.

Alert nursery to continue zidovudine.

Table 28-7

Meaures to Reduce Risk of Vertical Transmission

Avoid chorionic villus sampling, amniocentesis, percutaneous blood sampling

Avoid scalp electrode use

Avoid fetal scalp blood sampling

Avoid vacuum extractors

Avoid episiotomies

If possible, wash infant in antimicrobial bath *before* administering parenteral medications or obtaining blood

Avoid breast feeding

partum transmission. All gravidas, regardless of CD4 count, should be offered antepartum zidovudine after 14 weeks' gestation (Tables 28–6, 28–7).

Plasma HIV-1 RNA Measurements: "The Viral Load"

Recent advances have allowed us to measure the amount of virus circulating in a given patient. The test that reports the number of copies of RNA per milliliter is commonly referred to as "viral load." RNA measurements are obtained by DNA or reverse transcriptase PCR assays. Viral loads are increasingly being used to direct treatment. Lower viral loads are associated with improved outcome.

Limited data are available as to the interpretation of viral load in pregnant patients with regard to such factors as perinatal transmission or maternal outcome. A recent study showed that although perinatal transmission was less likely with decreasing viral load, transmission can and did occur even with undetectable plasma HIV-1 RNA levels.

Management of HIV Complications

As a rule, a pregnant patient with HIV infection should receive the same evaluation and treatment as nonpregnant patients, unless treatment (e.g., quinolones) poses unacceptable fetal risks. The three systems most often affected are pulmonary, gastrointestinal, and neurologic (Table 28–8).

Table 28–8

HIV Complications
Common Pneumonias in HIV-Infected Patients

Bacterial	Viral	Fungal	Parasitic
Staphylococcus pneumoniae	Cytomegalovirus	Histoplasmosis	Pneumocystis
H. influenzae	Herpes	Cryptococcus	
Gram-negative strains	Varicella	Aspergillus	
Tuberculosis	Influenza		
Legionella			
Mycobacterium avium complex			

Other pulmonary pathology: Lymphoma, Kaposi's sarcoma, etc.

Causes of Common Gastrointestinal Complications

↓ Oral Intake	Nausea/Vomiting	Diarrhea
Oral thrush	Medications	Medications
Oral ulcers		Salmonella
Poor dentition		Shigella
Nausea/vomiting		Parasites
Drug reactions		Cytomegalovirus
Depression		Fungi
Dementia		Proctitis

Common Neurologic Complications

Headache	Seizures	Neuropathy
HIV infection of CNS	Meningitis	Drugs (dapsone, DDC)
Sinusitis	CNS lymphoma/toxoplasmosis	Vitamin B_{12} deficiency
Meningitis	Drug/alcohol withdrawal	
CNS lymphoma	Trauma	
Fever	Electrolyte imbalance	
Anemia	HIV infection	
Drugs (acyclovir, zidovudine, fluconazole, rifampin)		

Table 28–9

Body Fluids and Universal Precautions

Universal Precautions Necessary	Universal Precautions Not Necessary *Unless* Contaminated with Blood
Blood	Breast milk
Semen	Urine
Vaginal secretions	Sputum
Tissue	Sweat
Fluids	Vomitus
Amniotic	Feces
Peritoneal	Nasal secretions
Pericardial	Tears
Pleural	Saliva
Synovial	
Cerebrospinal	

■
Safety Precautions for the Labor and Delivery Team

The Centers for Disease Control and Prevention established "universal precautions" in 1987 (Table 28–9). At least one blood exposure can be documented in roughly 30% of surgical procedures, most (75%) of which may be preventable (Table 28–10).

Table 28–10

Recommendations to Reduce Risk of Exposure When Using Sharp Instruments

Observe universal precautions
Do not recap needles
Wear double gloves
Place "sharp boxes" near where sharps are used
Announce all sharp instruments prior to passing them
Pass sharp instruments in an emesis basin
Use instruments to load needles
"One wound, one surgeon"
Check hourly for disruptions of protective barriers

Table 28-11

Drugs Commonly Used in HIV Infection

Drug	FDA Class	Indication	Dose	Toxicity/Side Effects	Breast Feed
Acyclovir	C	Herpes or varicella	Varies depending on infection	Headache, nephrotoxicity, reaction at IV site	Probably
Amphotericin B	B	Esophageal *Candida*, *Cryptococcus*, histoplasmosis	Varies depending on infection	Nephrotoxicity, fever, GI effects, hypokalemia, hypomagnesemia, rigors	†
Dapsone	*	PCP prophylaxis	50–100 mg/d PO	Peripheral neuropathy, rash, GI effects, vertigo, methemoglobinemia, hemolytic anemia, nephrotic syndrome	†
Didanosine (DDI)	*	Primary HIV infection with AZT or alone if AZT intolerant	Maternal weight >75 kg: 300 mg b.i.d. Maternal weight 50–74 kg: 200 mg. b.i.d.	Pancreatitis, rash, neuropathy, diarrhea, increased uric acid levels	†
Dideoxycytidine (DDC)	*	Primary HIV infection with AZT or alone if AZT intolerant	0.375–0.75 mg t.i.d.	Peripheral neuropathy, stomatitis, anemia, pancreatitis, rash, headache, fatigue, increased LFTs, GI	†
Fluconazole	C	Oral or esophageal *Candida* Histoplasmosis	50–200 mg/qd 400 mg PO b.i.d.	Rash, GI	Probably
Foscarnet	*	CMV retinitis	60 mg/kg t.i.d.	Seizures, electrolyte disturbances, nephrotoxicity	†
Ganciclovir	*	Herpes, varicella CMV retinitis	40 mg/kg q 8 hr, then suppress 5 mg/kg b.i.d. 14–21 d, then suppress	Neutropenia	†

Ketoconazole	C	Candida	200 mg/d PO for 2 wk	GI, hepatotoxicity, rash, headache, inhibition of cortisol synthesis	†
Pentamidine aerosolized	*	PCP prophylaxis PCP pneumonia	300 mg/mo 3–4 mg/kg/d (w/steroids)	Neutropenia, azotemia, hypotension, increased/decreased glucose, elevated LFTs, pancreatitis	†
Pyrimethamine w/sulfadiazine	C	Toxoplasmosis, encephalitis	200 mg PO 1st day, then 50–100 mg/d thereafter (pyrimethamine); 1–4 gm/d PO sulfadiazine (supplement with folate)	Anemia, leukopenia, GI effects, methemoglobinemia	Yes
Trimethoprim sulfamethoxazole	C	PCP prophylaxis	15 mg/kg/d in 3–4 doses	Rash, GI effects, neutropenia	Yes
Zidovudine (AZT)	C	Reduced risk of vertical transmission; primary HIV infection	200 mg t.i.d. or 500 mg qd	Headache, anemia, GI effects, insomnia, malaise, nail discoloration, seizures, mania, increased creatinine phosphokinase	†

*No FDA Class.

†No data.

Multiple side effects/interactions/complications occur with all of these medications. Experienced consultation should be actively sought.

If exposure occurs, the contact area should be washed immediately with soap and water. Other solutions (e.g., bleach, iodine) are not superior. Eyes should be irrigated with sterile water. There are no data to support the use of postexposure zidovudine, but some choose it nevertheless (500–600 mg/day). Exposed persons should be monitored and offered confidential counseling. Drugs commonly utilized in patients with an HIV infection are outlined in Table 28–11.

■
Appendix: AIDS-Defining Conditions (Centers for Disease Control and Prevention)

Candida infection of esophagus, trachea, bronchi, lungs
Invasive cervical cancer*
Coccidioidomycosis, extrapulmonary
Cryptococcosis, extrapulmonary
Cryptosporidiosis with diarrhea >1 mo
Cytomegalovirus of any organ except liver, spleen, or lymph nodes
Herpes simplex with mucocutaneous ulcer >1 mo or bronchitis, pneumonitis, esophagitis
Histoplasmosis, extrapulmonary
HIV dementia; disabling cognitive and/or motor function interfering with occupation or activities of daily living
HIV wasting; involuntary weight loss >10% of baseline plus chronic diarrhea (2 stools/d >30 d) or chronic weakness and enigmatic fever >30 d
Isosporiasis with diarrhea >1 mo*
Kaposi's sarcoma if <60 yr (or >60 yr and HIV-positive)
Lymphoma of the brain if <60 yr (or >60 yr and HIV-positive)
Lymphoma, non-Hodgkin's of B-cell or unknown immunotype or immunoblastic sarcoma
Mycobacterium avium or *Mycobacterium kansasii,* disseminated
Mycobacterium tuberculosis, disseminated*
Mycobacterium tuberculosis, pulmonary*
Nocardiosis
Pneumocystis carinii pneumonia
Recurrent pneumonia*
Recurrent, nontyphoid *Salmonella* septicemia*
Extraintestinal strongyloidosis
Toxoplasmosis of any internal organ

---

*Must be HIV seropositive.

■ Bibliography

Bartlett J: The Johns Hopkins Hospital Guide to Medical Care of Patients with HIV Infection, ed 4. Baltimore: Williams & Wilkins, 1994.

Cohen PT, Sande M, Volberding P (eds): The AIDS Knowledge Base, ed 2. Boston: Little, Brown, 1994.

DeVita V, Hellman S, Rosenberg S (eds): AIDS: Etiology, Diagnosis, Treatment and Prevention, ed 3. Philadelphia: J.B. Lippincott, 1992.

Evaluation and Management of Early HIV Infection: Clinical Practice Guidelines. AHCPR No.94-0572: U.S. Department of Health and Human Services, 1994.

Johnson M, Johnstone F (eds): HIV Infection in Women. New York: Churchill Livingstone, 1993.

Minkoff H, DeHovitz J, Duerr A (eds): HIV Infection in Women. New York: Raven Press, 1995.

Peiperi L: Manual of HIV/AIDS Therapy. Fountain Valley, California: Current Clinical Strategies Publishing, 1993.

Sande M, Volberding P (eds): The Medical Management of AIDS, ed 4. Philadelphia: W.B. Saunders, 1995.

Index

Note: Page numbers in *italics* refer to illustrations.
Page numbers followed by t refer to tables,
and those followed by b to boxed material.